T0249040

Osteoporosis: Secondary Osteoporosis and Pediatric Concerns

Osteoporosis: Secondary Osteoporosis and Pediatric Concerns

Edited by **Dan Heller**

FOSTER
ACADEMICS

New Jersey

Published by Foster Academics,
61 Van Reypen Street,
Jersey City, NJ 07306, USA
www.fosteracademics.com

Osteoporosis: Secondary Osteoporosis and Pediatric Concerns
Edited by Dan Heller

International Standard Book Number: 978-1-63242-306-1 (Hardback)

Contents

Preface

Osteoporosis is a serious health problem across the globe. In the last few years, growth has been seen in the knowledge of the pathophysiological mechanism of the disease. Modern technologies have added significant information in bone mineral density measurements and, furthermore, mechanical and geometrical properties of bone. Novel bone indices have been formulated from hormonal and biochemical measurements for the investigation of bone metabolism. Although, it is evident that drugs are a crucial part of the therapy. However, beyond medication there are other interventions in the management of the disease. Prevention of this disease begins at young age and goes on with the process of aging for the purpose of prevention of fractures related to the impaired quality of life, mortality, physical decline, and high cost for the health system. Several distinct specialties are holding the scientific knowledge in this disease. In this book, information from scientific departments from across the world has been compiled. Updated information regarding pediatric issues and secondary osteoporosis has been compiled extensively in this book.

The information shared in this book is based on empirical researches made by veterans in this field of study. The elaborative information provided in this book will help the readers further their scope of knowledge leading to advancements in this field.

Finally, I would like to thank my fellow researchers who gave constructive feedback and my family members who supported me at every step of my research.

Editor

Part 1

Secondary Osteoporosis

Osteoporosis in Microgravity Environments

Bradley K. Weiner, Scott E. Parazynski and Ennio Tasciotti
Weill Cornell Medical College, Orthopaedic Surgery, Spinal Surgery,
The Methodist Hospital, Orthopaedic Spine Advanced Technology Laboratory
The Methodist Hospital Research Institute, Houston, Texas
USA

1. Introduction

All life on earth has evolved in, and via the adaption to, the presence of gravity. This includes humans who branched off from a distant ancestor about five to seven million years ago. On April 12, 1961, one such human---Yuri Gagarin of the Soviet Union---took off in Vostok 3KA for the first trip into outer space. Since then, numerous trips to the moon, the Skylab, and within the Space Shuttle have followed. With the recent completion of the International Space Station, the current focus is set on very long duration crewed missions to the station, the establishment of a potential lunar outpost, and possible exploration of Mars.

As more and more humans head to space for longer and longer periods of time---out of desire or necessity---significant challenges will be faced. The *technological* challenges will undoubtedly be met. The past fifty years have taught us that given adequate time and financial resources nearly any technological hurdle can be jumped. The *biological* challenges are far greater. As noted, all human life on earth has evolved via adaption to gravity and long-term exposure to microgravity takes its toll; especially on the musculoskeletal, cardiovascular, sensory-motor, and immune systems.

In this chapter, we will review the known effects of long-term microgravity on the skeletal system, examine what is as-yet unknown, and explore possible interventions that might be used to address these effects.

2. The impact of microgravity at the cellular level

2.1 Osteoporosis on earth

Osteoporosis occurring on earth in the presence of normal gravity is most often associated with aging and most significantly impacted by peak bone mass and the rate of bone loss thereafter. Peak bone mass is generally achieved while humans are in their early thirties and subsequent bone loss is impacted not only by aging and menopause (women), but by hereditary predispositions, exogenous factors (such as alcohol, smoking, inactivity, malnutrition, prescription medications, etc.), and disease states (such as endocrine disorders, renal disorders, rheumatologic disorders, etc.). Each of these causes results in a final common pathway leading to osteoporosis---an imbalance between bone formation and bone resorption. Fractures, primarily of the proximal femur ('hip'), vertebral bodies, and distal radius ('wrist') are significant risks and, as other chapters in this text have outlined, represent important causes of morbidity and potential mortality.

Osteoblast and osteoclast uncoupling is the primary source of this excessive resorption and biomechanical fragility of bone. If the cause can be determined, then reasonable solutions aimed at such uncoupling can be offered to address the problem. Bispohosphonates and, more primitively phosphate, can impede osteoclastic resorption. Calcium, Vitamin D, calcitonin, estrogen, exercise, smoking and alcohol restriction, and avoidance of particular medications can help halt bone loss. Fluoride (no longer used), parathytoid hormone, and aggressive exercise might result in bone mass gain.

2.2 Osteoporosis in microgravity
Osteoporosis occurring as a result of microgravity is, from the perspective of the organism down to the lowest biological level, *different* than that encountered on earth.

2.2.1 Cytoskeletal alterations
Microgravity appears to significantly alter the cellular cytoskeleton. Proper cytoskeletal structure allows intracellular proteins to participate in important functions such as mitosis, cell motility, intracellular transport, and organization of organelles. Actin filaments, intermediate filaments, and microtubules are the key elements and they serve as a highly organized dynamic scaffold on which intracellular processes take place.

In microgravity, cellular structure, intracellular organization, and micro-fluid dynamics are altered[1]. Disruption of normal biochemical and physiological processes follows. Clement and Slenzka[2] have demonstrated that the spatial relationships between cellular organelles and structures are abnormal. And He[3] and Crawford-Young[4] have demonstrated that cellular cytoskeletal and microfilament dynamics are anomalous and might well be the source. Thus DNA replication, RNA transcription, protein migration, and ionic and molecular transport are perturbed.

2.2.2 Mesenchymal stem cells
The impact of these intracellular changes is felt by mesenchymal stem cells (MSC). MSC---present in adult life in the periosteum of bones and within the bone marrow---differentiate into osteoblasts following appropriate signaling and presence within the proper mileau. Meyers[5], Yuge[6], Huang[7], and Pan[8] (in separate studies) have demonstrated via flow cytometry, transcriptional analyses, and proteomic analyses that MSCs ability to proliferate, to differentiate into osteoblasts, and to contribute to osteogenesis is inhibited by microgravity.

2.2.3 Osteoblasts
Osteoblasts are also directly compromised. Bucaro[9] has demonstrated findings that suggest that direct induction of osteoblast apoptosis occurs in microgravity. Apoptosis is differentiated from usual cell necrosis (where cells swell, burst and die) by characteristic intracellular changes including nuclear condensation and shrinkage and cytoplasmic vacuolization. Observed osteoblastic apoptosis likely results from cytoskeletal changes.

Additionally, Colleran[10] has noted that the cephallic fluid shift experienced by humans in microgravity might alter interstitial fluid pressures and flows and, given that osteoblasts survive somewhat tenuously in low flow areas, these shifts might result in cell functional compromise or death.

3. The impact of microgravity at the systemic level

Systemically, microgravity induces osteoporosis via the above noted unique cellular changes *coupled* with an environment of nearly non-existent mechanical stresses where normal weight-bearing and the normal response of bone to proliferate accordingly (Wolff's Law) is altered. And this alteration differs than, say, that seen with immobilization. While patients placed in body casts and on bed rest (fully non-weightbearing) will suffer from osteoporortic changes, the amount of calcified bony tissue lost over three months is generally about 3%, tends to then level off at about three months (no further loss), and tends to be reversed with resumption of weight-bearing. In microgravity, the loss occurs at four times the rate, does not appear to level off, and appears to be much less reversible. Thus, the one-year trip to Mars is estimated to potentially result in a (devastating) greater than 25% reduction of bone mass. And this is in astronauts; predominantly male, at an age where their bone mass is at peak levels, exposed to no exogenous factors (smoking, excessive alcohol, etc.), in prime physical condition, and with no underlying disease states.

Simply, the combination of altered cellular form and function coupled with differences in bony response to microgravity systemically means that this form of osteoporosis bears relatively little relation to that seen on earth and that astronauts experience early, aggressive, continual bone loss. Predictably, systemic markers of bone resorption are greatly increased, while markers of bone formation are decreased[11] to levels rarely seen in on-earth conditions. And, importantly, it is unclear whether these changes are fully reversible upon return to earth and 'normal' gravity conditions.

4. Bone health and present day human spaceflight

Since the earliest days of human spaceflight, physiologists and NASA flight surgeons recognized the importance of exercise to maintain musculoskeletal and cardiovascular health. Owing to prolonged exposure to microgravity, Astronaut crews returning from America's first space station, Skylab, were too weak to stand upon return to earth. Exercise equipment thus became a requirement for all long duration space missions. A series of devices, including treadmills, stationary bicycles, rowing ergometers, simple resistive exercise systems and complex, reconfigurable "weight machines" have evolved in the years since, both in the Soviet-turned-Russian space program and now in the US-led International Space Station (ISS) program.

Exercise devices designed to maintain cardiovascular fitness in the absence of gravity proved to be a more straightforward engineering goal: movement against a friction wheel can easily challenge the cardiopulmonary system. Providing resistive exercise challenge to the postural musculoskeletal system of sufficient intensity and quality has only recently been accomplished aboard the ISS. The Advanced Resistive Exercise Device (ARED) uses pistons to provide smooth exercise loads, and is highly reconfigurable for a wide array of concentric and eccentric exercises.

The world record duration in space is held by Dr. Valeri Polyakov, who spent 437 consecutive days in microgravity, landing in 1995. During his endurance mission he was required to exercise up to four hours a day. Human spaceflight is very costly, but is obviously undertaken to accomplish important scientific goals in life sciences, material science, fluid and combustion physics, global environmental monitoring and many other disciplines. Even with the improved exercise countermeasures and added knowledge of today, the overhead of spending up to two hours each and every day in space for the sole purpose of exercise is problematic.

ISS crewmembers actively work with strength and conditioning coaches throughout their preflight training. Using exercise monitoring hardware aboard ISS, these same coaches perform inflight assessments of the crew's conditioning while they are in space, and make exercise prescription modifications from Mission Control Houston, as required. Additionally, they oversee the crew's postflight physical rehabilitation, a process which may take several months to restore bone density to critical areas such as the hip and lumbar vertebral bodies.

Armed with an understanding of the whole body, cellular and subcellular processes involved in bone density maintenance in altered gravitational fields, more effective and efficient means to preserve musculoskeletal health is necessary to send humans beyond short stays aboard the ISS: Lunar outposts and expeditions to Mars are even more committing endeavors, and warrant substantial attention.

5. Future directions for research

Despite a reasonable foundation of information, much work is needed to further delineate the impact of microgravity on bones at the cellular and systemic levels. Clearly the best strategy is to conduct experimental in-vivo human studies in space, but limited access to spaceflights and limited time during flight available to dedicate to these studies renders extensive (but necessary) study unachievable[1]. Accordingly, microgravity simulation has been the primary source of basic biological scientific information including most of what has been discussed thus far in this chapter.

On the celular level, simulation can be carried out within the rotating-wall vessel (RWV); a NASA-designed tissue culture bioreactor which simulates microgravity[1]. The bioreactor rotates horizontally such that, at an ideal speed, the contents achieve relative suspension simulating microgravity via dynamic equalibrium of forces---the contained cells / tissues remain in a state of long-term, suspended free-fall. The cells / tissues retain viability by being contained along with cell-specific growth media and oxygenation via active or passive diffusion provided by a silicon rubber membrane. To date however, relatively few studies have been carried out and there is significant need for further study on the cellular level as this level may be the key to differences relative to earthly osteoporosis. Additionally, comparison with studies performed in space will be required to validate the model and to ensure that changes noted are not unique to the system itself---in-vitro cellular behavior does not always mirror real life.

On the system / organism level, research has focused on animal models; most commonly hind-limb unloading and head-down bed rest (which has also been used in human volunteer subjects)[1]. While such models provide some insight into rapid bone loss, they are not fully satisfactory given that they fail to incite the noted cellular changes associated with microgravity and gravitational forces still compress bodily tissues whereas, in true microgravity, there is negative pressure experienced by tissues. It is clear that better models need to be developed.

6. Potential future options for treatment and prevention

Current options for the prevention and treatment of osteoporosis have proven far more successful on earth than in microgravity and this is likely commensurate with the above noted cellular anomalies encountered. Aggressive exercise by astronauts---recommended at two hours per day of heavy resistance work---has made an impact; however, freeing up time for such activities is difficult given the operational needs during missions and, as space flight expands generally, the baseline cardiovascular capabilities of travelers will be more limited. Additionally, the aforementioned cellular changes render supplements (Calcium, vitamin D, etc.), medications (bisphosphonates, etc.) and hormones (testosterone, etc.) significantly less effective in astronauts despite having a minor effect in microgravity animal models.

6.1 Diagnostic platforms

The identification of new diagnostic or prognostic biomarkers has been gaining attention in the field of bone disease research leading to significant benefits in terms of efficient and timely treatment. Clearly novel strategies will need to be developed, and directed both at the molecular / cellular and bony systemic levels, and will need to be long lasting and simple to administer. In our minds, the ideal platform for the development of such novel strategies will rest upon nanotechnology. The size of nanomaterials mirrors that of most biological molecules and structures allowing size-matched communication and intervention important in diagnostics and therapeutics at the sub-cellular level and felt to be the source of bone cell dysfunction in microgravity.

In this context, particular emphasis is placed on study of circulating proteome. The proteome represent the functional picture of the state of the cells because it constantly changes through its biochemical interactions with the genome and the environment. Protein turnovers and tissue microenvironment create a rich and heterogenic circulating mixture of protein fragments (low molecular weight peptidome, LMWP) that reflects both physiological and pathological processes. Despite its potential in clinical applications, profiling of the LMWP has proven to be a significant technical challenge because of the extremely high dynamic range of protein concentrations in blood and body fluids. Development of technologies that enable controlled fabrication of structure with nanoscale dimension can address the issues of the intrinsic complexity of the circulating low molecular weight peptidome [12,13]. Our group has developed diagnostic nanochannel-based lab-on-a-chip technologies [Fig 1] that can allow for the detection of the earliest signs of disease, including osteoporosis, using penny-sized discs (satisfying the need for space preservation during space flight). This device is a size-exclusion method based on mesoporous silica thin film chips able to rapidly fractionate, and selectively enrich and protect peptides and proteins from enzymatic degradation. The mesoporous silica chip were produced by the evaporation-induced self –assembly procedure under acidic conditions using triblock copolymers as structural templates [14,15].

Physical properties of mesoporous silica such as pore dimension, pore texture, and chemical surface properties such as charge and further functionalization with selective ligands can be easily controlled and tuned to enhance the ability to detect traces of molecules. The ability to fabricate nanoscale devices and materials with a high degree of precision and accuracy, in combination with the recent advances in mass spectrometry, resulted in a powerful proteomic nanoscale platform for early disease diagnosis [16]. These lab-on-a-chip based diagnostic technologies can be either used as external devices or be implanted in the body of the astronaut. Implantable chips can feature molecularly driven sensors able to measure vital signs and readily respond to specific variation by releasing counteracting molecules. Diagnostics based on readily accessible body fluids can be also used to monitor in real time the efficacy of therapeutic interventions. In their most complex configuration these implantable devices can be considered as artificial glands that sense the status of the body and adjust to it trying to bring back homeostasis. Nanotechnology based diagnostics offer higher detection capabilities due to the reduction of the size of the sensors, the increase of their sensitivity, the absence of non-specific reactions, and the multiplexing of the multi-scale detectors that allow a wide range of intensities of the signal to be measured.

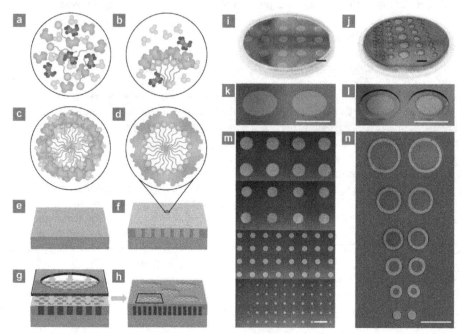

a-h, Schematic evolution of the chemical composition of the coating solution during the production of a mesoporous silica film. a, Fresh coating solution; b, Formation of micelles; c, Evaporation induced self assembly during spin-coating process; d, Zoomed in view of a pore after aging at elevated temperature. e, Bulk silicon wafer surface; f, Mesoporous silica film on a bulk silicon wafer. e-f, Cross-section of GX6 chip by SEM and TEM imaging respectively (scale bar is 500nm). i-n, images of the different chip surfaces and of the different masks that define the spotting areas.

Fig. 1. Production and assembly of MSC for proteomic applications

6.2 Delivery systems

We developed novel silicon-based theranostic nanoparticles [17-19] that have been used to achieve long-term, controlled, and targeted release of proteins and drugs that help halting or reversing osteoporosis. Among the molecules tested bone morphogenetic proteins (BMPs---which are differentiation factors that facilitate the transition of mesenchymal stem cells to osteoblasts thereby encouraging bone formation) and bisphosphonates (which inhibit osteoclasts mediated bone resorption). The finely-tuned, extended, local delivery allowed by the use of these particles means that a single treatment can be administered pre-flight with effects felt for months on end (no need to 're-dose') and might prove to prevent or treat osteoporosis of microgravity. Nanoporous silica and PLGA composites are capable of releasing molecules in a burst or steady fashion over the course of days, weeks, or even months. These systems can also be tuned to release their payload in response to environmental stimuli (pH, temperature, blood concentrations, exposure to radiation, bone degeneration, etc.). The local delivery of antibiotics, dexamethasone, and growth factors (BMP-2) to the bone defect areas by PLGA/pSi microspheres reduced inflammation and stimulated new bone formation whilke simultaneously fighting bacterial growth. A wide variety of therapeutic and imaging agents have been successfully loaded into and released from pSi particles such as steroids [21], hormones [22], proteins[23], cancer drugs [24], or even secondary drug delivery vehicles including iron oxide nanoparticles [25], quantum dots, liposomes [26] and carbon nanotubes loaded with therapeutic drugs[18,27] to the diseased areas. In order to achieve the level of control on the release dynamics, it is possible to tailor both the pore size of the pSi during particles' fabrication or vary polymer type, molecular weight and density. Finally, the overall size of the polymer/pSi composites can also be tuned from nano level to micro level to suit certain applications by changing the polymer concentration, surfactant concentration, or the stirring speed. This hybrid system not only can reduce or abolish burst release, and prolong release kinetics, but also protect biomolecules from denaturation both during the drug loading process and while implanted in vivo. These particles have been successfully tested in different orthopedic tissue engineering applications in small and large animal models of bone fracture repair (manuscripts in preparation).

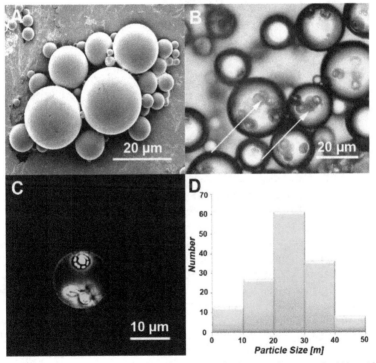

Fig. 2. Scanning electron microscopy (SEM) images of pSi particles reveals (A) uniform shape and size of particles, (B) the pore structure on the surface of the particles, and the (C) front and (D) rear surfaces of the particles.

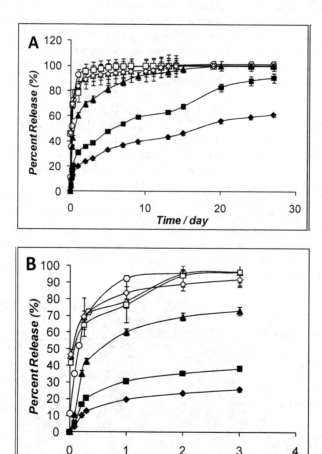

Fig. 3. Release profiles of FITC-BSA from various examined PLGA/pSi microsphere formulations. (A) Total FITC-BSA released over 27 days, (B) first three day release.

6.3 Injectable materials

Beyond these diagnostic and drug-delivery applications, our group has also developed injectable gels that employ nanotechnologies to deliver mesenchymal stem cells, platelet rich plasma, and osteogeneic factors directly to areas of bony weakness. Thus, astronauts identified to have focal osteoporosis of, say, the proximal femur, might be treated by simple focal injection affording the in-vivo, in-situ rapid regeneration of lost bony mass.

These composites have proved their osteogenic capacity in vitro and through in vivo subcutaneous implants where ectopic bone was formed. The use of bio-porogens synthesized from natural and biodegradable materials, encourages bone formation and vascularization in vivo. These porogens particles house and release MSC, recruit endogenous cells and create extracellular matrix, synergistically promoting bone formation

[28]. They also exhibit tremendous viability of MSC after cryo-preservation, allowing for long-term storage of prepared bio-porogens for immediate "on-demand" use in the clinic. Previously, we found that MSC isolated from compact bone (CB) tissue were more frequent in the total cell population and of greater colony-forming and tri-lineage differentiation potential than MSC in bone marrow (BM) (Figure 4).

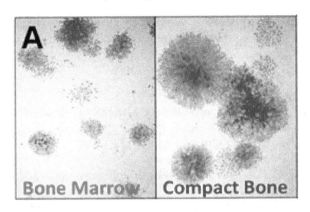

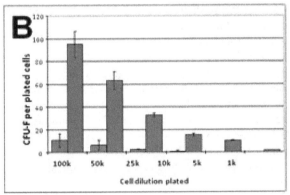

Fig. 4. MSC from compact bone (CB) produce larger and more defined colonies than those from bone marrow (BM) (A). The incidence of MSC from bulk cell populations is also nearly 10x higher in CB than BM (B).

All these biomaterials were based on the unique combination of I) nanostructured biomaterials able to mimic the extracellular matrices of either bone or cartilage with II) chemical and biochemical cues able to direct, control and preserve the phenotypes of both osteoblasts in their histological compartments. These biomaterials are made available as injectable hydrogel formulations thus reducing surgical invasiveness and improving the accuracy of the delivery to the targeted anatomical sites. Injectable composite hydrogels/pastes can be used for the spinal regions weakened by OP, with appropriate biomimetic and biomechanical characteristics.

These biomaterials can be functionalized and/or doped with chemical (e.g. strontium ions, oxygen transporters/scavangers) and biochemical (e.g. bioactive/biodocking peptides, genes) agents able to control cell phenotype and activity. Hydrogel formulations to be examined include collagen, gelatin, alginate, self-assembling peptides, or combinations thereof. The nano-features include peptides that bind to integral growth factors such as BMP-2 and VEGF and PRP. The scaffolds may be co-implanted with mesenchymal stem cells obtained from bone marrow and adipose aspirates. Finally, we have developed ways to reinforce biocompatible polymers with nanoparticles / nanowires that greatly increase their strength allowing for the replacement of bulky, heavy metallic devices currently used for fracture repair---the light-weight, injectable polymers ideal for transport on space flights and use for the repair of osteoporotic fractures once they occur.

7. References

[1] Blaber E, Marcal H, Burns B: Bioastronautics. Astrobiology 10: 463-473, 2010.

[2] Clement G, Slenzka K. Fundamentals of space biology. Springer, New York 2006.

[3] He J, Zhang X, Gao Y, et al.: Effects of altered gravity on the cell cycle. Acat Astronaut. 63: 915-922, 2008.

[4] Crawford-Young SJ: Effects of microgravity on cell cytoskeleton and embryogenesis. Int J Dev Biol 50: 183-191, 2006.

[5] Meyers VE, Zayzafoon M, Douglas JT, et al.: RhoA and cytoskeletal disruption mediate reduced osteoblastogenesis of human mesenchymal stem cells in modeled microgravity. J Bone Min Res 20: 1858-1866, 2005.

[6] Yuge L, Kajiume T, Tahara H, et al.: Microgravity potentiates stem cell proliferatio while sustaining the capability of differentiation. Stem Cell Dev 15:921-929, 2006.

[7] Huang Y, Dai ZQ, Ling SK, et al.: Gravity, a regulation factor in the differentiation of rat bone marrow mesenchymal stem cells. J Biomed Sci 16: 87, 2009.

[8] Pan Z, Yang J, Guo C, et al.: Effects of hindlimb unloading on ex vivo growth and osteogenic potential of bone-marrow derived mesenchymal stem cells in rats. Stem Cell Dev 17: 795-804, 2008.

[9] Bucaro MA, Zahm AM, Risbud MV, et al.: The effect of simulated microgravity on osteoblasts is independent of the induction of apoptosis. J Cell Biochem 102: 483-495, 2007.

[10] Colleran PN, Wilkerson MK, Bloomfield SA, et al.: Alterations in skeletal perfusion with simulated microgravity. J Appl Physiol 89: 1046-1054, 2000.

[11] Callot-Augusseau A, Lafage MH, Soler C, et al.: Bone formation and resorption biological markers in cosmonauts during and after a 180 day space flight. Clin Chem 44: 578-585, 1998

[12] Sakamoto JH, van de Ven AL, Godin B, Blanco E, Serda RE, Grattoni A, Ziemys A, Bouamrani A, Hu T, Ranganathan SI, De Rosa E, Martinez JO, Smid CA, Buchanan RM, Lee SY, Srinivasan S, Landry M, Meyn A, Tasciotti E, Liu X, Decuzzi P, Ferrari M. Enabling individualized therapy through nanotechnology. Pharmacol Res. 2010 Aug; 62(2):57-89. Epub 2010 Jan 5.

[13] Ye Hu, Daniel H. Fine, Ennio Tasciotti, Ali Bouamrani and Mauro Ferrari, Nanodevices in diagnostics, 2010.

[14] Hu, Y.; Bouamrani, A.; Tasciotti, E.; Li, L.; Liu, X.; Ferrari, M. Tailoring of the Nanotexture of Mesoporous Silica Films and their functionalized derivatives for

selectively harvesting low molecular weight protein. acs nano. 2010; vol. 4 n 1, 439–451.

[15] Bouamrani A, Hu Y, Tasciotti E, Li L, Chiappini C, Liu X, et al. Mesoporous silica chips for selective enrichment and stabilization of low molecular weight proteome. Proteomics. 2009; 10, 496–505.

[16] Ye Hu, Yang Peng, Louis Brousseau, Ali Bouamrani, Xuewu Liu, and Mauro Ferrari, Nanotexture Optimization by Oxygen Plasma of Mesoporous Silica Thin Film for Enrichment of Low Molecular Weight Peptides Captured from Human Serum, Sci China Chem. 2010 November 1; 53(11): 2257–2264.

[17] Tasciotti E, Liu X, Bhavane R, Plant K, Leonard AD, Price BK, Cheng MM, Decuzzi P, Tour JM, Robertson F, Ferrari M. Mesoporous silicon particles as a multistage delivery system for imaging and therapeutic applications. Nat Nanotechnol. 2008 Mar;3(3):151-7. Epub 2008 Mar 2.

[18] Tanaka T, Mangala LS, Vivas-Mejia PE, Nieves-Alicea R, Mann AP, Mora E, Han HD, Shahzad MM, Liu X, Bhavane R, Gu J, Fakhoury JR, Chiappini C, Lu C, Matsuo K, Godin B, Stone RL, Nick AM, Lopez-Berestein G, Sood AK, Ferrari M. Sustained small interfering RNA delivery by mesoporous silicon particles. Cancer Res. 2010 May 1;70(9):3687-96.

[19] Serda RE, Gu J, Bhavane RC, Liu X, Chiappini C, Decuzzi P, Ferrari M. he association of silicon microparticles with endothelial cells in drug delivery to the vasculature. Biomaterials. 2009 May; 30(13):2440-8. Epub 2009 Feb 12.

[20] D. Fan, E. DeRosa, M. B. Murphy, Y. Peng, C. A. Smid, C. Chiappini, X. Liu, P. Simmons, B. K. Weiner, M. Ferrari, and E. Tasciotti. Accepted by Advanced Functional Materials.

[21] E. J. Anglin, M. P. Schwartz, V. P. Ng, L. A. Perelman, M. J. Sailor, Langmuir. 2004, 20, 11264.

[22] A. B. Foraker, R. J. Walczak, M. H. Cohen, T. A. Boiarski, C. F. Grove, P. W. Swaan, Pharm. Res. 2003, 20, 110.

[23] C. A. Prestidge, T. J. Barnes, A. Mierczynska-Vasilev, W. Skinner, F. Peddie, C. Barnett, phys. status solidi A. 2007, 204, 3361.

[24] L. Vaccari, D. Canton, N. Zaffaroni, R. Villa, M. Tormen, E. di Fabrizio, Microelectron. Eng. 2006, 83, 1598.

[25] R. E. Serda, S. Ferrati, B. Godin, E. Tasciotti, X. Liu, M. Ferrari, Nanoscale. 2009, 1, 250.

[26] E. Tasciotti, B. Godin, J. O. Martinez, C. Chiappini, R. Bhavane, X. Liu, M. Ferrari, Mol Imaging. 2010, In press.

[27] J. S. Ananta, B. Godin, R. Sethi, L. Moriggi, X. Liu, R. E. Serda, R. Krishnamurthy, R. Muthupillai, R. D. Bolskar, L. Helm, M. Ferrari, L. J. Wilson, P. Decuzzi, Nano Tech. 2010, 5, 815.

[28] Buchanan, R.M., Klein, J.S., DeJong, N.S., Murphy, M.B., Yazdi, I.K., Weiner, B.K., Ferrari, F., and Tasciotti E. Platelet-rich Plasma/ Alginate Composite Microspheres for the Encapsulation, Cryopreservation, Delivery, and Proliferation of MSC. Submitted to Advanced Functional Materials

[29] Murphy, M.B., Blashki, D., Buchanan, R.M., Yazdi, I.K., Ferrari, M., Simmons, P.Jl, and Tasciotti, E. Characterization of Umbilical Cord Blood-Derived and Adult Platelet-Rich Plasma for Mesenchymal Stem Cell Proliferation, Chemotaxis, and Cryo-preservation. Submitted to Biomaterials.

2

Neurological Osteoporosis in Disabilities

Yannis Dionyssiotis
Physical and Social Rehabilitation Center Amyntæo
University of Athens, Laboratory for Research of the Musculoskeletal System
Greece

1. Introduction

Osteoporosis is characterized by low bone mass and destruction of the micro architecture of bone tissue, resulting in increased bone fragility and susceptibility to fractures (NIH 2001). The clinical usefulness of T-score at disabled people on the recognition of people with low BMD remains unclear according to ranking system of the World Health Organization (WHO 1994). Despite the increased number of risk factors in people with disabilities no guidelines are available on BMD measurements; so it would be more appropriate to use the term low bone mass instead of osteoporosis or osteopenia and also take into account the Z-score obtained from the measurement of bone densitometry which is the number of standard deviations above or below that normally expected for someone of similar age, sex, weight and race in question (Dionyssiotis, 2011c, 2011d).

In disabled subjects there are differences according to the type of injury (i.e. lesion with a level of injury vs. upper motor neuron pyramidal lesion), the type of lesion; complete (an absence of sensory or motor function below the neurological level, including the lowest sacral segment) vs. incomplete lesion (partial preservation of motor and/or sensory function below the neurological level, including the lowest sacral segment), the progression or not of the disease (i.e. progressive multiple sclerosis vs. complete paraplegia), life expectancy, the residual mobility and functionality, the ability to walk and stand (i.e. incomplete paraplegia vs. quadriplegia vs. high-low paraplegia), drug treatment (i.e. frequent corticosteroid therapy in multiple sclerosis vs. long-term therapy with anticoagulants in paraplegia), the degree of spasticity (i.e. flaccid vs. spastic paralysis) and it is necessary to take into account the issue of fatigue and muscle weakness. Depression in these subjects is usual; complicates the proposed treatments and limits mobility. Complete and incomplete disabled differ also in physical abilities. Moreover, subjects with complete injuries have greater bone loss than those with an incomplete injury (Garland et al., 1994) and as has already been shown in Brown-Sequard subjects (incomplete spinal cord lesion) where BMD of the more paretic knee was lower than that of the stronger knee (Lazo et al., 2001).

However, there are also similarities; for example the clinical equivalence of diseases with different physiopathology, location, evolution, etc. A severe form of multiple sclerosis (MS) can result in a wheelchair bound patient having a clinical figure equivalent to spinal cord injury paraplegia. One patient with MS may have better walking gait pattern in comparison with a patient with incomplete paraplegia but may also be unable to walk, bedridden and vice versa (Dionyssiotis, 2011c, 2011d).

In addition the role of factors which do not change, i.e.: race or gender is inadequately clarified. Studies in disabled women debate that bones are more affected compared to disabled men. In chronic spinal cord injured women a tendency to have lower bone mass than men (Coupaud et al., 2009) and higher rates of lower bone mass with lower T-scores compared to women with other disabilities have been reported (Smeltzer et al., 2005).

2. Spinal cord injury

Bone loss in spinal cord injury (SCI) is a multifactorial disease in acute and chronic phase and can be enhanced by the lack of weight bearing, muscular tension on bone or other neural factors associated with the injury. Moreover, differentiation of the sympathetic nervous system after SCI is leading to venous and capillary vascular stasis. Some additional non-mechanical factors to stimulate bone loss include poor nutritional adequacy, gonadal changes and other endocrine disorders (Chantraine 1978; Chantraine et al., 1979b; Jiang et al., 2007; Maimoun et al., 2006).

2.1 Bone mineral density

In individuals with SCI bone loss begins immediately after injury (Bauman et al., 1997; Uebelhart et al., 1995). SCI related bone impairment below the level of injury is much greater compared with other conditions (i.e. age, immobilization, bed rest, lack of gravity environment). A reduction of bone mineral content (BMC) during the first years after the injury of 4% per month in regions rich in cancellous bone, and 2% per month on sites containing mainly cortical bone is reported (Wilmet et al., 1995). According to another study 25 out of 41 patients with SCI (61%) met WHO's criteria for osteoporosis, eight (19.5%) were osteopenic and only eight (19.5%) showed normal values (Lazo et al., 2001). In SCI children (boys and girls) values for bone mineral density (BMD) at the hip were approximately 60% of normal, or had a Z-score that indicated a 1.6-1.8 SD reduction in BMD compared with age- and sex-matched peers (Lauer et al., 2007).

In studies with peripheral quantitative computed tomography (p QCT) in spinal cord injured subjects bone loss in the epiphyses was 50% in the femur and 60% in the tibia, while in the diaphyses of these bones was 35% and 25%, respectively, meaning that bone loss in the epiphyses almost doubled the loss in the diaphyses (Eser et al., 2004). This study also showed that bone loss between trabecular and cortical bone compartment differs in mechanism, i.e. in the epiphyses bone is lost due to the decrease in trabecular, while in diaphysis, the cortical bone density is maintained and bone is lost due to endocortical resorption. In line with the previous study another p QCT study, performed in complete paraplegics with high (thoracic 4-7) and low (thoracic 8-12) neurological level of injury at the tibia, found a loss of trabecular (57.5% vs. 51%, in high vs. low paraplegics, respectively) and cortical bone (3.6% and 6.5%, respectively), suggesting that trabecular bone is more affected during the years of paralysis in comparison with cortical bone (Dionyssiotis et al., 2007). In the same study both paraplegic groups had a similar loss of total BMD (46.90% vs. 45.15%, in high vs. low paraplegics, respectively) suggesting that a homogenously deficit pattern occurs in the epiphyseal area, especially in the group of low paraplegics because the central and the peripheral of the cross sectional area of bone were similarly affected. On the contrary, in high paraplegics' group trabecular bone loss was higher suggesting an increasing endocortical remodeling keeping the total BMD similar. Concerning cortical geometric properties the results had shown an increased endosteal circumference between both paraplegic groups vs. controls leading to reduction of cortical thickness, 19.78% vs. 16.98% in paraplegic groups respectively, whereas periosteal circumference was comparable to controls (Fig. 1).

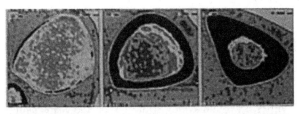

p QCT in the tibia of control subject 39 years old man, slices: 4%,14%,38%

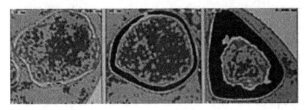

p QCT in the tibia in chronic complete AIS A paraplegic man thoracic 12 NLol 24 years old, slices: 4%,14%, 38%

Fig. 1. Peripheral quantitative computed tomography (p QCT) tibia slices in control (a) and paraplegic subject (b), (scanner XCT 3000 Stratec, Medizintechnik, Pforzheim, Germany). Areas in red represent trabecular bone, while areas in grey represent fat; pQCT allows the measurements of true volumetric densities at a minimum exposure to X-rays, assess cortical and trabecular bone density separately as well as to evaluate the geometrical properties of long bones non-invasively, adapted from Dionyssiotis, 2011c, 2011d, with permission.

Regarding tetraplegic patients statistically significant differences were found in BMD of the spine, trochanteric region and upper limbs between paraplegic and tetraplegic patients but not in the femoral neck, pelvis, and lower extremities (Tzuzuku et al., 1999). Indeed, the effects on spinal BMD differed from previously published work in which the investigation was mainly focused in paraplegics (Biering-Sorensen et al., 1988, 1991; Leslie & Nance, 1993).

The importance of mechanical loading and site specificity to maintain or increase BMD is already shown (Lanyon, 1986). According to bone loss there are some interesting features in spinal cord injured subjects; demineralization is area dependent, occurs exclusively in the areas below the level of injury (Dauty et al., 2000), affecting mainly paralyzed extremities and increasing from proximal to distal regions i.e. in paraplegics weight bearing skeleton regions, as the distal end of femur and proximal tibia, which are rich in cancellous bone, while region of the diaphysis of the femur and tibia, rich in cortical bone is reserved (Eser et al., 2004; Kiratli et al., 2000; Dionyssiotis et al., 2007). Moreover, bone loss between trabecular and cortical bone compartment differs in mechanism, i.e. in the epiphyses is due to decrease in trabecular but in diaphysis cortical bone is maintained and bone is lost through endocortical resorption by reducing cortical wall thickness (Dionyssiotis et al., 2007; Eser et al., 2004).

Women with disabilities have a higher risk of losing bone mass compared to men because of the inevitable reduction in estrogen levels that occurs at menopause. Findings that women with serious disabilities have low bone density are not surprising and are probably related to the lack of activity (reduced mobility, reduced loading on bone) and worsening of the disability. Regarding women with complete SCI, the initial bone loss in the lumbar spine is negligible. Post injury over a period of years BMD in SCI women is maintained or increases compared with non-injured age-matched women, in whom BMD decreases during aging (Dionyssiotis, 2011c).

2.2 Duration of paralysis and bone steady state

The duration of paralysis affects the degree of bone loss in regions below the level of injury. A study of 21 men with SCI with an average duration of 10.6 years, using dual-energy X-ray absorptiometry (DXA), expressed at various levels of injury an inverse relationship between BMD in the legs and the duration of the lesion (Clasey et al., 2004), while others found a weaker relationship regarding the microarchitecture of the distal end of tibia (Modlesky et al., 2004).

In a study which included paraplegics with duration of paralysis of 14 ± 11.5 years a positive correlation between the duration of paralysis and the degree of bone loss was found (Eser et al., 2004). The length of immobilization in the acute posttraumatic period increased bone loss in the legs, particularly in the proximal tibia; over 50% of bone mass was lost (in the affected areas) in the period of ten years after the injury (Dauty et al., 2000). When subjects categorized depending on the length of the lesion (0-1, 1-5, 6-9, 10-19, 20-29, 30-39, 40-49, and 50-59 years after the injury), in all age groups bone loss to the hip area occurs a year after the injury (Szollar et al., 1998).

Using DXA and QUS (quantitative ultrasound) measurements in 100 men with SCI, aged 18 to 60 years, it was found that bone density decreases over time in all measured points, while bone loss followed a linear pattern in the femoral neck and distal epiphysis, stabilized within three years after the injury. On the contrary, Z-scores of the distal region of the diaphysis of the tibia continued to decrease even beyond ten years after the injury (Zehnder et al, 2004). Duration of paralysis related bone loss in the legs of monozygotic twins with chronic paraplegia in comparison with their able-bodied co-twins has also been reported (Bauman et al., 1999).

The results of a comparison of chronic complete paraplegic men vs. controls in another study found a reduction of BMD in paraplegics' legs independent of the neurological level of lesion. BMD of the legs was negatively correlated with the duration of paralysis in the total paraplegic group, but after investigation according to the neurological level this correlation was due to the strong correlation of high paraplegics' legs BMD with the duration of paralysis, suggesting a possible influence of the neurological level of injury on the extent of bone loss (Dionyssiotis et al., 2008). A significant inverse relationship between percentage-matched in BMD leg, arm and trunk values and time since injury was found when varying levels of SCI were analyzed (Clasey et al., 2004).

Studies are supporting the concept of a new bone steady state at 16-24 months after injury, especially for bone metabolic process (Bauman WA 1997; Demirel et al., 1998; Szollar et al., 1998), but BMD decreases over the years at different areas and is inversely related to the time of the injury, which means continuous bone loss beyond the first two years after the injury (Coupaud et al., 2009; Dionyssiotis et al., 2008; Eser et al., 2004) (Fig. 2).

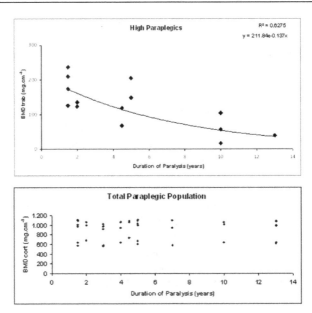

Fig. 2. The duration of paralysis was inversely related with trabecular bone loss in spinal cord injured subjects. Exponential correlation between volumetric trabecular bone mineral density BMD trab and duration of paralysis in high paraplegics was found to fit best. On the contrary no significant decrease in BMD cort of the diaphyses was found in total paraplegic group. BMD parameters were measured by pQCT in 31 paraplegic men in chronic stage (>1.5 years of injury). Spinal cord injury paraplegic men were allocated into 2 subgroups based on the neurological level of injury; subgroup A (n=16, Thoracic (T)4-T7 neurological level of injury) and subgroup B (n=15, T8-T12 neurological level of injury). BMDtrab: BMD trabecular; BMDcort: BMD cortical; (adapted from Dionyssiotis et al., 2011a, with permission).

The role played by factors such as race or gender of patients is not yet clear documented, but studies indicated more loss in women than men (Garland et al., 2001). Loss of bone is closing fracture threshold from 1 to 5 years after injury (Szollar et al., 1998) and risk factors for fractures after spinal cord injury are gender (women are more at risk than men), age and duration of injury (increasing age and duration of injury increases the risk of fracture with a statistically significant increase in 10 years after injury), the type of injury (complete SCI subjects have more fractures than incomplete), low body mass index (BMI) and low bone density in the tibia (Garland et al., 2004a,b; Garland et al., 1992; Lazo et al., 2001).

2.3. The role of central nervous system
2.3.1 Sympathetic denervation in SCI
Spinal cord injury is a dynamic process that is related to alterations in both the central and peripheral sympathetic nervous system (SNS). Sympathetic denervation in SCI may cause arteriovenous shunts and a slowdown of intraosseous blood flow, thus increasing bone resorption (Chantraine et al., 1979). With high-level spinal cord lesions the SNS is disproportionately involved when compared with the parasympathetic nervous system. In a complete high-level SCI, functioning in the isolated spinal cord below the lesion becomes

independent of supraspinal control and has been termed "decentralization" of the SNS (Karlsson et al., 1998).

Loss of supraspinal control leads to dysregulation of those homeostatic mechanisms normally influenced by the SNS through loss of facilitation or lack of inhibition (Teasell et al., 2000). Today there is clinical evidence that the sympathetic regulation of bone does exist in humans and plays a clinically important role in diseases characterized by excessive sympathetic activity (Schwartzman, 2000). The scientific finding about sympathetic innervations of bone tissue (Takeda et al., 2002; Kondo et al., 2005) and its role in the regulation of bone remodelling is of major interest in situations where uncoupling between osteoclasts and osteoblasts occurs (Levasseur et al., 2003).

2.3.2 Spasticity

Controversial results have also been reported regarding the effect of spasticity on BMD in SCI paraplegics. A cross-sectional study of 41 SCI paraplegics reported less reduction of BMD in the spastic paraplegics SCI patients compared to the flaccid paraplegic SCI patients (Demirel et al., 1998). Others reported that spasticity may be protective against bone loss in SCI patients, however, without any preserving effect in the tibia (Dionyssiotis et al., 2011; Eser et al., 2005). A possible explanation for that could lie in the fact that in the present study all paraplegics were above thoracic (T)12 level with various degrees of spasticity according to the Ashworth scale. In addition, muscle spasms affecting the lower leg would mainly be extension spasms resulting in plantar flexion thus creating little resistance to the contracting muscles. Furthermore, the measuring sites of the tibia did not include any muscle insertions of either the knee or the ankle extensor muscles (Dionyssiotis et al., 2011a; Dionyssiotis, 2011c). Other investigators also have not been able to establish a correlation between BMD and muscle spasticity (Lofvenmark et al., 2009).

3. Multiple sclerosis

Reduced mobility has been implicated as an important factor in bone loss in patients suffering from multiple sclerosis (MS) and it seems to greatly influence the BMD of the femur. However, the high proportion of ambulatory patients with bone loss suggest additional non-mechanical factors (Cosman et al., 1998; Dionyssiotis, 2011b).

There is a high incidence of vitamin D deficiency in MS patients and is determined by levels of 25-hydroxy vitamin D <20ng/ml (Nieves et al., 1994). The reasons might be due to a combination of low dietary vitamin D intake and avoiding of sun exposure, and that because of MS symptoms may worsen after sun exposure (fatigue-related heat) leading these patients to avoid sun. Low testosterone alone in these populations does not explain bone loss and no clear effect of smoking or alcohol abuse to decreased bone mass could be established (Weinstock-Guttman et al., 2004).

Glucocorticoid (GC)-induced osteoporosis (OP-GC) is the main type of secondary osteoporosis (Canalis et al., 2004; Canalis et al., 2007; Lakatos et al., 2000; Mazziotti et al., 2006; Schwid et al., 1996; Shuhaibar et al., 2009). The mechanism is that excess GC causes a rapid and significant damage to bone quality. Now days we know that GCs act direct on bone mainly to the stromalosteoblastic lineage and at high concentrations alter differentiation, survival, and function of them causing a shift from osteoblastic to adipocytic differentiation of precursors; inducing apoptosis of mature osteoblasts; and inhibition of synthesis and secretion of bone components (Manolagas, 2000; Pereira et al., 2002). Finally, GCs promote ostoclasts and stimulate bone resorption (Weinstein et al., 2002). The mechanisms of GCs action in bone has been studied extensively. In patients receiving chronic per os GC, bone loss is admitted rapidly and is evident within 6 or even 3 months (Cosman et al., 1998). A study investigated the effect of intravenously (i.v.) administration of glucocorticoids in MS patients found no clear effect on bone loss: on the contrary they reported an increase in BMD of the lumbar spine (Schwid et al., 1996). Prolonged treatment with glucocorticoids results in increased risk of fractures, evident at 3 months, regardless of changes in BMD. High dose, short-term i.v. treatment with GCs leads directly to reduction of bone formation and increased bone resorption, as indicated by markers of bone turnover (De Vries et al. 2007; Van Staa et al., 2000). Osteopenia not osteoporosis was significantly more frequent in patients with MS compared with controls, especially in women who received high dose methylprednisolone pulses (HDMP) in relapses period making important the regularly monitoring of BMD in these patients. The authors concluded that disability and the subsequent immobilization osteoporosis is the more serious factor in this group and treatment with repeated HDMP pulses did not cause osteoporosis in MS subjects followed-up for almost 8 years unlike chronic corticosteroid therapy which induces osteoporosis and/or recovery of BMD is permitted without permanent skeletal damage (Zorzon et al., 2005). The lack of physical activity exacerbates osteoporosis. All MS patients should be considered high risk for osteoporosis. Prevention with calcium rich foods and dietary supplements containing vitamin D and antiosteoporotic drugs is necessary for these patients. Particular attention should be paid to transfers and falls prevention in this population to prevent fractures which occur easily and heal slowly (Cattaneo et al., 2007; Dionyssiotis, 2011b).

In osteoporosis molecular mechanisms leading to bone loss are inadequately explained. There is evidence of interaction between bone and immune system. T cells' activity could stimulate bone loss under certain circumstances such as estrogen deficiency. Women with post-menopausal osteoporosis have higher T cell activity than healthy post-menopausal subjects which could be also the case in inflammatory or autoimmune disorders like MS: receptor activator of nuclear factor kappa B ligand (RANKL) stimulates osteoclastogenesis and the same do cytokines, such as TNF-a, IL-1, or IL-11, all produced by T-cells activation, leading to bone destruction. On the contrary osteoprotegerin (OPG) is an osteoclastogenesis inhibitory factor preventing the function from RANKL. A balanced system of RANKL/OPG regulates bone metabolism. In MS this system is disturbed in favour of RANKL (Zhao et al., 2008; Kurban et al., 2009).

4. Stroke

Disuse has been suggested as the main cause for loss of bone mass in patients immobilized because of stroke (Takamoto et al., 1995). However, this was not confirmed in a prospective study, in which only weak associations between bone loss and motor function, activities of daily living (ADL), or ambulation were found (Ramnemark et al., 1999a). This could be explained by the selected severely affected patients, but it does raise questions about other risk factors for the development of hemiosteoporosis apart from paresis and immobilization (Ramnemark et al., 1999b).

The critical role in pathogenesis of osteoporosis is attributed to hormonal processes and osteoporosis itself is often defined as generalized skeletal disorder. Findings of tibial bone changes in hemiplegic patients are not compatible with this view. The adaptations are found in trabecular bone in the epiphysis as well as in cortical bone in the diaphysis. They represent an individually different distribution of local changes which can be explained by the feedback principles of the muscle-bone-unit, in which bone strength is controlled by the muscle forces that act upon the bone. Muscle forces acting habitually on the paretic limb are considerably less than on the opposite side. This reduction of forces reduces the strain on bones. This leads to loss of bone mass and bone strength (Runge et al., 2004).

Determinants of bone mineral loss have been identified as duration of hemiplegia-induced immobilization and severity of palsy (Sato, 1996). A rapid and pronounced loss of BMD in the paretic extremities that progressed during the first year after stroke (Ramnemark et al., 1999a) more pronounced during the first few months after stroke onset (Hamdy et al., 1993). The lower extremities lost BMD bilaterally, but the losses were significant after 12 months in the affected femur, proximal femur and trochanter. In immobile patients, this could explain the loss of BMD in the nonaffected leg as compared with the nonaffected arm, which even increased in BMD, probably due to increased compensatory activity (Ramnemark et al., 1999a).

Hemiosteoporosis has previously been described as being caused by disuse and vitamin D deficiency (Sato et al, 1996), and in a randomized study a significant decrease in the rate of bone loss in stroke patients with a mean duration of 4.8 years after stroke when supplemental vitamin D was given (Sato et al., 1997). Bone mineral loss was more pronounced in the upper than in lower limbs, and the difference between sides was more marked in long-standing poststroke hemiparesis. The upper versus lower difference may reflect that hemiparesis from stroke is commonly more severe in the upper limb. Notably, BMD on the nonhemiplegic side is intermediate between that for the hemiplegic side and that in control subjects. The decrease in mobility of the intact limb, resulting from stroke-related need for assistance with activities of daily living, presumably results in mild osteoporosis paralleling the patient's overall degree of immobilization (Sato et al., 1998, 2000).

5. Myelomeningocele and cerebral palsy

Previous studies suggest that the level of neurological injury and mobility affect BMD in myelomeningocele (MMC). Studies concluded that loading of the lower limbs rather than child's potential ability to walk because of the level of neurological lesion or residual motor capacity of lower limbs is a prognostic criterion for the BMD (Apkon et al., 2009; Ausili et al., 2008; Quan et al., 1998). This theory is probably challenged by other studies that revealed low values of forearm BMD in individuals and indicate that in this patient osteoporosis can be caused by neurogenic and metabolic mechanisms. The fact is that these patients are loading the arms through the use of crutches and wheelchairs and BMD values in the upper extremities are expected to be higher in relation to immobilized people (Quan et al., 1998). Subjects with MMC may have hypercalciuria associated with immobilization and an additional risk factor for osteoporosis in these patients group (Quan et al., 2003). Others support that low-energetic fractures in MMC children may result from metabolic disturbances that are a consequence of excessive renal calcium loss or excessive fatty tissue content (Okurowska-Zawada et al., 2009).

Children with cerebral palsy (CP) are growing slowly. The impact of this altered growth on skeletal development and bone density is a difference in linear growth which becomes more accentuated over time compared with their typically growing peers. In addition, as growth slows, the bone mineral density also falls further outside the normal range (Houlihan et al., 2009). Significantly decreased bone density is virtually universal in non-ambulatory children with moderate to severe CP after the age of 10 years (Henderson et al., 2002); Bone-mineral content and density were measured in a study by dual energy X-ray absorptiometry in the proximal femur, femoral neck, and total body of nutritionally adequate children (n=17; 11 girls, six boys; aged 7.6 to 13.8 years) with spastic cerebral palsy (CP) and found that non-independent ambulators had lower z scores for total body BMD, femoral neck BMD, and BMC than independent ambulators (Chad et al., 2000). The potential causes of deficient bone mineralization in this population are multiple, including poor nutrition and abnormal vitamin D metabolism. Findings from recent studies (Shaw et al. 1994, Henderson et al. 1995, Wilmhurst et al. 1996) suggest that non-nutritional factors, such as ambulation, may contribute to the alterations in body composition observed in children with CP.

5.1 Interventions to prevent bone loss
5.1.1 Weight bearing activities-cycling-body weight supported treadmill
The effect of standing in bone after SCI has been investigated by many researchers. A beneficial effect on bone mass using passive mechanical loading has been shown on preservation of bone mass in the region of the femoral shaft, but not at the proximal hip of standing and non-standing patients and relatively better-preserved densities in patients standing with braces than in those using a standing frame or standing wheelchair (Goemaere et al., 1994). A slower rate of bone loss in paraplegic subjects who did standing was expressed in a prospective study of 19 patients in acute SCI phase participated in early standing training program showed benefits concerning the reduction of cancellous bone loss compared to immobilized subjects (de Bruin and others 1999; Frey-Rindova and others 2000), while no correlation for passive standing-training to bone status was found in another p QCT study (Eser et al., 2005). Protection afforded by standing in the femoral diaphysis stands in contrast with the loss of bone in the proximal femur. This suggests that the transmission of forces through trabecular and cortical bone varies; so the less effective strain for the initiation of bone remodeling reaches faster cortical bone (Frost, 1992, 2001, 2003). Others also supported the concept of different strain thresholds bone remodeling control (Gutin & Kasper, 1992; LeBlanc et al., 2007; Smith et al., 2009). There is level 2 evidence (from 1 non-randomized prospective controlled trial) that Functional Electrical Stimulation (FES) - cycling did not improve or maintain bone at the tibial midshaft in the acute phase (Eser et al., 2003). Moreover, there is level 4 evidence (from 1 pre-post study) that 6 months of FES cycle ergometry increased regional lower extremity BMD over areas stimulated (Chen et al., 2005). Body weight supported treadmill training (BWSTT) did not alter the expected pattern of change in bone biochemical markers over time and bone density at fracture-prone sites (Giangregorio et al., 2009).

5.1.2 Whole body vibration
At a meeting of the American Society for Bone and Mineral Research results of a small randomised, placebo-controlled study among 20 children with cerebral palsy who used a similar, commercially available vibrating platform for 10 min per day, 5 days per week for 6 months were reported (Ward et al., 2001). A significant increase in tibial, but not lumbar-

spine bone density in the treated group was found despite the simplicity, short duration of the "vibration", the young age of the children and the poor compliance (Eisman, 2001).

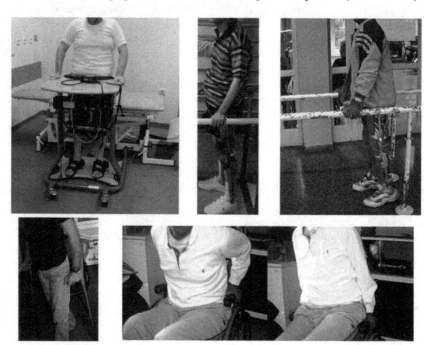

Fig. 3. Weight bearing in disabled subjects; using standing frames, functional walking with orthoses between bars and crutches, even push-ups in the wheelchair (in case of multiple sclerosis with a clinical equivalent like tetraplegia) bone can be loaded and bone loss rate would be slower (unpublished photos of Dionyssiotis Y).

After 6 months of whole body vibration (WBV) therapy in twenty children with cerebral palsy (age 6.2 to 12.3 years; 6 girls) randomized to either continue their school physiotherapy program unchanged or to receive 9 minutes of side-alternating WBV (Vibraflex Home Edition II®, Orthometrix Inc) not effect on areal BMD at the lumbar spine was observed, while areal BMD seemed to decrease somewhat in the cortical region of the femoral diaphysis. Authors explained that mechanical stimulation increases intracortical bone remodeling and thereby cortical porosity; moreover changes occurred in ways that are not reflected by areal BMD, but might be detectable by more sophisticated techniques such as such as peripheral quantitative computed tomography (Ruck et al., 2010). Low-intensity vibration (LIV) has shown to be associated with improvement in bone mineral density in post-menopausal women and children with cerebral palsy. Seven non-ambulatory subjects with SCI and ten able-bodied controls underwent transmission of a plantar-based LIV signal (0.27 +/- 0.11 g; 34 Hz) from the feet through the axial skeleton as a function of tilt-table angle (15, 30, and 45 degrees). SCI subjects and controls demonstrated equivalent transmission of LIV, with greater signal transmission observed at steeper angles of tilt which supports the possibility of the utility of LIV as a means to deliver mechanical signals in a form of therapeutic intervention to prevent/reverse skeletal fragility in the SCI population (Asselin et al., 2011).

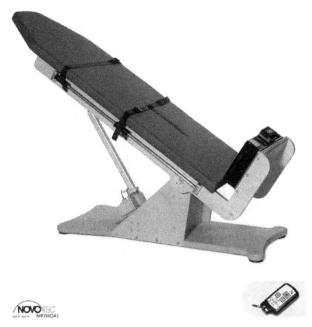

Fig. 4. The Galileo Delta A TiltTable offers a wide variety of applications from relaxation to muscle training for a diverse range of patients who are unable to stand without support. The motor driven adjustable tilt angle of the Galileo Delta TiltTable (90°) allows vibration training with reduced body weight from 0 to 100%. This is ideal for deconditioned and disabled patients for gradually increasing training weights up to full body weight. System for application in adults (max. body height: 1.90 m) and children (max. body height: 1.50 m).The Galileo Delta A TiltTable is exclusively available from the manufacturer Novotec Medical GmbH., (with permission).

5.1.3 Drugs

Calcitonin in varying doses and methods of administration has given variable results in paraplegia (preferred dosage regimen, treatment duration, and administration route for adequate efficacy in SCI patients' remains unclear) (Chantraine et al., 1979a; Minaire, 1987). Likewise, the outcome using bisphosphonates has been variable. Etidronate produced long-term benefit in lower limb bone mineral density (BMD) in selected walking SCI patients (Roux et al., 1998); whereas tiludronate appeared effective in reducing bone resorption and preserving bone mass in a histomorphometric study in 20 paraplegic patients (Chappard et al., 1995). Intravenous pamidronate has been shown to attenuate bone loss in SCI and normalize serum calcium in immobilization hypercalcemia (Bauman et al., 2005). Alendronate (1000 times more potent than etidronate), in an open observational study, reversed BMD loss in men with established SCI increased both axial and trabecular bone density and has proven efficacy and safety in men treated for osteoporosis, prevents hypercalciuria and bone loss after bed rest and lower leg fracture (Moran de Brito et al., 2005; Zehnder et al., 2004). Six months after using zolendronic acid in the treatment group BMD showed differences in the response to treatment between the mixed trabecular/

cortical regions (narrow neck and intertrochanteric) and the purely cortical shaft. With respect to cross-sectional geometry, bone cross-sectional area and sectional modulus (indices of resistance to axial and bending loads, where higher values would indicate a positive effect of treatment) increased at the hip and buckling ratio (an index of the instability of thin-walled cross sections, where lower values would suggest that the treatment is improving stability) decreased consistent with improved bone outcomes; at 12 months, narrow-neck femur values declined and intertrochanteric and femoral shaft BMD was maintained vs. placebo group which showed a decrease in bone outcomes and an increase in buckling ratio at the hip at 6 and 12 months, while with respect to bone prevention 4 mg i.v. were effective and well-tolerated to prevent BMD loss at the total hip and trochanter for up to 12 months following SCI (Bubbear et al; Shapiro et al., 2007).

Clinical examination and management of bone loss in SCI	
• history of the patient (co morbidities, neurologic complications, use of drugs which impair bone metabolism, alcohol, smoking and information about the level of injury, duration of paralysis, immobilization period, onset of rehabilitation, use of assistive devices and orthoses).	• pharmacological treatment with bisphosphonates p.os and i.v. that have been studied in patients with spinal cord injuries and had positive effects on bone parameters. • Use of calcium supplements (monitoring renal function) and vitamin D.
• anthropometric parameters (age, weight, body mass index, BMI) • clinical examination (level of injury according to American Spinal Injury Association Impairment Scale, AIS) and assessment of spasticity)	• Education on falls prevention • Counseling regarding osteoporosis and related factors and identification of fractures in regions of impaired sensation.
• imaging (bone densitometry by DXA at the hip and spine, and if possible, p QCT at the the tibia or femur)	• physical therapy including: a) range of motion exercises, b) loading of the skeleton to reduce bone loss, d) therapeutic standing-walking with orthoses, e) passive-active cycling
• measurement of bone turnover indices in the serum (parathyroid hormone, alkaline phosphatase, calcium, vitamin D, PINP molecule, osteocalcin) and urinary excretion of 24 hour (calcium, hydroxyproline, aminoterminal (NTx) and carboxylterminal (CTx) intermolecular cross-linking domain of bone type-1 collagen), which provide a good indicator of bone resorption.	• dietary interventions to improve dietary intake of calcium and nutrition indices.

Table 1. An algorithm for the screening and management of osteoporosis in subjects with spinal cord injury (should be read top to bottom starting with the left column); adapted from: Dionyssiotis Y. (2009). Bone loss in paraplegia: A diagnostic and therapeutic protocol. Osteoporos Int Vol. 20 (Suppl 1):S23-S176 (with permission).

6. References

Apkon, S.D., Fenton, L., & Coll, J.R. (2009). Bone mineral density in children with myelomeningocele. *Dev Med Child Neurol*, Vol. 51, No. 1, pp. 63-67.

Asselin, P., Spungen, A.M., Muir, J.W., Rubin, C.T., & Bauman, W.A. (2011). Transmission of low-intensity vibration through the axial skeleton of persons with spinal cord injury as a potential intervention for preservation of bone quantity and quality. *J Spinal Cord Med*, Vol.34, No. 1, pp. 52-59.

Ausili, E., Focarelli, B., Tabacco, F., Fortunelli, G., Caradonna, P., Massimi, L., Sigismondi, M., Salvaggio, E., & Rendeli, C. (2008). Bone mineral density and body composition in a myelomeningocele children population: effects of walking ability and sport activity. *Eur Rev Med Pharmacol Sci*, Vol. 12, No.6, pp. 349-354.

Bauman, W.A., & Schwartz E. (1997). Calcium metabolism and osteoporosis in individuals with spinal cord injury. *Top Spinal Cord Inj Rehabil*, Vol. 2, pp. 84-96.

Bauman, W.A., Spungen, A.M., Morrison, N., Zhang, R.L., & Schwartz, E. (2005). Effect of a vitamin D analog on leg bone mineral density in patients with chronic spinal cord injury. *J Rehabil Res Dev*, Vol. 42, No. 5, pp. 625-634.

Bauman, W.A., Wecht, J.M., Kirshblum, S., Spungen, A.M., Morrison, N., Cirnigliaro, C, & Schwartz, E. (2005). Effect of pamidronate administration on bone in patients with acute spinal cord injury. *J Rehabil Res Dev*, Vol. 42, No. 3, pp. 305-313.

Bauman, W.A., Schwartz, E., Song, I.S., Kirshblum, S., Cirnigliaro, C., Morrison, N. & Spungen, A.M. (2009). Dual-energy X-ray absorptiometry overestimates bone mineral density of the lumbar spine in persons with spinal cord injury. *Spinal Cord*, Vol. 47, No 8, pp. 628-633.

Biering-Sorensen, F., Hansen, B., & Lee, B.S. (2009). Non-pharmacological treatment and prevention of bone loss after spinal cord injury: a systematic review. *Spinal Cord*, Vol. 47, No. 7, pp. 508-518.

Biering-Sorensen, F., Bohr, H.H., & Schaadt, O.P. (1991). Longitudinal study of bone mineral content in the lumbar spine, the forearm and the lower extremities after spinal cord injury. *Europ J Clin Invest*, Vol.20, pp. 330-335.

Biering-Sorensen, F., Bohr, H.H., & Schaadt, O.P. (1988). Bone mineral content of the lumbar spine and lower extremities years after spinal cord lesions. *Paraplegia*, Vol. 26, pp. 293- 301.

Bikle, D.D., Halloran, B.P., & Morey-Holton, E. (1997). Spaceflight and the skeleton: lessons for the earthbound. *Gravi Space Biol Bull*, Vol. 10, No. 2, pp. 119-135.

Bubbear, J.S., Gall, A., Middleton, F.R., Ferguson-Pell, M., Swaminathan, R., & Keen, R.W. (2011). Early treatment with zoledronic acid prevents bone loss at the hip following acute spinal cord injury. *Osteoporos Int*, Vol. 22, No. 1. pp. 271-279.

Cavanagh, P.R., Licata, A.A., & Rice, A.J. (2005). Exercise and pharmacological countermeasures for bone loss during long-duration space flight. *Gravit Space Biol Bull*, Vol. 18, No. 2, pp. 39-58.

Chad, K.E., McKay, H.A., Zello, G.A, Bailey, D.A., Faulkner, R.A., Snyder, R.E. (2000). Body composition in nutritionally adequate ambulatory and non-ambulatory children with cerebral palsy and a healthy reference group. *Dev Med Child Neurol*, Vol. 42, No. 5, pp. 334-339.

Chantraine, A. (1978). Actual concept of osteoporosis in paraplegia. *Paraplegia*, Vol. 16, No 1, pp. 51-58.

Chantraine, A., Heynen, G., & Franchimont, P. (1979). Bone metabolism, parathyroid hormone, and calcitonin in paraplegia. *Calcif Tissue Int*, Vol. 27, No. 3, pp. 199-204.

Chantraine, A., van Ouwenaller, C., Hachen, H.J., Schinas, P. (1979). Intra-medullary pressure and intra-osseous phlebography in paraplegia. *Paraplegia*, Vol. 17, No. 4, pp. 391-399.

Chantraine, A., Nusgens, B., & Lapiere, C.M. (1986). Bone remodeling during the development of osteoporosis in paraplegia. *Calcif Tissue Int*, Vol. 38, No. 6, pp. 323-327.

Chen, S.C., Lai, C.H., Chan, W.P., Huang, M.H., Tsai, H.W., & Chen, J.J. (2005). Increases in bone mineral density after functional electrical stimulation cycling exercises in spinal cord injured patients. *Disabil Rehabil*, Vol. 27, No. 22, pp. 1337-1341.

Cosman, F., Nieves, J., Komar, L., Ferrer, G., Herbert, J., Formica, C., Shen, V., & Lindsay, R. (1998). Fracture history and bone loss in patients with MS. *Neurology*, Vol. 51, No. 4, pp. 1161-1165.

Coupaud, S., McLean, A.N., & Allan, D.B. (2009). Role of peripheral quantitative computed tomography in identifying disuse osteoporosis in paraplegia. *Skeletal Radiol*, Vol. 38, No. 10, pp. 989-995.

Clasey, J.L., Janowiak, A.L., & Gater, D.R. (2004). Relationship between regional bone density measurements and the time since injury in adults with spinal cord injuries. *Arch Phys Med Rehabil*, Vol. 85, pp. 59-64.

Dauty, M., Perrouin-Verbe, B., Maugars, Y., Dubois, C., & Mathe, J.F. (2000). Supralesional and sublesional bone mineral density in spinal cord-injured patients. *Bone*, Vol. 27, No. 2, pp. 305-309.

de Bruin, E.D., Frey-Rindova, P., Herzog, R.E., Dietz, V., Dambacher, M.A.,& Stussi, E. (1999). Changes of tibia bone properties after spinal cord injury: effects of early intervention. *Arch Phys Med Rehabil*, Vol. 80, No. 2, pp. 214-220.

Demirel, G., Yilmaz, H., Paker, N, & Onel S. (1998). Osteoporosis after spinal cord injury. *Spinal Cord*, Vol. 36, No. 12. pp. 822-825.

Dionyssiotis, Y, Trovas, G., Galanos, A., Raptou, P., Papaioannou, N., Papagelopoulos, P., Petropoulou, K., & Lyritis, G.P. (2007). Bone loss and mechanical properties of tibia in spinal cord injured men. *J Musculoskelet Neuronal Interact* Vol.7, No. 1, pp. 62-68.

Dionyssiotis, Y., Petropoulou, K., Rapidi, C.A., Papagelopoulos, P., Papaioannou, N., Galanos, A., Papadaki, P., & Lyritis, G.P. (2008). Body composition in paraplegic men. *J Clin Densitom*, Vol.11, No.3, pp. 437-443.

Dionyssiotis, Y., Lyritis, G.P., Papaioannou, N., Papagelopoulos, P., & Thomaides, T. (2009). Influence of neurological level of injury in bones, muscles, and fat in paraplegia. *J Rehabil Res Dev*, Vol. 46, No 8, pp. 1037-1044.

Dionyssiotis, Y. (2009). Bone loss in paraplegia: A diagnostic and therapeutic protocol. *Osteoporos Int*, Vol. 20, (Suppl 1):S23-S176.

Dionyssiotis, Y., Lyritis, G.P., Mavrogenis, A.F., & Papagelopoulos, P.J. (2011a). Factors influencing bone loss in paraplegia. *Hippokratia*, Vol.15, No. 1, pp. 54-59.

Dionyssiotis, Y. (2011b). Bone loss and fractures in multiple sclerosis: focus on epidemiologic and physiopathological features. *Int J Gen Med*, Vol. 4, pp. 505-509.

Dionyssiotis, Y. (2011c). Spinal cord injury-related bone impairment and fractures: An update on epidemiology and physiopathological mechanisms. *J Musculoskelet Neuronal Interact*, Vol.11, No. 3, pp. 257-265

Dionyssiotis Y. (2011d). Bone Loss in Spinal Cord Injury and Multiple Sclerosis. In: JH Stone, M Blouin, editors. *International Encyclopedia of Rehabilitation*. Available online: http://cirrie.buffalo.edu/encyclopedia/en/article/340/

Doty, S.B., & DiCarlo, E.F. (1995). Pathophysiology of immobilization osteoporosis. *Curr Opin Orthop*, Vol.6, No. 5, pp. 45-49.

Dovio, A., Perazzolo, L., Osella, G., Ventura, M., Termine, A., Milano, E., Bertolotto, A., & Angeli, A. (2004). Immediate fall of bone formation and transient increase of bone resorption in the course of high-dose, short-term glucocorticoid therapy in young patients with multiple sclerosis. *J Clin Endocrinol Metab*, Vol. 89, No. 10, pp. 4923-4928.

Dudley-Javoroski, S., & Shields, R.K. (2008). Dose estimation and surveillance of mechanical loading interventions for bone loss after spinal cord injury. *Phys Ther*, Vol. 88, No 3, pp. 387-396.

Dudley-Javoroski, S., & Shields, R.K. (2008). Muscle and bone plasticity after spinal cord injury: review of adaptations to disuse and to electrical muscle stimulation. *J Rehabil Res Dev*, Vol. 45, No. 2, pp. 283-296.

Dudley-Javoroski, S., & Shields, R.K. (2010). Longitudinal changes in femur bone mineral density after spinal cord injury: effects of slice placement and peel method. *Osteoporos Int*, Vol. 21, No. 6, pp. 985-995.

Eisman, J.A. (2001). Good, good, good... good vibrations: the best option for better bones? *Lancet*, Vol. 358, No. 9297, pp. 1924-1925.

Eser, P., de Bruin, E.D., Telley, I., Lechner, H.E., Knecht, H., & Stussi, E. (2003). Effect of electrical stimulation-induced cycling on bone mineral density in spinal cord-injured patients. *Eur J Clin Invest*, Vol. 33, No 5, pp. 412-419.

Eser, P., Frotzler, A., Zehnder, Y., Wick, L., Knecht, H., Denoth, J, & Schiessl H. (2004). Relationship between the duration of paralysis and bone structure: a pQCT study of spinal cord injured individuals. *Bone*, Vol. 34, No. 5, pp. 869-880.

Eser, P., Frotzler, A., Zehnder, Y., & Denoth, J. (2005). Fracture threshold in the femur and tibia of people with spinal cord injury as determined by peripheral quantitative computed tomography. *Arch Phys Med Rehabil*, Vol. 86, No. 3, pp. 498-504.

Eser, P., Frotzler, A., Zehnder, Y., Schiessl, H., & Denoth, J. (2005). Assessment of anthropometric, systemic, and lifestyle factors influencing bone status in the legs of spinal cord injured individuals. *Osteoporos Int*, Vol. 16, No. 1, pp. 26-34.

Fattal, C., Mariano-Goulart, D., Thomas, E., Rouays-Mabit, H., Verollet, C., & Maimoun, L. (2011). Osteoporosis in persons with spinal cord injury: the need for a targeted therapeutic education. *Arch Phys Med Rehabil*, Vol. 92, No. 1, pp. 59-67.

Faulkner, M.A., Ryan-Haddad, A.M., Lenz, TL, & Degner, K. (2005). Osteoporosis in long-term care residents with multiple sclerosis. *Consult Pharm*, Vol. 20, No. 2, pp. 128-136.

Frotzler, A., Coupaud, S., Perret, C., Kakebeeke, T.H., Hunt, K.J., Donaldson, Nde. N., & Eser, P. (2008). High-volume FES-cycling partially reverses bone loss in people with chronic spinal cord injury. *Bone*, Vol. 43, No. 1, pp. 169-176.

Frotzler, A., Coupaud, S., Perret, C., Kakebeeke, T.H., Hunt, K.J., & Eser, P. (2009). Effect of detraining on bone and muscle tissue in subjects with chronic spinal cord injury after a period of electrically-stimulated cycling: a small cohort study. *J Rehabil Med*, Vol. 41, No. 4, pp. 282-285.

Garland, D.E., Stewart, C.A., Adkins, R.H., Hu, S.S., Rosén, C., Liotta, F.J., & Weinstein, D.A. (1992). Osteoporosis after spinal cord injury. *J Orthop Res*, Vol. 10, No. 3, pp. 371-378.

Garland, D.E., Foulkes, G.D., Adkins, R.H., Stewart, C.A., & Yakura, J.S. (1994). Regional osteoporosis following incomplete spinal cord injury. *Contemporary Orthopaedics*, Vol. 28, pp. 134-139.

Garland, D.E., Adkins, R.H., Matsuno, N.N., & Stewart, C.A. (1999). The effect of pulsed electromagnetic fields on osteoporosis at the knee in individuals with spinal cord injury. *J Spinal Cord Med*, Vol. 22, No 4, pp. 239-245.

Garland, D.E., Adkins, R.H., Stewart, C.A., Ashford, R., & Vigil, D. (2001). Regional osteoporosis in women who have a complete spinal cord injury. *J Bone Joint Surg Am*, Vol. 83-A, No. 8, pp. 1195-200.

Garland, D.E., Adkins, R.H., Kushwaha, V., & Stewart, C. (2004a). Risk factors for osteoporosis at the knee in the spinal cord injury population. *J Spinal Cord Med*, Vol. 27, No. 3, pp. 202-206.

Garland, D.E., Adkins, R.H., Scott, M., Singh, H., Massih, M., & Stewart, C. (2004b). Bone loss at the os calcis compared with bone loss at the knee in individuals with spinal cord injury. *J Spinal Cord Med*, Vol. 27, No. 3, pp. 207-211.

Giangregorio, L.M., & Blimkie, C.J. (2002). Skeletal adaptations to alterations in weight-bearing activity: a comparison of models of disuse osteoporosis. *Sports Med*, Vol. 32, No 7, pp. 459-476.

Giangregorio, L.M., & Webber, C.E. (2004). Speed of sound in bone at the tibia: is it related to lower limb bone mineral density in spinal-cord-injured individuals? *Spinal Cord*, Vol. 42, No 3, pp. 141-145.

Giangregorio, LM, Craven, B.C., & Webber, C.E. (2005). Musculoskeletal changes in women with spinal cord injury: a twin study. *J Clin Densitom*, Vol. 8, No. 3, pp. 347-351.

Giangregorio, L.M., Thabane, L., Debeer, J., Farrauto, L., McCartney, N., Adachi, J.D., & Papaioannou, A. (2009). Body weight-supported treadmill training for patients with hip fracture: a feasibility study. *Arch Phys Med Rehabil*, Vol. 90, No. 12, pp. 2125-2130.

Griffiths, H.J., Bushueff, B.,& Zimmerman, R.E. (1976). Investigation of the loss of bone mineral in patients with spinal cord injury. *Paraplegia*, Vol.14, No. 3, pp. 207-212.

Gutin, B., & Kasper, M.J. (1992). Can vigorous exercise play a role in osteoporosis prevention? A review. *Osteoporos Int*, Vol. 2, No. 2, pp. 55-69.

Hamdy, R.C., Krishnaswamy, G., Cancellaro, V., Whalen, K., & Harvill, L. (1993). Changes in bone mineral content and density after stroke. *Am J Phys Med Rehabil*, Vol. 72, pp. 188–191.

Henderson, R.C., Lin, P.P., & Greene, W.B. (1995). Bone-mineral density in children and adolescents who have spastic cerebral palsy. *Journal of Bone and Joint Surgery*, Vol. 77A, pp. 1671–1681.

Henderson, R.C., Lark, R.K., Gurka, M.J, Worley, G., Fung, E.B., Conaway, M., Stallings, V.A., & Stevenson, R.D. (2002). Bone density and metabolism in children and adolescents with moderate to severe cerebral palsy. Pediatrics Vol. 110, No.1, p.5.

Houlihan, C.M., & Stevenson RD. (2009). Bone density in cerebral palsy. *Phys Med Rehabil Clin N Am*, Vol. 20, No. 3, pp. 493-508.

Jiang, S.D., Jiang, L.S., & Dai, L.Y. (2007). Changes in bone mass, bone structure, bone biomechanical properties, and bone metabolism after spinal cord injury: a 6-month longitudinal study in growing rats. *Calcif Tissue Int*, Vol. 80, No.3, pp. 167-175.

Jiang, S.D., Jiang, L.S., & Dai, L.Y. (2007). Effects of spinal cord injury on osteoblastogenesis, osteoclastogenesis and gene expression profiling in osteoblasts in young rats. *Osteoporos Int*, Vol. 18, No 3, pp. 339-349.

Jones, L.M., Legge, M., & Goulding, A. (2002). Intensive exercise may preserve bone mass of the upper limbs in spinal cord injured males but does not retard demineralisation of the lower body. *Spinal Cord*, Vol. 40, No. 5, pp. 230-235.

Kannisto, M., Alaranta, H., Merikanto, J., Kroger, H., & Karkkainen, J. (1998). Bone mineral status after pediatric spinal cord injury. *Spinal Cord*, Vol. 36, No 9, pp. 641-646.

Karlsson, A.K., Friberg, P., Lonnroth, P., Sullivan, L., & Elam, M. (1998). Regional sympathetic function in high spinal cord injury during mental stress and autonomic dysreflexia. *Brain*, Vol. 121, pp. 1711–1719.

Kiratli, B.J., Smith, A.E., Nauenberg, T., Kallfelz, C.F., & Perkash, I. (2000). Bone mineral and geometric changes through the femur with immobilization due to spinal cord injury. *J Rehabil Res Dev*, Vol. 37, No. 2, pp. 225-233.

Kondo, H., Nifuji, A., Takeda, S., Ezura, Y., Rittling, S.R., Denhardt, D.T., Nakashima, K., Karsenty, G., & Noda, M. (2005). Unloading induces osteoblastic cell suppression and osteoclastic cell activation to lead to bone loss via sympathetic nervous system. *J Biol Chem.*, Vol. 280, pp. 30192-30200.

Kurban, S., Akpinar, Z., & Mehmetoglu, I. (2008). Receptor activator of nuclear factor kappa B ligand (RANKL) and osteoprotegerin levels in multiple sclerosis. *Mult Scler*, Vol.14, pp. 431-432.

Lakatos, P., Nagy, Z., Kiss, L., Horvath, C., Takacs, I., Foldes, J., Speer, G., & Bossanyi, A. (2000). Prevention of corticosteroid-induced osteoporosis by alfacalcidol. *Z Rheumatol*, Vol. 59, Suppl 1, pp. 48-52.

Lanyon, L.E., Rubin, C.T., & Baust, G. Modulation of bone loss during calcium insufficiency by controlled dynamic loading. (1986). *Calcif Tissue Int*, Vol. 38, pp. 209-216.

Lazo, M.G., Shirazi, P., Sam, M., Giobbie-Hurder, A., Blacconiere, M.J., & Muppidi, M. (2001). Osteoporosis and risk of fracture in men with spinal cord injury. *Spinal Cord*, Vol. 39, No 4, pp. 208-214.

LeBlanc, A.D., Evans, H.J., Engelbretson, D.A., & Krebs, J.M. (1990). Bone mineral loss and recovery after 17 weeks of bed rest. *J Bone Miner Res*, Vol. 5, pp. 843-850.

LeBlanc, A.D., & Schneider, V. (1992). Countermeasures against space flight related bone loss. *Acta Astronaut*, Vol. 27, pp. 89-92.

LeBlanc, A.D., Spector, E.R., Evans, H.J., & Sibonga, J.D. (2007). Skeletal responses to space flight and the bed rest analog: a review. *J Musculoskelet Neuronal Interact*, Vol. 7, No. 1, pp. 33-47.

Leslie, W.D., & Nance, P.W. Dissociated hip and spine demineralization: a specific finding in spinal cord injury. *Arch Phys Med Rehabil*, Vol.74, pp. 960-964.

Leeds, E.M., Klose, K.J., Ganz, W., Serafini, A., & Green, B.A. (1990). Bone mineral density after bicycle ergometry training. *Arch Phys Med Rehabil* Vol. 71, No. 3, pp. 207-209.

Levasseur, R., Sabatier, J.P., Potrel-Burgot, C., Lecoq, B., Creveuil, C., & Marcelli, C. (2003). Sympathetic nervous system as transmitter of mechanical loading in bone. *Joint Bone Spine*, Vol. 70, pp. 515-519.

Lofvenmark, I., Werhagen, L., & Norrbrink, C. (2009). Spasticity and bone density after a spinal cord injury. *J Rehabil Med*, Vol. 41, No 13, pp. 1080-1084.

Maimoun, L., Couret, I., Micallef, J.P., Peruchon, E., Mariano-Goulart, D., Rossi, M., Leroux, J.L., & Ohanna, F. (2002). Use of bone biochemical markers with dual-energy x-ray absorptiometry for early determination of bone loss in persons with spinal cord injury. *Metabolism*, Vol. 51, No.8, pp. 958-963.

Maimoun, L., Couret, I., Mariano-Goulart, D., Dupuy, A.M., Micallef, J.P., Peruchon, E., Ohanna, F., Cristol, J.P., Rossi, M., & Leroux, J.L. (2005). Changes in osteoprotegerin/RANKL system, bone mineral density, and bone biochemicals markers in patients with recent spinal cord injury. *Calcif Tissue Int*, Vol. 76, No. 6, pp. 404-411.

Maimoun, L., Fattal, C., Micallef, J.P., Peruchon, E, & Rabischong, P. (2006). Bone loss in spinal cord-injured patients: from physiopathology to therapy. *Spinal Cord* Vol. 44, No. 4, pp. 203-210.

Marrie, R.A., Cutter, G., Tyry, T., & Vollmer, T. (2009). A cross-sectional study of bone health in multiple sclerosis. *Neurology*, Vol. 73, No 17, pp. 1394-1398.

Modlesky, C.M., Bickel, C.S., Slade, J.M., Meyer, R.A., Cureton, K.J., & Dudley, G.A. (2004). Assessment of skeletal muscle mass in men with spinal cord injury using dual-energy X-ray absorptiometry and magnetic resonance imaging. *J Appl Physiol* Vol. 96, pp. 561-565.

Moran de Brito, C.M., Battistella, L.R., Saito, E.T., & Sakamoto, H. (2005). Effect of alendronate on bone mineral density in spinal cord injury patients: a pilot study. *Spinal Cord*, Vol. 43, No. 6, pp. 341-348.

Nieves, J., Cosman, F., Herbert, J., Shen, V., & Lindsay R. (1994). High prevalence of vitamin D deficiency and reduced bone mass in multiple sclerosis. *Neurology*, Vol. 44, No. 9, pp. 1687-1692.

NIH. (2001). NIH Consensus Development Panel on Osteoporosis Prevention, Diagnosis, and Therapy. *JAMA*. pp. 785-795.

Okurowska-Zawada, B., Konstantynowicz, J., Kulak, W., Kaczmarski, M., Piotrowska-Jastrzebska, J., Sienkiewicz, D., & Paszko-Patej, G. (2009). Assessment of risk factors for osteoporosis and fractures in children with meningomyelocele. *Adv Med Sci*, Vol. 54, No 2, pp. 247-252.

Ozgocmen, S., Bulut, S., Ilhan, N., Gulkesen, A., Ardicoglu, O., & Ozkan, Y. (2005). Vitamin D deficiency and reduced bone mineral density in multiple sclerosis: effect of ambulatory status and functional capacity. *J Bone Miner Metab*, Vol. 23, No 4, 309-313.

Parfitt, A.M. (1981). Bone effects of space flight: analysis by quantum concept of bone remodelling. *Acta Astronaut*, Vol. 8, No. (9-10), pp. 1083-1090.

Perez Castrillon, J.L., Cano-del Pozo, M., Sanz-Izquierdo, S., Velayos-Jimenez, J., & Dib-Wobakin, W. (2003). Bone mineral density in patients with multiple sclerosis: the effects of interferon. *Rev Neurol* Vol. 36, No. 10, pp. 901-903.

Phaner, V., Charmetant, C., Condemine, A., Fayolle-Minon, I., Lafage-Proust, M.H., & Calmels, P. Osteoporosis in spinal cord injury. Screening and treatment. Results of a survey of physical medicine and rehabilitation physician practices in France. Proposals for action to be taken towards the screening and the treatment. *Ann Phys Rehabil Med*, Vol. 53, No. 10, pp. 615-620.

Pouilles, J.M., Ribot, C., Tremollieres, F., & Guell, A. (1992). Vertebral, femoral and radial bone density in simulation of prolonged weightlessness. Experience with healthy volunteers. *Presse Med*, Vol. 21, No 4, pp. 160-164.

Quan, A., Adams, R., Ekmark, E., & Baum, M. (1998). Bone mineral density in children with myelomeningocele. *Pediatrics*, Vol. 102, No. 3, E34.

Quan, A., Adams, R., Ekmark, E., & Baum, M. (2003). Bone mineral density in children with myelomeningocele: effect of hydrochlorothiazide. *Pediatr Nephrol* Vol. 18, No 9, pp. 929-933.

Ramnemark, A., Nyberg, L., Lorentzon, R., Englund, U., & Gustafson, Y. (1999).Progressive hemiosteoporosis on the paretic side and increased bone mineral density in the nonparetic arm the first year after severe stroke. *Osteoporos Int*, Vol. 9, No. 3, pp. 269-275.

Ramnemark, A., Nyberg, L., Lorentzon, R., Olsson, T., & Gustafson, Y. (1999). Hemiosteoporosis after severe stroke, independent of changes in body composition and weight. *Stroke*, Vol. 30, No. 4, pp. 755-760.

Reiter, A.L., Volk, A., Vollmar, J., Fromm, B.,& Gerner, H.J. (2007). Changes of basic bone turnover parameters in short-term and long-term patients with spinal cord injury. *Eur Spine J*, Vol.16, No. 6, pp. 771-776.

Roberts, D., Lee, W., Cuneo, R.C., Wittmann, J., Ward, G., Flatman, R., McWhinney, B., & Hickman, P.E. (1998). Longitudinal study of bone turnover after acute spinal cord injury. *J Clin Endocrinol Metab*, Vol. 83, No. 2, pp. 415-422.

Runge, M., Rehfeld, G., & Schiessl, H. Skeletal adaptations in hemiplegic patients. (2004). *J Musculoskelet Neuronal Interact*, Vol. 4, No 2, pp. 191-196.

Rubin, C., Xu, G., & Judex, S. (2001). The anabolic activity of bone tissue, suppressed by disuse, is normalized by brief exposure to extremely low-magnitude mechanical stimuli. *Faseb J*, Vol. 15, No 12, pp. 2225-2229.

Ruck, J., Chabot, G., & Rauch, F. Vibration treatment in cerebral palsy: A randomized controlled pilot study. *J Musculoskelet Neuronal Interact*. Vol.10, No 1, pp. 77-83.

Sabo, D., Blaich, S., Wenz, W., Hohmann, M., Loew, M., & Gerner, H.J. (2001). Osteoporosis in patients with paralysis after spinal cord injury. A cross sectional study in 46 male patients with dual-energy X-ray absorptiometry. *Arch Orthop Trauma Surg*, Vol.121, No. (1-2), pp. 75-78.

Sato, Y., Maruoka, H., Oizumi, K., & Kikuyama, M. (1996). Vitamin D deficiency and osteopenia in the hemiplegic limbs of stroke patients. *Stroke*, Vol. 27, pp. 2183-2187.

Sato, Y., Maruoka, H., Honda, Y., Asoh, T., Fujimatsu, Y., & Oizumi, K. Development osteopenia in the hemiplegic finger in patients with stroke. *Eur Neurol*, Vol. 36, pp. 278-283.

Sato, Y., Maruoka, H., & Oizumi, K. Amelioration of hemiplegia associated osteopenia more than 4 years after stroke by 1 alphahydroxyvitamin D3 and calcium supplementation. *Stroke*, Vol. 28, pp. 736-739.

Sato, Y., Fuiimatsu, Y., Kikuvama, M., Kaii, M., & Oizumi, K. (1998). Influence of immobilization on bone mass and bone metabolism in hemiplegic elderly patients with a long-standing stroke. *J Neural Sci*, Vol. 156, pp. 205-210.

Sato, Y., Kaji, M., & Oizomi, K. (1999). An alternative to vitamin D supplementation to prevent fractures in patients with MS. *Neurology*, Vol. 53, No. 2, pp. 437.

Sato, Y. (2000). Abnormal bone and calcium metabolism in patients after stroke. *Arch Phys Med Rehabil*, Vol. 81, pp. 117-121.

Schwarzman, R.J. (2000). New treatments for reflex sympathetic dystrophy. *N Engl J Med*, Vol. 343, pp. 654–656.

Shaw, N.J., White, C.P., Fraser, W.D., & Rosenbloom L. (1994) Osteopenia in cerebral palsy. *Archives of Disease in Childhood*, Vol. 71, pp. 235–238.

Schwid, S.R., Goodman, A.D., Puzas, J.E., McDermott, M.P., & Mattson, D.H. (1996). Sporadic corticosteroid pulses and osteoporosis in multiple sclerosis. *Arch Neurol* Vol. 53, No. 8, pp. 753-757.

Shields, R.K. (2002). Muscular, skeletal, and neural adaptations following spinal cord injury. *J Orthop Sports Phys Ther, Vol.* 32, No 2, pp. 65-74.

Shojaei, H., Soroush, M.R., & Modirian, E. (2006). Spinal cord injury-induced osteoporosis in veterans. *J Spinal Disord Tech*, Vol. 19, No.2, pp. 114-117.

Shuhaibar, M., McKenna, M.J., Au-Yeong, M., & Redmond, J.M. (2009). Favorable effect of immunomodulator therapy on bone mineral density in multiple sclerosis. *Ir J Med Sci* Vol. 178, No. 1, pp. 43-45.

Sioka, C., Kyritsis, A.P., & Fotopoulos, A. (2009). Multiple sclerosis, osteoporosis, and vitamin D. *J Neurol Sci*, Vol. 287, No (1-2), pp. 1-6.

Smeltzer, S.C., Zimmerman, V., & Capriotti, T. (2005). Osteoporosis risk and low bone mineral density in women with physical disabilities. *Arch Phys Med Rehabil*, Vol. 86, pp. 582-586.

Smith, E.M., Comiskey, C.M., & Carroll, A.M. (2009). A study of bone mineral density in adults with disability. *Arch Phys Med Rehabil*, Vol. 90, No 7, pp. 1127-1135.

Smith, S.M., Zwart, S.R., Heer, M.A., Baecker, N., Evans, H.J., Feiveson, A.H., Shackelford, L.C., & Leblanc, A.D. (2009). Effects of artificial gravity during bed rest on bone metabolism in humans. *J Appl Physiol, Vol.*107, No 1, pp. 47-53.

Sniger, W., & Garshick, E. (2002). Alendronate increases bone density in chronic spinal cord injury: a case report. *Arch Phys Med Rehabil*, Vol. 83, No.1, pp. 139-140.

Spector, E.R., Smith, S.M., & Sibonga, J.D. (2009). Skeletal effects of long-duration head-down bed rest. *Aviat Space Environ Med* Vol. 80, No. (5 Suppl):A23-8.

Stenager, E., Jensen, K. (1991). Fractures in multiple sclerosis. *Acta Neurol Belg* Vol. 91, No 5, pp. 296-302.

Szollar, S.M., Martin, E.M., Sartoris, D.J., Parthemore, J.G., & Deftos, LJ. (1998). Bone mineral density and indexes of bone metabolism in spinal cord injury. *Am J Phys Med Rehabil*, Vol. 77, No. 1, pp. 28-35.

Takamoto, S., Masuyama, T., Nakajima, M., Seikiya, K., Kosaka, H., Morimoto, S., Ogihara, T., & Onishi T. (1995). Alterations of bone mineral density of the femurs in hemiplegia. *Calcif Tissue Int*. Vol. 56, pp. 259 –262.

Takata, S., & Yasui, N. (2001). Disuse osteoporosis. *J Med Invest*, Vol. 48, No. (3-4), pp. 147-156.

Takeda, S., Elefteriou, F., Levasseur, R., Liu, X., Zhao, L., Parker, K.L., Armstrong, D., Ducy. P., & Karsenty, G. (2002). Leptin regulates bone formation via the sympathetic nervous system. *Cell, Vol.* 111, pp. 305-317.

Teasell, R.W., Arnold, J.M., Krassioukov, A., & Delaney, G.A. (2000). Cardiovascular consequences of loss of supraspinal control of the sympathetic nervous system after spinal cord injury. *Arch Phys Med Rehabil,* Vol. 81, pp. 506-516.

Tsuzuku, S., Ikegami, Y., & Yabe, K. Bone mineral density differences between paraplegic and quadriplegic patients: a cross-sectional study. *Spinal Cord,* Vol. 37, pp. 358-361.

Uebelhart, D., Demiaux-Domenech, B., Roth, M., & Chantraine, A. (1995). Bone metabolism in spinal cord injured individuals and in others who have prolonged immobilisation. A review. *Paraplegia,* Vol. 33, No 11, pp. 669-673.

Ward, K.A., Alsop, C.W., Brown, S., Caulton, J., Adams, J.E., & Mughal Z. (2001). A randomized, placebo controlled, pilot trial of low magnitude, high frequency loading treatment of low bone mineral density in children with disabling conditions. *J Bone Miner Res,* Vol.16: S173.

Wilmshurst, S., Ward, K., Adams, J.E., Langton, C.M., & Mughal, M.Z. (1996) Mobility status and bone density in cerebral palsy. *Archives of Disease in Childhood,* Vol. 75, pp. 164-165.

Weinstock-Guttman, B., Gallagher, E., Baier, M., Green, L., Feichter, J., Patrick, K., Miller, C., Wrest, K., & Ramanathan, M. (2004). Risk of bone loss in men with multiple sclerosis. *Mult Scler,* Vol. 10, No. 2, pp. 170-175.

Whalen, R.T. A.S., & Grindeland, R.E. Proceedings of the NASA symposium on the influence of gravity and activity on muscle and bone; 1991. pp. 1-178.

Whedon, G.D. (1984). Disuse osteoporosis: physiological aspects. *Calcif Tissue Int,* Vol.36, Suppl 1:S146-150.

WHO. (1994). Assessment of fracture risk and its application to screening for postmenopausal osteoporosis. Report of a WHO Study Group. Geneva, pp. 1-129 .

Wilmet, E., Ismail, A.A., Heilporn, A., Welraeds, D., & Bergmann, P. (1995). Longitudinal study of the bone mineral content and of soft tissue composition after spinal cord section. *Paraplegia,* Vol. 33, No 11, pp. 674-677.

Wronski, T.J., & Morey, E.R. (1983). Alterations in calcium homeostasis and bone during actual and simulated space flight. *Med Sci Sports Exerc,* Vol.15, No. 5, pp. 410-414.

Zehnder, Y., Risi, S., Michel, D., Knecht, H., Perrelet, R., Kraenzlin, M., Zach, G.A., & Lippuner, K. (2004). Prevention of bone loss in paraplegics over 2 years with alendronate. *J Bone Miner Res,* Vol. 19, No 7, pp. 1067-1074.

Zehnder, Y., Lüthi, M., Michel, D., Knecht, H., Perrelet, R., Neto, I., Kraenzlin, M., Zäch, G., & Lippuner, K. (2004). Long-term changes in bone metabolism, bone mineral density, quantitative ultrasound parameters, and fracture incidence after spinal cord injury: a cross-sectional observational study in 100 paraplegic men. *Osteoporos Int,* Vol. 15, pp. 180-189.

Zhang, H.,& Wu, J. (2010). A cross-sectional study of bone health in multiple sclerosis. *Neurology* Vol. 74, No. 19, pp. 1554; author reply 1555.

Zhang, P., Hamamura, K., & Yokota, H. (2008). A brief review of bone adaptation to unloading. *Genomics Proteomics Bioinformatics,* Vol. 6, No.1, pp. 4-7.

Zhao, W., Liu, Y., Cahill. C.M., Yang. W., Rogers. J.T. & Huang. X. (2009). The role of T cells in osteoporosis, an update. *Int J Clin Exp Pathol*, Vol.20, No.2, pp.544-552.

Zorzon, M., Zivadinov, R., Locatelli, L., Giuntini, D., Toncic, M., Bosco, A., Nasuelli, D., Bratina, A., Tommasi, M.A., Rudick, R.A & Cazzato, G. (2005). Long-term effects of intravenous high dose methylprednisolone pulses on bone mineral density in patients with multiple sclerosis. *Eur J Neurol*, Vol. 12, No. 7, pp. 550-556.

3

Patchy Osteoporosis in Complex Regional Pain Syndrome

Geun-Young Park, Sun Im and Seong Hoon Lim
College of Medicine,
The Catholic University of Korea
Republic of Korea

1. Introduction

Complex regional pain syndrome (CRPS), formerly known as "reflex sympathetic dystrophy" and "causalgia", is a syndrome that refers to a chronic pain condition associated with autonomic disturbances of vasomotor and sudomotor origin (Birklein et al., 1998), along with trophic skin changes and patchy demineralization of the bones (Poplawski et al., 1983). CRPS is classified into type I and II; the former can develop after minor or remote trauma like stroke, spinal cord injury or myocardial infarction (Wasner et al., 1998); the latter can develop after a large peripheral nerve lesion (Janig & Baron, 2003). The syndrome corresponding to what was formerly described as reflex sympathetic dystrophy is now termed as CRPS type I; causalgia is now termed as CRPS type II (Merseky & Bogduk, 1994). Although the mechanism of CRPS has not been elucidated yet, recent studies indicate that it is a complex disorder that involves both the central and peripheral nervous systems (Daemen et al., 1998; Huygen et al., 2001). CRPS pathogenesis is heterogeneous and complex, which makes its treatment challenging. Pharmacological therapies of CRPS include anti-inflammatory drugs, systemic corticosteroid (Kingery, 1997), antidepressants, opioid (Mackey & Feinberg, 2007), anticonvulsants, free-radical scavengers, vasodilatory medication (Perez et al., 2010) and even bisphosphonate agents (Adami et al., 1997; Manicourt et al., 2004; Robinson et al., 2004; Varenna et al., 2000). In addition, vitamin C is recommended to prevent the occurrence of CRPS type I after wrist fracture (Perez et al., 2010).

However, there is yet no single pharmacological agent or treatment algorithm that can resolve all of its heterogenic features. The efficacy for most pharmacological agents remains largely empirical, with the exception of bisphosphonate agents, which are the only agents with proven efficacy for CRPS based on multiple controlled trials (Adami et al., 1997; Brunner et al., 2009; Mackey & Feinberg, 2007;, Manicourt et al., 2004, Robinson et al., 2004, Varenna et al., 2000).

In order to understand how these bisphosphonate agents are useful in CRPS treatment, it is imperative to understand the pathogenesis of patchy osteoporosis in CRPS. This section will first review CRPS, then it will introduce the different experimental animal models. Finally this section will discuss the different treatment agents that have been studied for patchy osteoporosis.

2. Clinical findings of CRPS

2.1 Overview of CRPS

CRPS is painful and it can affect one or more extremities (de Mos et al., 2008). It usually occurs following a physical injury, such as, after fracture or surgery. But spontaneous onset without any triggering factor may occur as well (Veldman et al., 1993). According to a case control study (de Mos et al., 2008), fracture was the most common precipitating injury in 49% of the cases. The mixed etiologies of CRPS are evidenced in its heterogeneous constellation of clinical symptoms. In the acute stages, hallmarks include mechanical hyperalgesia, edema, increased sweating, skin temperature and hair growth (Doury, 1988; Janig & Baron, 2003). After some time, CRPS symptoms progress from a warm to a cold stage, with decrease of skin temperature, formation of skin atrophy and bony osteoporotic changes (van der Laan et al., 1998).

2.2 Diagnosis

CRPS diagnosis is based on its clinical presentation, whereby the diagnostic criteria as developed by the International Association for the Study of Pain (IASP) is most widely accepted (Stanton-Hicks et al., 1995). The IASP task force proposed a definition based on four criteria (Harden et al., 2007). (Table 1) In addition, involuntary movements, muscle spasm, paresis, pseudoparalysis, skin, muscle and bone atrophy, hyperhidrosis and changes in hair and nail growth, can also be observed (Perez et al., 2010; Veldman et al., 1993).

General definition of the syndrome:
CRPS describes an array of painful conditions that are characterized by a continuing (spontaneous and/or evoked) regional pain that is seemingly disproportionate in time or degree to the usual course of any known trauma or other lesion. The pain is regional (not in a specific nerve territory or dermatome) and usually has a distal predominance of abnormal sensory, motor, sudomotor, vasomotor, and/or trophic findings. The syndrome shows variable progression over time

To make the clinical diagnosis, the following criteria must be met:
1. Continuing pain, which is disproportionate to any inciting event
2. Must report at least one symptom in three of the four following categories:
   Sensory: Reports of hyperesthesia and/or allodynia
   Vasomotor: Reports of temperature asymmetry and/or skin color changes and/or skin color asymmetry
   Sudomotor/Edema: Reports of edema and/or sweating changes and/or sweating asymmetry
   Motor/Trophic: Reports of decreased range of motion and/or motor dysfunction (weakness, tremor, dystonia) and/or trophic changes (hair, nail, skin)
3. Must display at least one sign at time of evaluation in two or more of the following categories:
   Sensory: Evidence of hyperalgesia (to pinprick) and/or allodynia (to light touch and/or temperature sensation and/or deep somatic pressure and/or joint movement)
   Vasomotor: Evidence of temperature asymmetry (>1°C) and/or skin color changes and/or asymmetry
   Sudomotor/Edema: Evidence of edema and/or sweating changes and/or sweating asymmetry
   Motor/Trophic: Evidence of decreased range of motion and/or motor dysfunction (weakness, tremor, dystonia) and/or trophic changes (hair, nail, skin)
4. There is no other diagnosis that better explains the signs and symptoms

---

For research purposes, as a rule, CRPS is diagnosed when least one of the symptoms in all of the four symptom categories and at least one sign (observed at evaluation) in two or more sign categories is manifested.

Table 1. Proposed clinical diagnostic criteria for CRPS

Plain radiographs can be used to evaluate the demineralization status, but these show positive findings only in the chronic stages. Three-phase bone scintigraphy is a highly specific and sensitive test for CRPS (Demangeat et al., 1998). The classical finding on bone scintigraphy is increased periarticular activity in the affected limb (Todorovic-Tirnamic et al., 1995). Autonomic function can be tested by infrared thermography. Also, skin temperature differences may be helpful for the diagnosis of CRPS; however, these typical temperature side differences are not static descriptors but comprise changes that can be critically dependent on environmental temperature (Wasner et al., 2001).

2.3 Pathomechanism

The complex cascade of CRPS is postulated to initiate after the sensitization of C-nociceptive fibers and release of neuropeptides, which are linked to vasodilatation and hypersensitization of nerve endings (Guo et al., 2004; Kurvers, 1998; Schurmann et al., 1999). Osteoclasts are also activated and this in turn leads to nociceptor stimulation and sensitization (Mach et al., 2002; Sevcik et al., 2004) leading to a vicious cycle.

A medical history of asthma, migraine, osteoporosis, a recent history of menstrual cycle-related problems or preexisting neuropathies are common pre-existing problems or conditions often concomitantly found in CRPS patients. Therefore finding a common mediator that is both present in these conditions and CRPS could help to reveal the possible triggering factors. The mediators (de Mos et al., 2008; Karacan et al., 2004; Toda et al., 2006) that have been linked among asthma, migraine and CPRS are the neuropeptides calcitonin-gene related peptide, substance P (de Mos et al., 2008), mast cell products (Bradding et al., 2006) and transcription factors such as nuclear factor kappa B (Barnes, 2006; Reuter et al., 2002). Inflammatory cytokines such as interleukin 1, tumor necrosis factor alpha have also been suggested to be common denominators among CRPS, osteoporosis and menstrual cycle related disorders, but their definite roles need to be established through continuous studies (Marie et al., 1993; Zarrabeitia et al., 1991).

3. Patchy osteoporosis

3.1 Pathomechanism

Why does bone loss occur in CRPS? Some have postulated that immobilization plays a role in CRPS. Suyama et al, have (Suyama et al., 2002) observed a reduction in BMD 1 to 7 weeks postsurgery with an increase in the number of osteoclasts at 2, 3, and 5 weeks in their CRPS model. They have suggested that one possible mechanism would be the increase of bone resorption with immobilization. Another possible mechanism suggested by others (Whiteside et al., 2006) would be that bone loss in CRPS models may be due to altered nerve signaling and not attributable to limb disuse or reduced mechanical loading associated with pain. Experimental studies have shown that substance P release is involved in the pathogenesis of bony changes induced by CRPS (Gaus et al., 2003).

The exact pathological mechanism of patchy osteoporosis in CRPS and altered nerve signaling is still poorly understood, some consider to be attributable to a regional sympathetic hyperactivity of sympathetic dysfunction (Goldstein et al., 2000; He et al., 2011; Kurvers et al., 1998; Laroche et al., 1997). Sympathetic deregulation causes vasomotor irregularities, and an imbalance between vasoconstriction and vasodilatation, which in turn influences the blood supply to the bone. Other studies have shown that the immune and skeletal systems are closely related to maintain the homeostasis of the bone but when this interaction is disrupted in CRPS; the balance favors bone loss. This complex cascade is postulated to initiate after sensitization of C-nociceptive fibers and release of neuropeptides, which are linked to vasodilatation, hypersensitization of nerve endings (Guo et al., 2004; Kurvers et al., 1995; Schurmann et al., 1999), and osteoclasts activation, which increase bone resorption, lead to nociceptor stimulation and sensitization (Mach et al., 2002; Sevcik et al., 2004).

3.2 Characteristics

Bone loss in CRPS occurs regionally with loss of the trabecular bone (Bickerstaff et al., 1991; Doury, 1988) with marked bone demineralization observed at the subchondral regions. Epiphyseal regions are predominantly affected, however no narrowing of joint space or bony sclerosis is observed. Recovery of lost bone mineral content is slow and may persist after several years from the initial diagnosis (Nilsson, 1966) and this persistent regional osteoporosis can predispose to other future fractures after minor injuries (Sarangi et al., 1993). Same as the clinical manifestation, studies that have used rat models of CRPS have shown that bone mineral density significantly decrease from the second week (Suyama et al., 2002) and this loss is known to persist for at least 20 weeks (Kingery et al., 2003).

3.3 Radiographic findings

Bone changes can be observed by typical roentgenography but these changes are known to occur only after several months. However periarticular bone loss can be observed in radiograhs of CRPS limbs even within 3 weeks after injury (Bickerstaff et al., 1993). Bone mineral density, measured by dual energy xray abosorpotometry is reduced in the CRPS limbs in a periarticular distribution (Gue et al., 2004).

3.4 Neuropeptides in patchy osteoporosis

Substance P (Bianchi et al., 2008), one of the neuropeptides closely linked to the pathogenesis of CRPS, binds to NK1 receptors of postcapillary venules and causes vasodilation, increasing vascular permeability. The increased activity of this neuropeptide, which are elevated in serum samples from CRPS patients (Schinkel et al., 2006), are deemed to be responsible for the subsequent warmth and interstitial edema observed in CRPS through vasodilation and increased protein extravasation.

This substance P is also postulated to play a role in the development of patchy osteoporosis in CRPS. Studies have shown that substance P is known to stimulate osteoclast formation and active bone resorption through NK1-receptor found in the bone cells (Goto et al., 1998; Liu et al., 2007).

The exact mechanism of how substance P induces bone loss needs to be elucidated; substance P not only has osteoclastic effects but is known to have an osteogenic effect on bone marrow cells and to directly stimulate osteoblastic bone formation (Imai & Matsusue, 2002). The mechanism that favors osteoclastic activation, instead of osteoblastic activation, to result in bone loss in CRPS needs further studies. But in line with the current literature that supports abnormal osteoclastic activation through substance P in CRPS, it is reasonable to theorize that an agent that inhibits substance P would help to reduce osteoclast activation and its ensuing bone loss. This topic was evaluated in a study that used a substance P antagonist LY303870 (Kingery et al., 2003) and determined whether it was efficient in controlling osteoporosis. Although this antagonist was effective in the nociceptive and vascular abnormalities (Kingery et al., 2003), it proved to be ineffective in preserving bone loss. Its use instead enhanced the widespread osteoporotic effects (Kingery et al., 2003). The dual and dichotomous roles of substance P in maintaining bone integrity in CRPS needs to be further elucidated.

Substance P activation also leads to the over-expression of the inflammatory cytokines (Wei et al., 2009). Some of these cytokines play a role in the development of patchy osteoporosis in CRPS. Nerve growth factor is one of the cytokines activated by the substance P, and its activity leads to nociceptive sensitization, enhanced osteopenia with increased cytokine content (Sabsovich et al., 2008). Tumor necrosis factor alpha is another pro-inflammatory cytokine postulated to play a role in the development of CRPS changes after trauma and its expression is increased in CRPS patients (Huygen et al., 2001). Although the increased level of the tumor necrosis factor is an important mediator of regional nociceptive sensitization, it does not contribute to the enhanced bone loss (Sabsovich et al., 2008).

4. Current laboratory research in osteoporosis related with CRPS

4.1 Overview of laboratory research in CRPS

In order to unravel the mechanisms underlying osteoporosis in CRPS, many animal models have been introduced. There are two broad categories of mechanisms underlying CRPS: (1) peripheral mechanisms: CRPS is primarily an inflammatory disease in the periphery (CRPS I) or a consequence of nerve damage (CRPS II), (2) central mechanisms that involve reorganization of the somatosensory, somatomotor and autonomic systems in the central nervous system triggered by a peripheral input (Drummond et al., 2001; Turner-Stokes, 2002; Wasner et al., 2003). Both the peripheral and central nervous systems play a role in the pathogenesis of CRPS. The peripheral mechanisms includes immune cell mediated inflammatory, autoimmune inflammatory processes, neurogenic inflammation and tissue hypoxia. (Daemen et al., 1998a; Daemen et al., 1998b; Kingery et al., 2003b; Kurvers et al., 1998; Offley et al., 2005; Schurmann et al., 2000). However, the amount of contribution of these two mechanisms and how they interact with each other to manifest in CPRS has not been determined yet. Keeping in mind of these two different mechanisms, and that CRPS can be either type I or II, several animal models that represent these features have been introduced but because of the inherent heterogenic features of CRPS, there is no absolute model that shows and reproduces all CRPS features.

Depending on the presence of peripheral nerve injury, three animal models will be discussed. For CRPS type I, the tibia fracture model and chronic ischemic model will be presented (Coderre et al., 2004; Guo et al., 2006; Ludwig et al., 2007). The chronic constriction injury (CCI) model of the sciatic nerve will be presented for CRPS type II (Bennett and Xie, 1988). Choosing the type of experimental model may depend on the objective of the research or researcher's habit. The methodologies of these different animal models are discussed to provide detail reference for the readers.

4.2 Tibia fracture and cast rat model

Tibia fracture and cast rat model had been introduced for the animal model of CRPS type I, and is popularly used in laboratory studies (Guo et al., 2004; Guo et al., 2006; Sarangi et al., 1993). The method of induction for tibia fracture model is as follows: the hind limb of rat is wrapped in stockinet and the distal tibia is fractured. The hind limb is then wrapped in casting tape with the hip, knee, and ankle in flexed position. The cast extends from the metatarsals of the hindpaw up to a spica formed around the abdomen. At 4 weeks the cast is removed. This rat model shows changes in volume, temperature, nociception and osteoporosis of the hind limb.

This tibia fracture and cast model has several benefits. Most of all, this animal model represents the CRPS type 1. This model is theorized to induce post-junctional facilitation of substance P signaling. Because this model reproduces the typical symptoms of CRPS such as mechanical allodynia, paw thickness (edema), vasodilation and bone mineralization, it is commonly used in research studies that focus on the treatment and pathomechanism of CRPS. The exact mechanisms of how the intact peptidergic primary afferent neurons are activated after fracture and casting has not elucidated yet. Although there are many studies that have used this model to investigate the pathomechanism of CRPS type I, there are yet no studies that have exclusively focused on patchy osteoporosis with this model.

4.3 Ischemic – Reperfusion injury model

Another typical animal model for CRPS type I is the chronic ischemic model (Coderre et al., 2004; Xanthos et al., 2004). The femoral artery is dissected and ligated above the origin of the profunda femoris artery for the 3 hours with a small polyethylene tube. Ligation is performed tightly with the vessel walls pressed together and complete arterial occlusion is ensured under microscope. This method completely interrupts the arterial blood supply to the lower leg and hindpaw. The wound is closed by means of five sutures put on the skin. To prevent thrombosis of the artery, two subcutaneous injections of heparin are given subcutaneously, one at the beginning and one at the end of the period of ischemia. This ischemic injury shows change of skin temperature, spontaneous pain behavior, mechanical and cold allodynia and edema, and are consistent with CRPS type I.

Previous research revealed that CRPS type I may depend on chronic tissue ischemia that is dependent on, or exacerbated by, an indirect sympathetic–afferent coupling with an intervening role of enhanced a-adrenoceptor mediated vasoconstriction. The ischemia-reperfusion injury model is another animal model for CRPS type I that is produced based on this mechanism.

4.4 Chronic constriction injury (CCI) model

The CCI model; first introduced by Bennett and Xie (1998); is a classic model for CRPS and has been commonly used in various studies. In this model the common sciatic nerve is exposed at the level of the middle of the thigh by blunt dissection through the biceps femoris. Proximal to the sciatic's trifurcation, about 7 mm of nerve is freed from adhering tissue and 4 ligatures are loosely tied loosely around it with 1 mm spacing. The length of the ligated nerve is approximately 4-5 mm long.

This model is known to represent CRPS type II. This model shows changes of skin thickness, temperature, mechanical sensitivity and bony changes such as patchy osteoporosis. This model has been the model most frequently used to study the patchy osteoporosis in CRPS. Patchy osteoporosis resembling that of CRPS can also be induced by the sciatic nerve trans-section (Kingery et al., 2003a; Kingery et al., 2003b). This model is also used for studies on CRPS type II. However, the CCI model had shown several benefits for weight bearing than the sciatic nerve trans-section model. Many of the laboratory researches on patchy osteoporosis in CRPS are mostly based on the CCI model.

5. Treatment of patchy osteoporosis in CRPS

5.1 Overview of medication for patchy osteoporosis

Pharmacological therapy of CRPS encompasses a wide spectrum of medication; from anti-inflammatory drugs, systemic corticosteroid (Kingery, 1997), antidepressants, opioid (Mackey & Feinberg, 2007), to anticonvulsants agents. Because the activation of bony osteoclasts is known to play significant role in CRPS pain generation, it is not surprising that aside from these central pain modulating medications, bone modulating agents are used in CRPS. These agents are known not only to alleviate pain but also to reverse and inhibit CRPS associated osteopenia (Whiteside et al., 2006). The two bone modulating agents in reference are calcitonin and bisphosphonate agents.

5.2 Calcitonin

Calcitonin has been traditionally used in bone pathologic conditions due to its efficacy on microvasculature, bone resorption and analgesic action (Friedman & Raisz, 1965). The use of calcitonin in CRPS has been shown through its possible mechanism in controlling bone pain. The results of calcitonin in clinical practice are still controversial; while some have questioned the efficacy (Kingery, 1997), others support its efficacy in CRPS pain (Perez et al., 2001). A recent review analysis also describes positive results for calcium-regulating drugs, including calcitonin, administered to CRPS patients (Fofouzanfar et al., 2002). Although calcitonin has some efficacy in pain, range of motion, with a rapid onset of action (Gobelet et al., 1992), whether its use has effect on the patchy osteoporosis in CRPS has not been validated through animal or clinical studies.

5.3 Bisphosphonate

5.3.1 Mechanism of bisphosphonate through experimental studies

Bisphosphonates are analogues of inorganic pyrophosphates and are inhibitors of bone resorption. They act on the bone and inhibit the action of osteoclasts, thereby limiting bone resorption. Due to this mechanism, they have been found to be effective in the treatment of osteoporosis and other bone conditions. Bisphosphonates have been used traditionally for pathological bone conditions, such as osteoporosis, Paget's disease, cancer related bone pain, metastatic cancer, tumor related hypercalcemia, myeloma and vertebral fracture (Adami et al., 1997; Brunner et al., 2009; Bonabello et al., 2001; Fleisch, 1997; Fulfaro et al., 1998; Fulfaro et al., 2005). In CRPS, bisphosphonates have shown more promising results than calcitonin and many studies supports itse use in CRPS (Adami et al., 1997; Breuer et al., 2008; Manicourt et al., 2004; Robinson et al., 2004; Varenna et al., 2000), in fact, bisphosphonates are the only pharmacological agents with beneficial analgesic results confirmed through placebo controlled trials (Adami et al., 1997; Manicourt et al., 2004; Varenna et al., 2000). However, there is yet no consensus on the optimum dosage, frequency, and duration of treatment in CPRS.

The role of bisphosphonate in the regulation of the substance P and hyperalgesia has been shown in an experimental study using ibandronate (Bianchi et al., 2008), a bisphosphonate agent. As stated earlier, substance P sensitizes afferent fibers and increases the sensitivity to nociceptive stimuli. It has been hypothesized that ibandronate prevents proton production by osteoclasts, and reduce the activation of specific ion channels and consequent production of substance P by primary afferents (Bianchi et al., 2008), thereby limiting hyperalgesia and bone loss. Also bony calcium homeostasis can influence the Ca^{2+} dependent endogenous regulation of pain sensitivity (Bonabello et al., 2001). Bisphosphonates can effect bone tissue by alternation of the calcium/phosphate product. It is postulated that it is through these mechanisms that bisphosphonate administration inhibits the release of neuropeptides that are responsible for the pain and other vasomotor changes in CRPS. Also, it is postulated that it is through these same mechanisms that bisphosphonate agents are useful in limiting bone loss. In fact, animal studies have shown bisphosphonates are effective in preserving CRPS associated bone loss. Chronic administration of zoledronate acid can lead to increased BMD in CCI animal models (Whiteside et al., 2006). The efficacy of alendronate in limiting bone loss in CCI rat model has been shown in a recent study (Im et al., 2010). In both the acute and chronic stages after CCI induction, alendronate treatment preserved bone mass with sustained efficacy in bone preservation, which was demonstrated through in vitro tibia BMD and tibia strength results.

5.3.2 Clinical studies of bisphosphonate
The role of bisphosphonates in CRPS is well supported by many clinical studies but most were focused on their efficacies in pain. There are already many reports that have advocated the use of bisphosphate agents for CRPS related hyperalgesia and pain (Adami et al., 1997; Breuer et al., 2008; Mackey & Feinberg, 2007; Manicourt et al., 2004; Robinson et al., 2004; Varenna et al., 2000). Results from clinical studies have postulated that alendroate reduces local bone resorption and is effective in CRPS pain by its nociceptive effects in bone. (Adami et al., 1997; Manicourt et al., 2004). For example, Varenna et al. have shown in their randomized, double blind placebo controlled study that a 10 day intravenous clondronate course is effective in the treatment of CRPS (Varenna et al., 2000). A recent clinical study of ibandronate, a potent bisphosphonate agent, has shown that its analgesic effects (Bianchi et al., 2008). However, most studies focused on their analgesic effects for bone pain rather than on their bone preserving effects.

Bone loss in CRPS predominate the chronic stages of CRPS and is accompanied by trophic changes. This patchy bone loss is difficult to reverse and as stated earlier, can lead to fractures even from trivial stress. Therefore, alongside with the management of pain, management of CRPS associated patchy osteoporosis is important to prevent such detrimental consequences.

The efficacy of bisphosphonate agents in patchy osteoporosis have been shown in some studies. A theraupetic role of bisphosphonates on clinical and densiometric recovery was shown in transient hip osteoporosis; a condition considered by many to be a prestage of CRPS (Mailis et al., 1992) with similar features commonly observed in CRPS. Administration of bisphosphonate in transient hip osteoporosis led to the recovery of bone densiometry along with complete pain resolution (Varenna et al., 1996). Similary, the efficacy of bisphosphonate therapy in the recovery of bone mineral content was also shown in CRPS (Adami et al., 1997). Adami et al. used intravenous alendronate and evaluated their pain, tenderness, swelling and bone mineral content of the affected arm. Although a change of bone mineral content was not observed in the unaffected side, the affected side bone mineral content rose significantly in comparison to baseline values. These results show that bisphosphonates are helpful in limiting CRPS associated pathcy osteoporosis.

5.4 Dosage and administration of bisphosphonate in patchy osteoporosis
With bisphosphonates as the agent with much clinical and experimental evidence to support its use in CRPS, the best dosage and timing of administration is an issue that has gained much focus. A study of dosage differentiation was previoulsy carried out with doses of pamidronate

varying from 30mg/day to 1mg/Kg/day, provided for three consecutive days. However no dose correlation was observed in these clinical trials (Maillefert et al., 1995). In contrast, some animal studies have shown a dose dependent antinociceptive effects (Bonabello et al., 2001)with pamidronate and clodronate. Etidronate and alendronate have not shown this dose dependent response and their analgesic effects were observed only with the highest dose.

Similar to these experiments, in their study with CCI models, Im et al. has shown that different dosage and time of administration of oral alendronate leads to different results in bone mineral density of the tibia and tibia bone strength (Im et al., 2010). The high dosage group received 1mg/kg/day while the low dosage group received 0.1mg/kg/day. To determine whether the time of administration lead to significant differences, the high and low dosage groups were further divided into the early and late administered group. The early group received alendronate treatment immediately after CCI induction, while the late group received alendronate at the 14th day. Both groups received alendronate treatment until the 6th week of CCI induction. The results showed that different dosages and time of administration leads to different efficacies across different CRPS signs. While the hind paw thickness and temperature were significantly reduced only with high dosage administered immediately after CCI induction (Fig. 1, Fig. 2), bone strength and bone mineral density was significantly increased in the high dosage group, with both in the early and late admistered group (Fig. 3, Fig. 4). Bone loss in CRPS becomes manifest in the chronic stages and is known to progress over several months. Because bone loss predominates the later course of CRPS, the authors suggested that the high dosage alendronate, whether admnistred in the early or late course of CRPS, can show significant efficacy in bone metabolism.

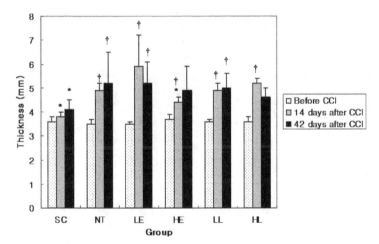

*P<0.001 as compared with NT group, †P<0.001 as compared with SC group.
Abbreviations: CCI, chronic constriction injury; SC, sham control; NT, no treatment; LE, low dosage early treatment; HE, high dosage early treatment; LL, low dosage late treatment; HL, high dosage late treatment

Fig. 1. Efficacy of oral alendronate in different dosage and time of administration in dorsal-ventral thicknesses of the affected hind-paw from Sprague-Dawley rats. (Adapted from Im, S., Lim, S.H., Lee, J.I., Ko, Y.J., Park, J.H., Hong, B.Y. & Park, G.Y. Effective dosage and administration schedule of oral alendronate for non-nociceptive symptoms in rats with chronic constriction injury. Journal of Korean Medical Science 2010; 25(6): 938-944)

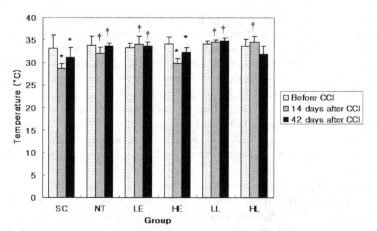

*P<0.001 as compared with NT group, †P<0.001 as compared with SC group.
Abbreviations: CCI, chronic constriction injury; SC, sham control; NT, no treatment; LE, low dosage early treatment; HE, high dosage early treatment; LL, low dosage late treatment; HL, high dosage late treatment

Fig. 2. Efficacy of oral alendronate in different dosage and time of administration in skin temperature of the affected hind-paw from Sprague-Dawley rats. (Adapted from Im, S., Lim, S.H., Lee, J.I., Ko, Y.J., Park, J.H., Hong, B.Y. & Park, G.Y. Effective dosage and administration schedule of oral alendronate for non-nociceptive symptoms in rats with chronic constriction injury. Journal of Korean Medical Science 2010; 25(6): 938-944)

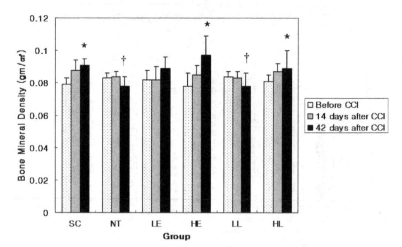

*P<0.001 as compared with NT group, †P<0.001 as compared with SC group.
Abbreviations: CCI, chronic constriction injury; SC, sham control; NT, no treatment; LE, low dosage early treatment; HE, high dosage early treatment; LL, low dosage late treatment; HL, high dosage late treatment

Fig. 3. Efficacy of oral alendronate in different dosage and time of administration in BMD of the affected tibia from Sprague-Dawley rats. (Adapted from Im, S., Lim, S.H., Lee, J.I., Ko, Y.J., Park, J.H., Hong, B.Y. & Park, G.Y. Effective dosage and administration schedule of oral alendronate for non-nociceptive symptoms in rats with chronic constriction injury. Journal of Korean Medical Science 2010; 25(6): 938-944)

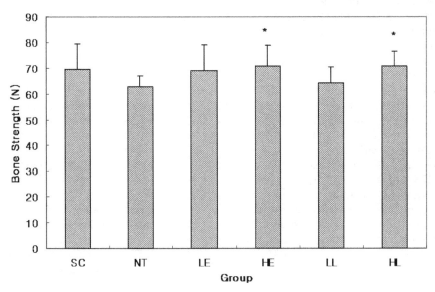

*P<0.001 as compared with NT group
†P<0.001 as compared with SC group.
Abbreviations: CCI, chronic constriction injury; SC, sham control; NT, no treatment; LE, low dosage early treatment; HE, high dosage early treatment; LL, low dosage late treatment; HL, high dosage late treatment

Fig. 4. Efficacy of oral alendronate in different dosage and time of administration in bone strength of the right tibia from Sprague-Dawley rats, obtained after the rats were sacrificed. (Adapted from Im, S., Lim, S.H., Lee, J.I., Ko, Y.J., Park, J.H., Hong, B.Y. & Park, G.Y. Effective dosage and administration schedule of oral alendronate for non-nociceptive symptoms in rats with chronic constriction injury. Journal of Korean Medical Science 2010; 25(6): 938-944)

Despite these results, studies that evaluate on the appropriate human dosage of bisphosphonates to alleviate CRPS associated bone loss are warranted in future studies. Although previous studies have shown variable efficacy of bisphosphonate agents with different dosages and time of administration for the different signs of CRPS, the dosage administered in the high dosage group was approximately 5–6 times higher than standard clinical dosages, thus, the high dosage used in experimental studies poses potential problems to directly administer to humans.

Responses to bisphosphonates can vary depending on which agent is used and also on when and how these agents are administered. More experimental studies that asses the efficacy of different bisphosphonate dosages and time of administration in pain and temperature are needed to translate these findings to clinical usage. Also, it would be of interest to determine if prophylactic high dosage bisphosphonate administration in CRPS are helpful in limiting the bone loss that continues until the later stages of CRPS. Finally long term follow-up clinical data are needed to evaluate the efficacy of bisphosphonates in limiting bone loss through objective evidence from bone densiometry and bone markers.

5.5 Neuropeptide modulators

Because the pathogenesis of patchy osteoporosis is related to neurogenic inflammation and the production of substance P, many studies that targeted these neuropeptides have been published. As stated earlier, substance P activation also leads to the over-expression of the inflammatory cytokines (Wei et al., 2009), for example, nerve growth factor is one of the cytokines that leads to osteopenia. The use of a nerve growth factor antibody not only reduced nociception but to a modest degree, maintained further bone loss in the distal trabecular bone (Sabsovich et al., 2008). Pentoxifylline, a cytokine inhibitor, was used to evalute its effect in trabecular bone loss (Wei et al., 2009). Pentoxifylline had significant effects in the fracture induced up-regulation of inflammatory cytokines and reversed nociceptive sensitization and vascular abnormalities. However, it had insignificant effects on bone architecture as measured by microcomputed tomography in a tibia fracture model of CRPS. Although pentoxifylline treatment can induce osteoblastic differentiation, it had no significant effect on trabecular bone loss (Sabsovich et al., 2008).

Although the exact mechanism and relationship of osteoclastic activation, with subsequent activation of substance P and inflammatory cytokines needs further evaluation, most experimental studies have shown that only the agents that directly inhibit bone resorption through osteoclast inhibition have efficacy in preserving CRPS associated bone loss. To date, bisphosphonate agents are ideal for controlling the pain and for limiting bone loss in CRPS.

6. Conclusion

The main focus in CRPS both in clinical and experimental settings has been focused on hyperalgesia and vasomotor symptoms. The symptoms are manifest from the early stages of disease, are profound and affects patients' quality of life. In contrast, patchy osteoporosis in CRPS are not apparent until the later stages, and bone loss rarely causes any symptoms until a minor trauma leads to unexpected fractures. Despite the different clincal manifestations of hyperalgesia and osteoporosis, and the tendency to divide CRPS into different stages, all the signs of CRPS are in continuum and dependent on one another; one sign of CRPS does not stand alone and one can not exist without the other, therefore simply aiming the treatment focused on one aspect can not limit the heterogenic features of CRPS. Vasomotor and sudomotor signs and patchy osteoporosis in CRPS are triggered through similar pathways and neuropeptides are the mediators that link them together. To date, bisphosphonates in high dosages have been used with the aim to control these neuropeptides through osteoclastic modulation. Future studies and clinical trials are warranted for the treatment of CRPS patchy osteoporosis.

7. References

Brunner, F., Schmid, A., Kissling, R., Held, U. & Bachmann, L.M. (2009). Biphosphonates for the therapy of complex regional pain syndrome I--systematic review. European Journal of Pain, Vol.13, No.1, (January 2009),pp. 17-21, ISSN 1532-2149

Daemen, M., Kurvers, H., Bullens, P., Barendse, G., Van Kleef, M. & Van den Wildenberg, F. (1998). Neurogenic inflammation and reflex sympathetic dystrophy (in vivo and in vitro assessment in an experimental model). Acta Orthopaedica Belgica, Vol.64, No.4, (December 1998),pp. 441-447, ISSN 0001-6462 de Mos, M., Huygen, F.J., Dieleman, J.P., Koopman, J.S., Stricker, B.H. & Sturkenboom, M.C. (2008). Medical history and the onset of complex regional pain syndrome (CRPS). Pain, Vol.139, No.2, (October 15 2008),pp. 458-466, ISSN 1872-6623

Demangeat, J.L., Constantinesco, A., Brunot, B., Foucher, G. & Farcot, J.M. (1988). Three-phase bone scanning in reflex sympathetic dystrophy of the hand. Journal of Nuclear Medicine, Vol.29, No.1, (January 1988),pp. 26-32, ISSN 0161-5505

Doury, P. (1988). Algodystrophy. Reflex sympathetic dystrophy syndrome. Clinical Rheumatology, Vol.7, No.2, (June 1988),pp. 173-180, ISSN 0770-3198

Fleisch, H.A. (1997). Bisphosphonates: preclinical aspects and use in osteoporosis. Annals of Medicine, Vol.29, No.1, (February 1997),pp. 55-62, ISSN 0785-3890

Forouzanfar, T., Koke, A.J., van Kleef, M., Weber, W.E. (2002). Treatment of complex regional pain syndrome type I. European Journal of Pain, Vol.6, No.2, (April 2002), pp.105-122, ISSN 1090-3801

Friedman, J. & Raisz, L.G. (1965). Thyrocalcitonin: inhibitor of bone resorption in tissue culture. Science, Vol.150, No.702, (December 10 1965),pp. 1465-1467, ISSN 0036-8075

Fulfaro, F., Casuccio, A., Ticozzi, C. & Ripamonti, C. (1998). The role of bisphosphonates in the treatment of painful metastatic bone disease: a review of phase III trials. Pain, Vol.78, No.3, (December 1998),pp. 157-169, ISSN 0304-3959

Fulfaro, F., Leto, G., Badalamenti, G., Arcara, C., Cicero, G., Valerio, M.R., Di Fede, G., Russo, A., Vitale, A., Rini, G.B., Casuccio, A., Intrivici, C. & Gebbia, N. (2005). The use of zoledronic acid in patients with bone metastases from prostate carcinoma: effect on analgesic response and bone metabolism biomarkers. Journal of Chemotherapy, Vol.17, No.5, (October 2005),pp. 555-559, ISSN 1120-009X

Gaus, S., Moriwaki, K., Suyama, H., Kawamoto, M. & Yuge, O. (2003). Capsaicin treatment inhibits osteopenia and heat hyperalgesia induced by chronic constriction injury to the sciatic nerve in rats. Hiroshima Journal of Medical Sciences, Vol.52, No.3, (September 2003),pp. 43-51, ISSN 0018-2052

Gobelet, C., Waldburger, M. & Meier, J.L. (1992). The effect of adding calcitonin to physical treatment on reflex sympathetic dystrophy. Pain, Vol.48, No.2, (February 1992),pp. 171-175, ISSN 0304-3959

Goldstein, D.S., Tack, C. & Li, S.T. (2000). Sympathetic innervation and function in reflex sympathetic dystrophy. Annals of Neurology, Vol.48, No.1, (July 2000),pp. 49-59, ISSN 0364-5134

Guo, T.Z., Offley, S.C., Boyd, E.A., Jacobs, C.R. & Kingery, W.S. (2004). Substance P signaling contributes to the vascular and nociceptive abnormalities observed in a tibial fracture rat model of complex regional pain syndrome type I. Pain, Vol.108, No.1-2, (March 2004),pp. 95-107, ISSN 0304-3959

Guo, T.Z., Wei, T., Kingery, W.S. (2006). Glucocorticoid inhibition of vascular abnormalities in a tibia fracture rat model of complex regional pain syndrome type I. Pain, Vol.121, No.1-2, (March 2006),pp.158-167, ISSN 0304-3959

Harden, R.N., Bruehl, S., Stanton-Hicks, M. & Wilson, P.R. (2007). Proposed new diagnostic criteria for complex regional pain syndrome. Pain Medicine, Vol.8, No.4, (May-June 2007),pp. 326-331, ISSN 1526-2375

He, J.Y., Jiang, L.S. & Dai, L.Y. (2011). The roles of the sympathetic nervous system in osteoporotic diseases: A review of experimental and clinical studies. Ageing Research Reviews, Vol.10, No.2, (April 2011),pp. 253-263, ISSN 1872-9649

Huygen, F.J., de Bruijn, A.G., Klein, J. & Zijlstra, F.J. (2001). Neuroimmune alterations in the complex regional pain syndrome. European Journal of Pharmacology, Vol.429, No.1-3, (October 19 2001),pp. 101-113, ISSN 0014-2999

Im, S., Lim, S.H., Lee, J.I., Ko, Y.J., Park, J.H., Hong, B.Y. & Park, G.Y. (2010). Effective dosage and administration schedule of oral alendronate for non-nociceptive symptoms in rats with chronic constriction injury. Journal of Korean Medical Science, Vol.25, No.6, (June 2010),pp. 938-944, ISSN 1598-6357

Imai, S. & Matsusue, Y. (2002). Neuronal regulation of bone metabolism and anabolism: calcitonin gene-related peptide-, substance P-, and tyrosine hydroxylase-containing nerves and the bone. Microscopy Research and Technique, Vol.58, No.2, (July 15 2002),pp. 61-69, ISSN 1059-910X

Janig, W. & Baron, R. (2003). Complex regional pain syndrome: mystery explained? Lancet Neurology, Vol.2, No.11, (November 2003),pp. 687-697, ISSN 1474-4422

Karacan, I., Aydin, T. & Ozaras, N. (2004). Bone loss in the contralateral asymptomatic hand in patients with complex regional pain syndrome type 1. Journal of Bone and Mineral Metabolism, Vol.22, No.1, (January 2004),pp. 44-47, ISSN 0914-8779

Kingery, W.S. (1997). A critical review of controlled clinical trials for peripheral neuropathic pain and complex regional pain syndromes. Pain, Vol.73, No.2, (November 1997),pp. 123-139, ISSN 0304-3959

Kingery, W.S., Davies, M.F. & Clark, J.D. (2003). A substance P receptor (NK1) antagonist can reverse vascular and nociceptive abnormalities in a rat model of complex regional pain syndrome type II. Pain, Vol.104, No.1-2, (July 2003),pp. 75-84, ISSN 0304-3959

Kingery, W.S., Offley, S.C., Guo, T.Z., Davies, M.F., Clark, J.D. & Jacobs, C.R. (2003). A substance P receptor (NK1) antagonist enhances the widespread osteoporotic effects of sciatic nerve section. Bone, Vol.33, No.6, (December 2003),pp. 927-936, ISSN 8756-3282

Kurvers, H., Daemen, M., Slaaf, D., Stassen, F., van den Wildenberg, F., Kitslaar, P. & de Mey, J. (1998). Partial peripheral neuropathy and denervation induced adrenoceptor supersensitivity. Functional studies in an experimental model. Acta Orthopaedica Belgica, Vol.64, No.1, (March 1998),pp. 64-70, ISSN 0001-6462

Kurvers, H.A., Jacobs, M.J., Beuk, R.J., Van den Wildenberg, F.A., Kitslaar, P.J., Slaaf, D.W. & Reneman, R.S. (1995). Reflex sympathetic dystrophy: evolution of microcirculatory disturbances in time. Pain, Vol.60, No.3, (March 1995),pp. 333-340, ISSN 0304-3959

Laroche, M., Redon-Dumolard, A., Mazieres, B. & Bernard, J. (1997). An X-ray absorptiometry study of reflex sympathetic dystrophy syndrome. Revue du Rhumatisme England Ed, Vol.64, No.2, (February 1997),pp. 106-111, ISSN 1169-8446

Mach, D.B., Rogers, S.D., Sabino, M.C., Luger, N.M., Schwei, M.J., Pomonis, J.D., Keyser, C.P., Clohisy, D.R., Adams, D.J., O'Leary, P. & Mantyh, P.W. (2002). Origins of skeletal pain: sensory and sympathetic innervation of the mouse femur. Neuroscience, Vol.113, No.1, (August 2002),pp. 155-166, ISSN 0306-4522

Mackey, S. & Feinberg, S. (2007). Pharmacologic therapies for complex regional pain syndrome. Current Pain and Headache Reports, Vol.11, No.1, (February 2007),pp. 38-43, ISSN 1531-3433

Mailis, A., Inman, R. & Pham, D. (1992). Transient migratory osteoporosis: a variant of reflex sympathetic dystrophy? Report of 3 cases and literature review. The Journal of Rheumatology, Vol.19, No.5, (May 1992),pp. 758-764, ISSN 0315-162X

Maillefert, J.F., Chatard, C., Owen, S., Peere, T., Tavernier, C. & Tebib, J. (1995). Treatment of refractory reflex sympathetic dystrophy with pamidronate. Annals of Rheumatic Diseases, Vol.54, No.8, (August 1995),pp. 687, ISSN 0003-4967

Manicourt, D.H., Brasseur, J.P., Boutsen, Y., Depreseux, G. & Devogelaer, J.P. (2004). Role of alendronate in therapy for posttraumatic complex regional pain syndrome type I of the lower extremity. Arthritis and Rheumatism, Vol.50, No.11, (November 2004),pp. 3690-3697, ISSN 0004-3591

Nilsson, B.E. (1966). Post-traumatic osteopenia. A quantitative study of the bone mineral mass in the femur following fracture of the tibia in man using americium-241 as a photon source. Acta Orthopaedica Scandinavica, Vol.37, (January 1966),pp. Suppl 91:91-55, ISSN 0001-6470

Perez, R.S., Kwakkel, G., Zuurmond, W.W. & de Lange, J.J. (2001). Treatment of reflex sympathetic dystrophy (CRPS type 1): a research synthesis of 21 randomized clinical trials. Journal of Pain and Symptom Management, Vol.21, No.6, (June 2001),pp. 511-526, ISSN 0885-3924

Perez, R.S., Zollinger, P.E., Dijkstra, P.U., Thomassen-Hilgersom, I.L., Zuurmond, W.W., Rosenbrand, K.C. & Geertzen, J.H. (2010). Evidence based guidelines for complex regional pain syndrome type 1. BMC Neurology, Vol.10, (March 2010),pp. 20, ISSN 1471-2377

Poplawski, Z.J., Wiley, A.M. & Murray, J.F. (1983). Post-traumatic dystrophy of the extremities. The Journal of Bone and Joint Surgery American Volume, Vol.65, No.5, (June 1983),pp. 642-655, ISSN 0021-9355

Reuter, U., Chiarugi, A., Bolay, H. & Moskowitz, M.A. (2002). Nuclear factor-kappaB as a molecular target for migraine therapy. Annals of Neurology, Vol.51, No.4, (April 2002),pp. 507-516, ISSN 0364-5134

Robinson, J.N., Sandom, J. & Chapman, P.T. (2004). Efficacy of pamidronate in complex regional pain syndrome type I. Pain Medicine, Vol.5, No.3, (September 2004),pp. 276-280, ISSN 1526-2375

Sabsovich, I., Guo, T.Z., Wei, T., Zhao, R., Li, X., Clark, D.J., Geis, C., Sommer, C. & Kingery, W.S. (2008). TNF signaling contributes to the development of nociceptive sensitization in a tibia fracture model of complex regional pain syndrome type I. Pain, Vol.137, No.3, (July 31 2008),pp. 507-519, ISSN 1872-6623

Sarangi, P.P., Ward, A.J., Smith, E.J., Staddon, G.E. & Atkins, R.M. (1993). Algodystrophy and osteoporosis after tibial fractures. The Journal of Bone and Joint Surgery. British Volume, Vol.75, No.3, (May 1993),pp. 450-452, ISSN 0301-620X

Schurmann, M., Gradl, G., Andress, H.J., Furst, H. & Schildberg, F.W. (1999). Assessment of peripheral sympathetic nervous function for diagnosing early post-traumatic complex regional pain syndrome type I. Pain, Vol.80, No.1-2, (March 1999),pp. 149-159, ISSN 0304-3959

Sevcik, M.A., Luger, N.M., Mach, D.B., Sabino, M.A., Peters, C.M., Ghilardi, J.R., Schwei, M.J., Rohrich, H., De Felipe, C., Kuskowski, M.A. & Mantyh, P.W. (2004). Bone cancer pain: the effects of the bisphosphonate alendronate on pain, skeletal remodeling, tumor growth and tumor necrosis. Pain, Vol.111, No.1-2, (September 2004),pp. 169-180, ISSN 0304-3959

Stanton-Hicks, M., Janig, W., Hassenbusch, S., Haddox, J.D., Boas, R. & Wilson, P. (1995). Reflex sympathetic dystrophy: changing concepts and taxonomy. Pain, Vol.63, No.1, (October 1995),pp. 127-133, ISSN 0304-3959

Suyama, H., Moriwaki, K., Niida, S., Maehara, Y., Kawamoto, M. & Yuge, O. (2002). Osteoporosis following chronic constriction injury of sciatic nerve in rats. Journal of Bone and Mineral Metabolism, Vol.20, No.2, (March 2002),pp. 91-97, ISSN 0914-8779

Toda, K., Muneshige, H., Maruishi, M., Kimura, H. & Asou, T. (2006). Headache may be a risk factor for complex regional pain syndrome. Clinical Rheumatology, Vol.25, No.5, (September 2006),pp. 728-730, ISSN 0770-3198

Todorovic-Tirnanic, M., Obradovic, V., Han, R., Goldner, B., Stankovic, D., Sekulic, D., Lazic, T. & Djordjevic, B. (1995). Diagnostic approach to reflex sympathetic dystrophy after fracture: radiography or bone scintigraphy? European Journal of Nuclear Medicine, Vol.22, No.10, (October 1995),pp. 1187-1193, ISSN 0340-6997

van der Laan, L., Veldman, P.H. & Goris, R.J. (1998). Severe complications of reflex sympathetic dystrophy: infection, ulcers, chronic edema, dystonia, and myoclonus. Archives of Physical Medicine and Rehabilitation, Vol.79, No.4, (April 1998),pp. 424-429, ISSN 0003-9993

Varenna, M., Sinigaglia, L., Binelli, L., Beltrametti, P. & Gallazzi, M. (1996). Transient osteoporosis of the hip: a densitometric study. Clinical Rheumatology, Vol.15, No.2, (March 1996),pp. 169-173, ISSN 0770-3198

Varenna, M., Zucchi, F., Ghiringhelli, D., Binelli, L., Bevilacqua, M., Bettica, P. & Sinigaglia, L. (2000). Intravenous clodronate in the treatment of reflex sympathetic dystrophy syndrome. A randomized, double blind, placebo controlled study. The Journal of Rheumatology, Vol.27, No.6, (June 2000),pp. 1477-1483, ISSN 0315-162X

Veldman, P.H., Reynen, H.M., Arntz, I.E., & Goris, R.J. (1993). Signs and symptoms of reflex sympathetic dystrophy: prospective study of 829 patients. Lancet, Vol.342, No.8878, (October 1993),pp. 1012-1016, ISSN 0140-6736

Wasner, G., Backonja, M.M. & Baron, R. (1998). Traumatic neuralgias: complex regional pain syndromes (reflex sympathetic dystrophy and causalgia): clinical characteristics, pathophysiological mechanisms and therapy. Neurologic Clinics, Vol.16, No.4, (November 1998),pp. 851-868, ISSN 0733-8619

Wasner, G., Schattschneider, J., Heckmann, K., Maier, C. & Baron, R. (2001). Vascular abnormalities in reflex sympathetic dystrophy (CRPS I): mechanisms and diagnostic value. Brain, Vol.124, No.Pt 3, (March 2001),pp. 587-599, ISSN 0006-8950

Wei, T., Sabsovich, I., Guo, T.Z., Shi, X., Zhao, R., Li, W., Geis, C., Sommer, C., Kingery, W.S. & Clark, D.J. (2009). Pentoxifylline attenuates nociceptive sensitization and cytokine expression in a tibia fracture rat model of complex regional pain syndrome. European Journal of Pain, Vol.13, No.3, (March 2009),pp. 253-262, ISSN 1532-2149

Whiteside, G.T., Boulet, J.M., Sellers, R., Bunton, T.E. & Walker, K. (2006). Neuropathy-induced osteopenia in rats is not due to a reduction in weight born on the affected limb. Bone, Vol.38, No.3, (March 2006),pp. 387-393, ISSN 8756-3282

4

The Skeleton Abnormalities in Patients with Neurofibromatosis Type 1: Important Consequences of Abnormal Gene Function

Marek W. Karwacki and Wojciech Wozniak

Nf-1 Outpatients Clinic & Department of Oncological Surgery for Children and Youth,
Institute of Mother and Child
Poland

1. Introduction

Neurofibromatosis type 1 [Nf-1, OMIM #162200[1]], formerly known as von Recklinghausen disease, is one of the most frequent disorders affecting mankind, inherited as an autosomal dominant trait. The relatively high prevalence, with an incidence at birth of approximately one in 2500 to 3500 live births, and a progressive nature of the disorder, notable for its phenotypic variability with almost 100% penetrance, as well as high proportion of sporadic cases (almost 50% of de novo mutations), constitute for the clinical magnitude of this disease. Multiple café au lait spots [CALs], axillary and inguinal freckling, multiple discrete cutaneous neurofibromas [NFM] and more prominent plexiform neurofibromas [PNF], and iris Lisch nodules constituted for the cardinal signs of the disease. Learning disabilities and attention deficits states, but usually with normal intelligence in adulthood, are present in at least 50% of individuals with Nf-1. Neurofibromatosis type 1 belongs to the group of disorders with significantly increased risk of tumorigenesis. The other significant manifestations of Nf-1 include bone dysplasias, clinically presented as progressive dystrophic scoliosis, vertebral dysplasia, overgrowth and tibial dysplasia with pseudarthrosis, and vasculopathy. Pubertal development is usually normal, but precocious puberty, especially in those with an optic chiasm glioma, as well as delayed puberty, may commonly occur in children with Nf-1. The life expectancy of Nf-1 patients is assumed to be reduced by 15 years. The most important causes of early death in these patients are malignant peripheral nerve sheath tumors and severe complications of vasculopathy (Friedman et al., 1999; Jett & Friedman, 2010; Larizza et al., 2009).

Despite the possibility of molecular testing, the diagnosis of Nf-1 is still based on clinical findings and is usually unequivocal in all but the young children (DeBella et al., 2000b). The diagnostic criteria for Nf-1 (Tabl. 1) were developed by the US National Institutes of Health (National Institute of Health [NIH], 1988) and are generally accepted worldwide for routine clinical use (Ferner et al., 2007; Williams et al., 2009). The disease is characterizes by extreme clinical variability, not only between unrelated, but also among affected individuals within a

---

[1] Online Mendelian Inheritance in Man, OMIM (TM). Johns Hopkins University, Baltimore, MD. MIM Number: #162200, 07/06/2011. World Wide Web URL: http://www.ncbi.nlm.nih.gov/omim/

single family carrying the same type of mutation, and even within a single person with Nf-1 at different times in life. Penetrance of *NF1* gene mutation is virtually complete (100% of penetration) after childhood and the frequency of more serious complications increases with age. Various manifestations of Nf-1 have different characteristic times of appearance (DeBella et al., 2000b; Boulanger & Larbrisseau, 2005; Friedman ed., 1999; Williams et al., 2009). The clinical NIH diagnostic criteria are both highly specific and highly sensitive only in adults. Less than half of youngest children with no family history of Nf-1 meet NIH criteria, although almost all do by adolescence. Yet, neonates who inherited *NF1* mutation from one of the parents can usually be identified within the first year of life by the presence of numerous CALs (DeBella et al., 2000b).

The presence of two or more of the following features is required for the diagnosis of Nf-1:
1. Six or more café au lait macules over 5 mm in greatest diameter in prepubertal individuals and over 15 mm in greatest diameter in postpubertal individuals
2. Two or more neurofibromas of any type, or one plexiform neurofibroma
3. Freckling in the axillary or inguinal regions
4. Optic glioma
5. Two or more Lisch nodules (iris hamartomas)
6. A distinctive osseous lesion such as sphenoid dysplasia or tibial pseudarthrosis
7. A first-degree relative (parent, sib, or offspring) with Nf-1 as defined by the above criteria

Table 1. The NIH diagnostic criteria for neurofibromatosis type 1

Neurofibromatosis type 1 is caused by heterozygous mutations (intragenic or microdeletion) in *NF1* tumor suppressor gene, located at 17q11.2. Its product, neurofibromin, has different biochemical interactions, including association to microtubules and participation in several signaling pathways, especially as a member of the GTPase-activating proteins. Its main physiological function is inactivation of energized *ras* oncogene. *NF1* mutation extinguish a gene function and leads to aberrant *ras* activity. *NF1* gene belongs to the family of tumor suppressor genes and neurofibromatosis type 1 is thought to be a hereditary malignancy syndrome, which is highly influenced by complex action of other genes, required in signal transmission processing. In human diseases predisposing to cancer, cells usually carry heterozygous germline, what means inherited, mutations in growth regulator genes that are essential for organized cell growth and differentiation. Affected individuals, such as Nf-1 patients, are at significant risk for development of benign or malignant tumors early in life. In case of Nf-1, the most distinguished types of neoplasia are tumors arising from peripheral and optic nerves sheath (Schwann cells), usually benign neurofibroma and optic nerve glioma or seldom, malignant peripheral nerve sheath tumor [MPNST]. MPNST usually growths as a result of malignant transformation of plexiform neurofibroma [PNF], a specific, clinically distinguished type of neurofibroma. The risk of transformation of PNF into MPNST is not higher than 10%, and have been finally evaluated in recent clinical trials (Upadhyaya, 2011). The overall risk of cancer development in Nf-1 patients surpass the healthy general population risk by 2.7 times (Walker et al., 2006). The risk of malignancy is higher in those patients because inherited nature of the first mutation released the entire process, and in consequence, only one additional acquire genetic alteration, resulted in loss of the wild allele of affected gene, is further necessary to facilitate tumorigenesis. In healthy individual both mutations must be acquire in intact alleles, so the chance for that is much lower. Cells that have lost both copies of the tumor suppressor gene have a growth advantage over so called wild cells. In a susceptible environment, this 'second hit' may result in tumor formation (Larizza et al., 2009; Upadhyaya, 2011). This helps to explain the development of neurofibromas and other malignancies occurring in Nf-1 patients, but currently does not fully explain the role of neurofibromin on the development of other ailments, and osseous abnormalities in particular. However the precise role of neurofibromin is not yet fully elucidated, although neurofibromin deficiency causes multiple clinical effects, suggesting that this gene product has diverse functions in a variety of tissues. Distorted process is responsible not only for tumorigenesis, but also for memory processing (intellectual disability) and bone remodeling (typical bone deformity seen in Nf-1 patients) (Radtke et al., 2007).

Phenotype expression of *NF1* gene mutation is extremely variable, so even individuals from one family with identical germline mutation may have dramatically different clinical manifestations. Observed complexity and the diversity of constitutional *NF1* mutations occurring in Nf-1 patients will continue to make genotype-phenotype correlation almost impossible. Clinical variability of Nf-1 results most probably from a combination of founder mutation effect of *NF1* gene influenced by further action of other genes engaged in signal transduction, as well as other genetic, non-genetic, and stochastic factors (Jouhilahti et al., 2011). Till now more than 500 different mutations of the *NF1* gene have been identified, and most of them are unique to a particular family. Different, mostly loss-of-function mutations, have been observed repeatedly, but none has been found in more than a few percent of studied families (Radtke et al., 2007). In consequence, there are not so called hot spots sequences manifest along the entire gene length, what significantly complicated not only molecular testing but genetic counseling as well. Till now, only two clear correlations have been observed between particular mutant *NF1* alleles and consistent clinical phenotypes. In one, the whole *NF1* gene deletion is associated with more prominent presentation of the disease (Mensink et al., 2006). In another, characterized by 3-bp in-frame deletion of exon 17 (c.2970-2972 delAAT), the typical pigmentary features, but no cutaneous or surface plexiform neurofibromas, exist (Upadhyaya et al., 2007). Data concerning *NF1* mutation have accumulated slowly owing to the variability of the mutation types and the size and complexity of the gene, belongs to the longest in human genome. This also reflects the lack of a simple, inexpensive, highly accurate DNA-based test for Nf-1 at present (Radtke et al., 2007).

Currently no treatments dedicated specifically to Nf-1 patients exist. Because of the increased risk of cancer and multiorgan involvement, Nf-1 patients required extensive medical surveillance, provided on the regular bases by the specific, highly specialized Nf-1 clinics (Karwacki & Wozniak, 2006). It obey a comprehensive standards, comprises of regular physical examination by a Nf-1 specialist, regular blood pressure and ophthalmologic monitoring, anthropometric and developmental assessment of children and periodical imaging, warrants follow-up of clinically suspected intracranial and other internal tumors, done by USG and/or MR imaging. CT scans are hardly recommended in NF-1 patients, but children in particular, as the imaging exerts the risk of irradiation and is of limited diagnostic value, especially in visualization of Nf-1 brain specific lesions, called undifferentiated bright objects [UBO](DeBella et al., 2000a). According to specific ailment, patients are referred by Nf-1 clinic to other specialists as well.

The skeletal manifestations of a disease itself and the post-surgical bony complications occurred in Nf-1 patients, are common and have a prominent place in the orthopedic literature. The orthopedic complications of Nf-1, which usually appear early, include spinal deformities such as dystrophic scoliosis and kyphoscoliosis, congenital bowing and pseudoarthrosis of the tibia and the forearm, overgrowth phenomenon of the extremity, and soft tissue tumors, both benign and malignant (Crawford & Schorry, 1999, 2006).

2. Primary and secondary bone abnormalities in neurofibromatosis type 1

Although phenotype of Nf-1 patients is well described, the osseous manifestations are rarely emphasized in the clinical and genetic discussions concerning the diseases. In fact, one of the seventh diagnostic NIH criterion represents a distinctive osseous defect. Nf-1 is classically considers as a neurocutaneous disorder and clinical features of Nf-1 are classically thought of as neural crest in origin, but currently it is well accepted that mesodermally-derived abnormalities coexist as well. Restricted knowledge concerning the pathophysiology of Nf-1 skeletal abnormalities reflects the limited therapeutic modalities. Nf-1 is characterized by a multifaceted, polysystemic pathology. Among the other, bone involvement is representative for the majority of patients with Nf-1. The presentation of an ailment differs from patient to patient, but sometimes is extremely severe and appear from the birth or become evident either early in the childhood or further on and will accentuate with age. A number of skeletal involvements are highly morbid with a natural history distinct from that of the general population. A large proportion of patients with Nf-1 display primary skeletal involvement, including scoliosis and pseudoarthrosis, which are compounded by osteoporosis and poor bone healing (Crawford & Schorry, 1999). In considerable proportion of patients, these bone lesions can result in significant morbidity. The natural history and pathogenesis of the skeletal abnormalities, resulted from alter NF1 gene function, are poorly understood. Consequently, therapeutic options for these ailments are currently limited. Corrective orthopedic intervention quite often fails necessitating multiple revision surgeries followed by prolonged recovery periods (Crawford & Schorry, 2006).

Besides true dysplasia of bone, some of the skeletal changes observed in these patients are secondary to a tumor, compressing the bone through expansive growth, or its metastases. The most frequently, such tumors are plexiform neurofibromas, and rarely other malignancies occurred in Nf-1 more frequently than in general population, such as soft tissue sarcomas, notably rhabdomyosarcoma, and especially, malignant peripheral nerve sheath tumor [MPNST]. These tumors infiltrate easily in surrounding tissue, eroding the neighborhood bone, and frequently give rise to metastases, mostly to bones. Malignant peripheral nerve sheath tumor is an uncommon soft-tissue sarcoma [STS] that occurs at a higher incidence in patients with prior radiation exposure and Nf-1. MPNST resulted almost exclusively from the malignant transformation of PMF. It is assessed that every Nf-1 patient presenting PMF has a life time risk of 8 to 13% to develop a MPNST out of a pre-existing benign plexiform neurofibroma. In comparison to intragenic mutation, in patients with a NF1 microdeletion (5% of Nf-1 patients) this risk is twice as high. That risk is even greater in patients, in whom PMFs were incorporated into the field of therapeutic radiotherapy performed as an component of complex oncological treatment. Irradiation is linked with much higher risk of such a transformation, and in some STS therapeutic protocols introduced to the clinic by oncological treatment groups is either contraindicated or introduced with caution, when offered to children with Nf-1. Most of MPNST, especially arising in Nf-1 patients, are considered high-grade sarcomas with the tendency to recur as well as to metastasize, typically to the lungs. It belongs to a group of malignancies of particularly worse prognosis and due to its rarity, there is a paucity of data concerning chemotherapy response of MPNST.

As the overall understanding of bone growth, remodeling, and repair dependent on *NF1* gene function is critical to development of possible therapeutic interventions, in order to ensure continued collaboration and advancement toward better clinical management as well as effective drug therapies for Nf-1 related primary skeletal ailments, an International Nf-1 Bone Abnormalities Consortium have been convened in February 2008. The main goal of this Consortium is to identify barriers that might be impeding progression to future clinical trials for Nf-1 skeletal abnormalities and to highlights priorities for future research, based on animal model of Nf-1 related bone disease (Elefteriou et al., 2009).

2.1 Skeletal abnormalities in humans: Clinical presentation, diagnosis, complications

The Nf-1 skeletal phenotypes might be either generalized or focal. Manifestation of generalized skeletal abnormalities, mostly osteopenia or osteoporosis and short stature, are common, but of mild clinical implications. Focal lesions, such as tibial dysplasia, short angle scoliosis, and sphenoid wing dysplasia, are less common, but usually cause significant morbidity.

Skeletal Deformities:
- Short stature
- Macrocephaly
- Sphenoid wing dysplasia
- Cervical spine disorders
- Scoliosis
    - short-angle dystrophic
    - idiopathic non-dystrophic
- Spondylolisthesis
- Kyphoscoliosis
- Abnormalities of the rib cage and/or rib fusion
- Long bone dysplasia
- Osteosclerosis
- Congenital bone bowing
- Pseudoarthrosis
- Genu varum/valgum
- Absence of the patella
- Subperiosteal bone proliferation
- Partial overgrowth of an extremity
- Syndactyly
- Intra osseous-cysts and lytic bone lesions

Bone Metabolism Disorders:
- Osteopenia and frank osteoporosis
- Hypophosphatemic rickets
- Impaired bone healing

Table 2. Frequent manifestations of osseous abnormalities in patients suffering from Nf-1

2.1.1 Focal lesions: Spinal and chest wall deformations

Spinal deformities frequently occur in individuals with Nf-1. These changes result from intra or perispinal pathology, such as tumors, or either meningoceles or dural ectasia. However, the deformities may be also present in persons with entirely normal intraspinal contents. In such patients, primary bone dysplasia accounts for the dystrophic vertebral changes.

The most frequent is scoliosis, and the most devastating form – kyphoscoliosis of progressive course regardless the intensive physiotherapy. In various series of Nf-1 patients reported in the literature, frequency of scoliosis is assumed for 10 to 33% (Crawford & Herrera-Soto, 2007; Wang & Liu, 2010). Vice versa, in general population, Nf-1 could be confirm in app. 2% of children suffering from scoliosis (Vitale et al., 2002). Orthopedic surgeons distinguished two types of spinal curvature disturbances in children with Nf-1: dystrophic and non-dystrophic. The cause of spinal deformity in Nf-1 is still a matter of debate, but some have suggested that it is secondary to endocrine disturbances observed in these patients, mesodermal dysplasia probably resulted from *NF1* mutations, and osteomalacia, caused by a localized neurofibromatous tumor eroding and infiltrating adjacent bone.

The dystrophic scoliosis, usually associated with paravertebral neurofibromas, has a progressive nature and is associated with vertebral scalloping and wedging. Almost always develops before 10th year of life (Crawford & Herrera-Soto, 2007). Dystrophic scoliosis is often early onsetting, the shortsegmented, sharply angulated type of this ailment that includes fewer than 6 spinal segments. It has a tendency to progress to a severe deformity. The term dystrophic is usually used to describe a dysplastic vertebrae observed within scoliotic spine. Although there is no formal diagnostic criterion for such a form of scoliosis, Durrani et al. (2000) described nine specific radiographic features associated with dystrophic scoliosis (Tabl. 3).

1.	Scalloping of the posterior vertebral margins
2.	Severe rotation of the apical vertebra
3.	Widening of the spinal canal
4.	Enlargement of the neural foramina
5.	Defective pedicles
6.	A paraspinal mass
7.	Spindling of the transverse process
8.	Rotation of the ribs (the ribs resemble twisted ribbons)

Table 3. The radiologic appearance of the dystrophic scoliosis (Durrani et al., 2000)

Distinctive radiographic features of dystrophic scoliosis, usually presented in the preadolescent child, include a short-segment sharply angulated curve (involving four to six vertebrae), scalloping of vertebral margins, vertebral wedging, spinal canal widening, defective pedicles, and rib-penciling (Crawford et al., 2007). It is potentially debilitating and may rapidly progress to neurological impairment. This kind of scoliosis is frequently associated with paraspinal or other internal neurofibromas adjacent to the vertebrae, which could be seen in app. 70% of Nf-1 patients' MRI (Khong et al., 2003; Ramachandran et al., 2004). The complication of NFMs, or much frequently, PNFs penetrating into vertebral canal is dural ectasia, defined as widening of the dural sac surrounding the spinal cord, which might be seen in these patients (Khong et al., 2003; Schonauer et al., 2000; Tubbs and Oakes,

2002). However, dural ectasia may be a primary mesodermal dysplasia of the meninges as well (Casselman and Mandell, 1979). The vertebral column can further displace or erode, causing rib dislocation into the spinal canal, resulting in spinal cord injury. Weakening of spinal natural stabilizers, such as facets, pedicles, and ligaments, usually distorted in Nf-1, may lead to kyphosis. Kyphoscoliosis and humpback is a severe complication of advanced dystrophic scoliosis and finally can lead to cardiorespiratory insufficiency and failure. In this point, the best and well known touching description of Nf-1 patient's suffering, given by Victor Hugo in "The Hunchback of Notre Dame", is worth to be remembered. Dystrophic scoliosis in Nf-1 patients is particularly difficult to treat and necessitates early aggressive surgical stabilization very often.

The other, milder form of scoliosis occurring in Nf-1 children, is called non-dystrophic. It is diagnosed typically during adolescence and resembles idiopathic adolescent scoliosis in healthy population (Crawford & Herrera-Soto, 2007; Wang & Liu, 2010). This form usually involves 8-10 spinal segments. The deformity is most often convex to the right; however, this is not consistent. In rare instances, non-dystrophic scoliosis can progress to the dystrophic form.

The presence of neurofibroma or abnormal pressure phenomena in and around the spinal canal neuraxis resulted in meningoceles, pseudomeningoceles, dural ectasia, and dumbbell lesions development.

Kyphosis in individuals with Nf-1 might be distinguished by acute anteroposterior angulation. Severe deformity of vertebral bodies in Nf-1 might be confused even with congenital deformities.

Chest wall deformities in patients with Nf-1 are observed even more frequently than scoliosis, and are thought to be present in as many as 50% of patients (Riccardi, 2010). The relationship between chest wall deformities and scoliosis is not clear, but its existence exacerbates the course of dysplastic scoliosis in particular. It could happened, that chest wall deformities constitute the first clinical sign of tumor arising within the chest and quite often penetrating throughout the intervertebral foramina or dura mater. It resembles an hourglass shape, and is called spinal dumbbell tumor. This kind of growth is usually form by multiple tumors arose in the intradural and epidural spaces from one nerve root, occurring at the same time in different regions, such as the paravertebral, epidural and intradural spaces. Histopathological diagnosis is usually plexiform neurofibroma, but it still comprises the risk of malignant transformation into MPNST.

2.1.2 Focal lesions: Head and neck region

Increased head circumference is frequently observed in patients with Nf-1, and macrocephaly (head circumference >2 SD above the mean) occurs in about one-fourth of patients (Szudek et al., 2000). It is thought to be the consequence of brain enlargement (Greenwood et al., 2005). It is still not clear whether the skull growth contributes to macrocephaly. Contrariously, the association between macrocephaly and learning disabilities or underlying structural brain abnormalities has never been proof (Gutmann at al., 1997).

Sphenoid Wing Dysplasia Cranial defects attributed to the clinical pathology in Nf-1 with relatively lower frequency (eg. 11% had a dysplastic sphenoid wing in an observational study of Friedman and Birch (1997)). Sphenoid dysplasia usually is asymptomatic but occasionally can be associated with herniation through the bony defect. It is still under debate whether these type of changes reveal a primary bone dysplasia related to *NF1* mutation, or occur as secondary response of bone to the adjacent soft tissue abnormality. Most cranial defects are associated with plexiform neurofibromas of the eyelid or temporal region induced ipsilateral infiltration and decalcification of cranial bones adjacent to tumors (Jacquemin et al., 2002, 2003). Other lesions, including arachnoid cysts, dural ectasia, or buphthalmos, usually associate sphenoid wing defects. The suggestion of a bone cell-autonomous defect, accounted for the dysplastic sphenoid wing, is based on two meaningful observations: (1) Nf-1 sphenoid wing lesions have been associated with tibial and vertebral dysplasia (Alwan et al., 2007), and (2) formation of this skull structure proceeds through endochondral bone formation, which is defective in Nf-1 (Kolanczyk et al., 2007). Regardless the cause, a congenital malformation or secondary bony defect, the sphenoid wing dysplasia is not currently a primary target for therapeutic prevention. Nevertheless, it is imperious necessity to apply sensitive imaging techniques to screen patients with sphenoid wing dysplasia for adjacent tumors, which may be amenable to therapy (Jacquemin, 2002, 2003).

Increased caries and early primary tooth eruption as well as periapical cemental dysplasia have been quite often reported in patients with Nf-1 (Lammert et al., 2007; Tucker et al., 2007; Visnapuu et al., 2007). Dental abnormalities in Nf-1 patients still require more attention, yet everyday practice pointed unnecessary dental procedures performed in these patients, for instance when periapical cemental dysplasia is confused with chronic inflammation on radiographic analysis and precipitate dental surgery.

Cervical spine abnormalities are due to cervical spine instability or intraspinal pathology, caused mostly by benign tumor. These occur much more frequently when a scoliosis or kyphoscoliosis is present in the thoracolumbar region, but could be omitted as the examiner's attention is focused on the more obvious deformity. Severe cervical kyphosis is the most common abnormality, which itself is highly suggestive for Nf-1 diagnosis. Patients usually had either limited motion or pain in the neck, which were probably attributed to cervical instability. The numerous, minor to major neurologic deficits, such as paraplegia, are present.

2.1.3 Focal lesions: Long bones and extremities

Long bone dysplasia appears in a small percentage (3–4%) of patients with Nf-1 in clinic-based series (Friedman & Birch, 1997) and tibia is involved most often among other long bones, which can be affected sparsely. Infant with such an ailment usually presents with unilateral anterolateral bowing of the lower leg, notably tibial, although a child may be born with fracture and/or pseudarthrosis as well, or develop these shortly after birth. The deformity may appear before other protean manifestations of Nf-1, such as café-au-lait spots. The tibial bowing is usually evident within the first year of life, with a fracture not uncommonly occurring by age of 2-2.5 year. The tibial bowing associated with Nf-1 is always anterolateral. Affected bone is subject to pathologic fracture usually before age 3 years, often with minimal trauma. Subsequent healing may not occur normally, leading to consecutive non-union and pseudoarthrosis, sometimes requiring even amputation of affected extremity. As confirm histologically, the fibrous pseudarthrosis tissue seen at the fracture site is not a neurofibroma, but a fibrous overgrowth of unspecified cell origin. The ipsilateral fibula is often involved in association with tibial pseudoarthrosis and focal dysplasia of the ulna, radius, scapula, or vertebra may occur as well. The anterolateral bowing characterized patients with Nf-1 should be distinguished from the bilateral physiological bowing, exemplary common in children as they begin to walk or from the other type pathology.

Various radiographic classification systems for tibia bowing have been proposed, but they are still not rigorous and several subtypes represent rather changes over time, than the real variety. Nevertheless, tibial bowing in Nf-1 patients prior to fracture represents in radiograph a cortical thickening and medullary canal narrowing at the apex of the convexity, typically near the junction of the middle and distal thirds of the tibia (Stevenson et al., 2007).

In general, every bone of whatever kind and at any localization may usually be affected by the adjacent tumors as well, with all the consequences resemble the ones described above.

2.1.4 Generalized skeletal abnormalities

Although focal skeletal abnormalities, such as dystrophic scoliosis or tibial pseudoarthrosis and the like, can be severely disabling, they are uncommon among individuals with Nf-1. In contrary, generalized skeletal abnormalities are less severe but much more frequent in these patients. The osseous dysplasia result from disturbed bone growth, perhaps secondary to a mineralization disturbance. Findings such as decreased bone mineral density (BMD) and short stature reflect a generalized alteration of bone. The Nf-1 patients tend to be below average in height for age (below -2SD), although heights less than -3SD below the mean is seen hardly ever. Decreased BMD in both sexes at an early age has been reported in up to 50% of individuals with Nf-1. Reduced BMD in Nf-1 patients was initially recognized by Illes et al. (2001).

The exact pathogenesis of these bony changes is not understood, but patients with Nf-1 present lower than expected serum 25-hydroxyvitamin D (25OHD) concentrations, elevated serum parathyroid hormone concentration, and evidence of increased bone resorption. Defects in vitamin D metabolism, osteoclastogenesis or bone cell response to systemic signals regulating bone remodeling are likely involved. An inadequate increase in bone remodeling is also indirectly confirm by both bone histomorphometry and changes in circulating bone markers (Stevenson et al., 2008; Seitz et al., 2010). However, an increased incidence of fractures has not been firmly established. Still, generalized osteopenia and frank osteoporosis are more common than expected in patients with Nf-1. The results of one of the biggest series, in which Nf-1 children became the subject of multivariant analysis, indicate that the mean lumbar and whole body BMD z-scores were in the range of osteopenia and osteoporosis in 48% and 25% of subjects, respectively. BMD was reduced at multiple bone sites, while the lumbar spine being more severely affected (Brunetti-Pierri et al., 2008). A tumor inductive role has also been suggested (Ben-Baruch et al., 1994).

Several case reports from Nf-1 patients have identified histologically proven osteomalacia, which might be associated with hypophosphatemia due to renal phosphate wasting (Abdel-Wanis & Kawahara, 2002). Although the concentration of baseline vitamin D were in the normal range in these patients, researchers further found that the osteomalacia can be reversed independently of phosphate supplementation with oral treatment of 1-alpha-(OH)-vitamin D3 (Konishi et al., 1991). Moreover, a recently published comparative study reported that 25OHD serum concentration were about twofold lower in the Nf-1 patients than in healthy population and were inversely correlated with the number of neurofibromas (Lammert et al., 2006). The exact underlying mechanism of vitamin D deficiency in Nf-1 patients still remains unclear as well as the value of vitamin D supplementation for the treatment of the patients is still poorly understood.

Selected genetic disease populations, including Nf-1, display increased risks for osteoporosis, which is an emerging complication of utmost importance. Early diagnosis in the pediatric population is essential, since the highest contribution to peak bone mass is attained in the first three decades. Osteopenia or decreased bone mass accrual in the pediatric period can lead to frank osteoporosis and fractures in adulthood in the general population, as peak bone density is generally reached by late adolescence. Emerging evidence shows that vitamin D deficiency combined with a higher than normal bone turnover contributes to decreased bone mineral density in patients with Nf-1. The results of currently published studies suggest that the population of Nf-1 patient is at an increased risk for the development of clinical complications related to osteoporosis.

Seldom but yet published data revealed that significantly lower blood concentration of osteocalcin was observed in Nf-1 patients with, in comparison with patients without, skeletal abnormalities. Osteocalcin is secreted by osteoblasts, plays a role in mineralization and calcium ion homeostasis and its level reflects the rate of bone formation. Reduced blood concentration of osteocalcin in Nf-1 patients with skeletal deformity may indicate defect in osteoblasts functioning. Other biochemical markers of bone turnover usually do not exhibit any difference between these groups (Duman et al., 2008). When compared to healthy subjects, in Nf-1 patients BMD of the lumbar spine and femoral neck is significantly decreased. The same significant decrease apply to pubertal patients when compared to pubertal controls and in prepubertal patients when compared to prepubertal controls. The decrease in BMD is still more pronounced in Nf-1 patients with severe scoliosis, than those without spinal deformities. Duman et al. (2008) suggests that relevant predictors of skeletal abnormalities among Nf-1 patients are bone formation markers (exclusively osteocalcin) rather than imaging (conventional radiography, CT, MRI or quantitative ultrasonometry of the calcaneal bone) and densitometry techniques, especially dual-energy X-ray absorptiometry (DXA). In opposite to this report, the other published data suggest that both DXA and quantitative ultrasonometry of the calcaneal or other bones may prove useful to identify individuals with NF1 who are at risk for clinical osseous complications. These techniques and the logistics, introduced into pediatric practice quite recently, may also be appropriate for monitoring of therapeutic trials concerning skeletal ailments in Nf-1 children. However, many significant heterogeneities among the reports in the literature, such as patient groups (ages, variability of skeletal involvements, etc.) and methods (BMD assaying, comparison criteria such as T-score, Z-score, their cutoff points, etc.) make the comparisons amongst the studies very difficult. The densitometric criterion commonly used as a predictor of fracture risk for osteoporotic adults, called T-scores, derived from reference populations of young-adult women. While useful for evaluation of fracture risk in adults, but especially in postmenopausal women, is not applicable to the diagnosis of osteoporosis in children. In this age period the evaluation of osteoporotic risk of fracture is much more difficult. Densitometric data in children must be compared with age-matched control populations (z-scores). Currently, it is generally accepted that z-scores below −1.5 indicate low bone mass or osteopenia, and that osteoporosis is suspected strongly with z-scores below −2, especially followed by the episodes of fracturing. According to Writing Group for the ISCD Position Development Conference, z-score less than −2 define low bone density in children (2004).

According to unique published papers, children with Nf-1 had also statistically significant decreases in muscle mass compared to healthy controls regardless the presence or not of clinically proven osseous abnormalities (Stevenson et al., 2005). Muscle mass is important in the development of bone strength, as voluntary muscle forces (the largest physiological load) impact skeletal response. Combinations of extrinsic forces including decreased muscle mass could compromise potentially abnormal osseous matrix as well.

It is well known that *NF1* gene is widely expressed in chondrocytes, osteoblasts, osteoclast, and osteocytes (Kuorilehto et al., 2004). Kuorilehto et al. (2004) reported as well that neurofibromin is expressed in growing cartilage in areas where proliferation has ceased and the chondrocytes are undergoing differentiation, and in periostealosteoblasts of embryonic and mature mice and rats. However, mechanism of various skeletal deformities and bone metabolism defects in Nf-1 patients are not clearly understood. Experimental work done on animal models suggest that patients with Nf-1 suffers from a bone formation defect rather than bone resorption.

2.1.5 Other skeletal manifestations of neurofibromatosis type 1

Individuals with Nf-1 tend to be shorter than expected for their families (Szudek et al., 2000; Virdis et al., 2003), with 20–30% of adults with NF1 estimated to have a height below the 3rd centile. Growth velocity in these individuals is typically normal or near normal before puberty, then declines. Short stature in patients with NF1 is usually proportional. Scoliosis, growth hormone deficiency, and other Nf-1 related complications can contribute to short stature, but the cause of this in most patients with Nf-1 is unknown.

Bony abnormalities may be clinically silent, with radiographic evidence of long bone intramedullary fibrosis, cortical thinning, or vertebral dural ectasias often found incidentally.

Among the other bone abnormalities observed Nf-1 patients rarely, but with frequency a bit higher than in general populations, are cystic osseous lesions. They are usually identified incidentally during ongoing process of repeated imaging, reflecting the international recommendations. Found during radiographic knee exam, these cystic lesions are occasionally seen in the absence of tumors or long bone dysplasia (Colby & Saul, 2003; Lee & Cho, 2006). The lesions rarely fracture or show progressive deformity, and biopsy generally shows non-ossifying fibroma bone tumors. The association of multiple non-ossifying fibromas with cafe au lait skin patches are the fundamental signs of Jaffee-Campanacci syndrome (JCS) (Campanacci et al., 1983). The long bones affected more often are the femur, the humerus, and the tibia as well as the bones of the jaw. Other bones can be involved less frequently, especially the pelvis, the fibula, the radius, and the ulna. The lesions may be large enough to cause pathological fracture of the involved bone. Recent findings suggest that JCS may be a form of Nf-1 (Colby & Saul, 2003).

2.2 Pathophysiology of skeletal abnormalities in neurofibromatosis type 1: Experience from transgenic mouse models

Studies assessing the role of *NF1* gene not only in tumor formation and development, but also in pathogenesis of other multiple abnormalities, are to be a matter of numerous experimental work, which cannot be apply neither on living individuals, nor cell lines. These restrictions led to the development of transgenic mouse models allowing determination of the role of *NF1* gene and its product in affected systems and facilitate preclinical studies. Unfortunately, mice's embryos with inactivated both *NF1* alleles exhibit severe neural closure defect, namely exencephaly, and cardiovascular abnormalities including structural malformations of the outflow tract of the heart and enlarged endocardial cushions. These NF1-deficient embryos die between embryonic days 12.5 and 13.5, presumably due to the cardiac vessel defect. In contrast to completely defective organism, inactivation of only one allele of NF1 gene locally, in the neural crest only, does not cause cardiac defects but results in tumors of neural crest origin, resembling those seen in Nf-1 patients. Following this early experiments the another models of an experimental animal has been developed to determine the role of NF1 in bone cells and resolve difficulties in understanding the human pathophysiology of Nf-1 skeletal defects (Kolanczyk, 2007, 2008).

It has been well known that neurofibromin is a cytoplasmic protein that is predominantly expressed in neurons, Schwann cells, oligodendrocytes, astrocytes, and leukocytes. Due to early studies based on transgenic animal models of skeletal defective mice it is obvious currently that NF1-mRNA and neurofibromin are expressed in mouse bone and cartilage during development and adulthood (Kuorilehto et al., 2004), and more specifically in mesenchymal stem cells, chondrocytes, osteoblasts (Elefteriou et al., 2006; Kolanczyk et al., 2007), and osteoclasts (Yang et al., 2006a). Kuorilehto et al. (2004) reported the expression of neurofibromin in growth plate, periosteum, and tracebular bone of mice, and the expression in growth plate was mainly located in chondrocytes of the hypertrophic layer. Yu et al (2005) showed that upon the activation of ras signals, NF1+/- murine osteoprogenitor cells show increased proliferation and premature apoptosis; the osteoprogenitor cells also exhibit a lower rate of differentiation to osteoblasts. He considered neurofibromin and its role as ras signal regulator to be necessary for osteoblast function. Kolanczyk et al (2007) found that osteoblasts from NF1Prx1(NF1+/-) mice show increased proliferation and decreased abilities to differentiate and mineralize, whereas chondrocytes demonstrate a lower proliferation rate and defective differentiation. These results indicate that NF1 has multiple roles in skeletal development including joint formation, growth plate function, osteoblast differentiation, and control of vessel growth, and proved that NF1 is an important regulator of development and growth of the skeleton. The pattern of expression suggests that NF1-related skeletal abnormalities stem in part from primary osseous defects caused by bone cellular dysfunctions related to generalized NF1 heterozygosity, and/or to NF1 loss of function in specific bone cell types.

Investigations of affected skeletal tissue in tibial pseudarthrosis model created by inactivation of one of NF1 alleles during early mouse limb development, confirm that further mutation of the second NF1 allele, thus the homozygous loss of NF1 function, was detrimental for normal bone development. Thus, like in NF1-mediated tumorigenicity, a loss of both NF1 alleles is likely to be required to cause the skeletal abnormality phenotype.

Available mouse models recapitulate some, but not all, of the bone abnormalities in patients with Nf-1. Mouse data helped clarify that NF1 haploinsufficiency is likely related to the generalized Nf-1 bone remodeling defects, whereas total loss of NF1 function is likely related to the focal dysplastic events. Identifying neurofibromin cellular functions, target genes and downstream signaling pathways remains a priority to understand the etiology of the Nf-1 skeletal manifestations.

3. Present day and future treatment of skeletal dysplasia in neurofibromatosis type 1

Consensus guidelines for the treatment of the specific orthopedic manifestations in patients with Nf-1 do not exist and clinical management practices for each Nf-1 skeletal abnormality varied considerably.

At present, there are either no clinical trials to support the use of osteoporotic drugs in a population of Nf-1 patients or treatment guidelines. Thus, conservative therapy to promote bone health, such as treatment with calcium and vitamin D, and weight-bearing exercise forms the first line of therapy in children with Nf-1 and low bone mass. Correction of measured deficiencies in hormones (vitamin D, thyroid, estrogen, etc.) that are known to regulate skeletal growth and maturation is inevitable. Judicious vitamin D supplementation may prove beneficial for patients with Nf-1 who have vitamin D deficiency or evidence of osteopenia. Similarly, until further information is obtained, treatment of osteoporosis in adults with Nf-1 follow the recommendations developed for general population. Because low serum 25-OH-D and osteomalacia has been reported in patients with Nf-1 and low bone mass, osteoporotic adult patients over age 50 years should take supplemental 1,200 mg calcium and 800–1,000 IU vitamin D per day, and reduce clinical risk factors by regular weight bearing and muscle strengthening exercises and avoidance of smoking and excessive alcohol. Selection of approved anabolic or anti-resorptive drugs to prevent or treat osteoporotic fractures should follow the standard practice with exception of children. Children should be treated as well, as soon as fracture complicates the osteopenic/osteoporotic bone dysplasia (Elefteriou, 2009). Unfortunately, anabolic substances available currently upon two forms of parathyroid hormone pose the increased risk of osteosarcoma development, proven in rats, and are contraindicated in children (Tashjian & Gagel, 2006). Bisphosphonates and monoclonal antibodies that target osteoclasts, belonging to anti-resorptive drugs, have been used to reduce osteoporotic fractures in adults, but their effect on BMD and fracture risk in children with Nf-1 is unknown. Clinical trials are necessary to determine which of currently available therapies are most effective to treat patients with Nf-1 and reduces BMD, but especially frank osteoporosis.

In patients with Nf-1, the morbidity associated with either dystrophic scoliosis or tibial dysplasia is much greater than that of osteopenia and osteoporosis or even non-dystrophic scoliosis. This helps define priorities for current and future trials. Some of the ailments, particularly dystrophic scoliosis or tibial bowing, can lead to clinically significant consequences if neglected.

Children with dystrophic scoliosis require the extensive medical attention. In children who do not complete skeletal maturation, typically presented dystrophic form of scoliosis, bracing is routinely used when the spine curvature exceeded 25 up to 45 degrees. While the curvature progresses to more than 45 degrees before maturity or 55 degrees after maturity, surgery is commonly employed. Unique management approach due to progression is necessary in skeletally immature patients with dystrophic scoliosis in whom a curvature exciding 30 degrees. Exclusion of paravertebral tumors and dystrophic changes required MR or, less sensitive, CT imagings, as those finding may be missed on plain radiographs. Regarding possible complications of surgery, careful presurgical assessment is critical, as the lamina may be thin, the canal affected by dural ectasia or intraspinal tumors, and a rib may have displaced into the spinal canal, all of which express an increased risk of poor post-surgical outcome. Variables such as age, gender, associated neurofibromas, location and degree of the curve, and associated radiographic dystrophic features make the operation design difficult. Surgical treatment with fusion and growing rods is complex. Occasionally, intraspinal elements may directly compromise the cord when instrumentation and stabilization are attempted, or they may cause erosive changes in the bone, preventing primary fusion. The local condition may exclude the possibility of radical excision of tumor not infrequently, additionally worsen the postsurgical outcome. A lack of animal models of dystrophic scoliosis and consequently poor understanding of the natural history of this ailment, additionally hinder progress. As the pathogenesis of Nf-1 dystrophic scoliosis is still poorly understood, there are no clear pharmacologic adjunctive options. It is postulated, that prospective studies to determine the relationship of spinal neurofibromas in patients with dystrophic scoliosis may help to determine if early treatment of spinal tumors could prevent dystrophic scoliosis. Currently there is no effective treatment for Nf-1 related dural ectasia. If microfractures and vertebral wedging with subsequent development of scoliosis is diagnosed, then pharmacologic agents to increase vertebral strength may be appropriate (Elefteriou, 2009).

The dumbbell tumors, most of which are located unilaterally in the spinal canal and paravertebral space, are excised through a hemilaminectomy and a facetectomy, because these techniques provide large space for tumors excision. In addition, the spinal stability can be reconstructed by Rogers wiring and contralateral facet fusion, because the hemilaminectomy and facetectomy can minimize damage to spinal stability by leaving the spinous process, supra- and intraspinous ligaments, and contralateral facet joint.

Some dermal and most often internal plexiform neurofibromas, generally larger, more diffuse, and locally invasive to adjacent tissue and bone are seen in more than one fourth of patients with Nf-1 and can present a surgical or medical management conundrum. Besides pain, disfigurement, neurological and other clinical deficits complicated its growth, the wisdom of watchful waiting versus aggressive intervention is often debated (Wozniak & Karwacki, 2008). Complete resection of a PNF, radicalism of which is always controversial, without residual functional deficits is rarely possible, on the other hand, it must be remembered that app. 10% of them undergo malignant transformation. Thus debulking or partial resection of PNF may be undertaken not only for cosmetic purposes, but especially when progressive functional consequences are anticipated.

Surgical treatment of the chest wall deformities is usually not required, and the ailment, as well as short but proportional stature and not prominent macrocephaly, are assumed as principally cosmetic.

Sphenoid wing dysplasia, comprising a congenital malformation or a secondary bony defect, is not a primary target for therapeutic prevention. Although, it requires sensitive imaging techniques, particularly MRI, to screen patient for adjacent tumor, which may be amenable to therapy.

The management of anterolateral bowing deformity, characteristic for Nf-1, is most frustrating. Unlike scoliosis, treatment of congenital pseudarthrosis of the tibia does not appear to be more successful when it is initiated early. Anecdotally, early surgical intervention in children with Nf-1 and tibial pseudarthrosis results in poorer outcomes compared to later surgical management. The Consortium orthopedists recommended routine bracing of the dysplastic long bone upon diagnosis of bowing and agreed that prophylactic surgery should be avoided (Elefteriou, 2009). So, the current standard for treatment of long bone bowing in children is bracing to prevent fracture. The majority of members of the Consortium advocated early bracing until the child achieves maturity and, in some cases, continued even into adulthood. Evaluations of brace type, duration of use, or long-term benefits have not been obvious. Treatment of long bone pseudarthrosis is often unsatisfactory and very often require multiple surgeries or ultimate amputation. It is general belief that bracing after pathological fracture should continue, delaying surgery until mid-childhood, in fifth - eight year of age at earliest. Among the surgical procedures the most often applied are resection of the pseudarthrotic region and bone bridging with fixation via intramedullary stabilization devices, or free vascularized fibular grafting (contralateral or ipsilateral), or external fixation (e.g., Ilizarov technique), either alone or in combination with transankle fixation. Residual angular deformity, ankle stiffness, limb length discrepancy, refracture, and chronic pain are amongst the most severe complications of long bone pseudarthrosis. Attempts must been made to promote bone healing, always impaired in children with Nf-1 affected bones. Thus, electrical stimulation, varying periods of postoperative immobilization, supplemental bone grafting, and more sophisticated techniques, such as application of bone morphogenetic proteins and monocytic progenitors stem cells are under the routine or experimental options. Summarizing, tibial dysplasia with pseudarthrosis is still challenging Nf-1 skeletal manifestation required further extensive elaboration, on both scientific and everyday practice fields (Elefteriou, 2009).

Established transgenic mouse models of NF1 gene and its protein dysfunctions opens up new vistas for a better understanding of the natural history and the development of new therapies and long-term orthopedic management essential to improve patient care. Based on data from these models, a variety of cell types and signaling pathways are likely to be involved in Nf-1 patients with bone manifestations. Therefore, combination therapies, using both anabolic and anti-catabolic medications, will likely give optimal results. For example, use of locally applied biological mediators (e.g., bone morphogenetic protein) at the time of surgery in patients with pseudarthrosis is an attractive option in order to avoid complications of systemic administration of pharmacologic agents. Unfortunately, no mouse model, even closely resembles the human skeletal manifestations, is fully identical, despite similarities with the human condition, in part due to the limitations of the genetic manipulations. Nevertheless, NF1-deficient mice are currently the only and highly valuable project in preclinical testing of candidate therapies for Nf-1 skeletal defects.

Various studies have been initiated until now in preclinical mouse models to assess the potential efficacy of selected drugs on bone formation, repair and remodeling. Even when they represent just an initial approach, the most promising demonstrated potential of bisphosphonates (such as zolendronic acid) and recombinant human bone morphogenetic proteins (rhBMPs), which induces bone and cartilage formation, for improved net bone production in an in vivo model of heterotopic bone formation (Schindeler et al., 2008, Schindeler et al., 2011). Bisphosphonates are currently approved for other applications, so they could transition rapidly to Nf-1 clinical trials. Kolanczyk et al. (2008) quite recently published data concerning lovastatin, which improves cortical bone injury healing defects observed in the NF1-deficient mice. The inhibition of Ras/Erk signaling by lovastatin and other statins in mouse model counteracts the Ras/Erk constitutive activation occurred in NF1-deficient osteoblasts (as in Schwann cells), and improves bone healing defects. His work established the base for future experiments aimed at the treatment of the focal Nf-1 bone changes with local statin's delivery (Weixi et al., 2010).

4. Final remarks and conclusions for the future

Although neurofibromatosis type 1 is associated with marked clinical variability, most affected children do well from the standpoint of their growth and development. Some features of Nf-1 are present at birth, and others are age related abnormalities of tissue proliferation, which necessitate periodic monitoring to address ongoing health and developmental needs and to minimize the risk of serious medical complications. Among the most important and often debilitating are skeletal abnormalities. The skeleton is frequently affected in individuals with Nf-1, and some of these bone manifestations can result in significant morbidity and even profound invalidism. The natural history and pathogenesis of these skeletal abnormalities are still poorly understood and consequently therapeutic options for these manifestations are currently limited. Lately established transgenic mouse models as well as continuously developing new and improved imaging techniques warrants further achievements either in basic science concerning the complications of *NF1* mutation or clinical availability of diagnostic tools. The ongoing investigational trials, both preclinical and clinical as well as observational, gather significant number of participants, strengthen patient's belief for future improved care and therapy potentially freed them from often burdensome complications of disease course.

5. References

Abdel-Wanis, M. & Kawahara, N. (2002). Hypophosphatemic osteomalacia in neurofibromatosis type 1: hypotheses for pathogenesis and higher incidence of spinal deformity. Med Hypotheses. Vol. 59, No. 2, pp. 183–185

Alwan, S., Armstrong, L., Joe, H., Birch, P.H., Szudek, J. & Friedman, J.M. (2007). Associations of osseous abnormalities in Neurofibromatosis 1. Am J Med Genet, Part A. Vol. 143A, No. 12, pp. 1326–1333

Ben-Baruch, D., Ziv, Y., Sandbank, J. & Wolloch, Y. (1994). Oncogenic osteomalacia induced by schwannoma in a patient with neurofibromatosis. Eur J Surg Oncol. Vol. 20, No. 1, pp. 57-61

Boulanger, J.M. & Larbrisseau, A. (2005). Neurofibromatosis type 1 in a pediatric population: Ste-Justine's experience. Can J Neurol Sci. Vol. 32, No. 2, pp. 225–231

Brunetti-Pierri, N., Doty, S.B., Hicks, J., Phan, K., Mendoza-Londono, R., Blazo, M., Tran, A., Carter, S., Lewis, R.A., Plon, S.E., Phillips, W.A., O'Brian Smith, E., Ellis, K.J. & Lee, B. (2008). Generalized metabolic bone disease in neurofibromatosis type I. Mol Genet Metab. Vol. 94, No. 1, pp. 105–111

Campanacci, M., Laus, M. & Boriani, S. (1983). Multiple non-ossifying fibromata with extraskeletal anomalies: a new syndrome? J Bone Joint Surg Br. Vol. 65, No. 5, pp. 627-32

Casselman, E.S. & Mandell, G.A. (1979). Vertebral scalloping in neurofibromatosis. Radiology. Vol. 131, No. 1, pp. 89–94

Colby, R.S. & Saul, R.A. (2003). Is Jaffe-Campanacci syndrome just a manifestation of neurofibromatosis type 1? Am J Med Genet. Vol. 15, No. 1, pp. 60-3

Crawford, A.H. & Schorry, E.K. (1999). Neurofibromatosis in children: The role of the orthopaedist. J Am Acad Orthop Surg.Vol. 7, No. 4, pp. 217–230

Crawford, A.H. & Schorry, E.K. (2006). Neurofibromatosis update. J Pediatr Orthop. Vol. 26, No. 3, pp. 413-23

Crawford, A.H. & Herrera-Soto, J. (2007). Scoliosis associated with neurofibromatosis. Orthop Clin North Am. Vol. 38, No. 4, pp. 553-62

Crawford, A.H., Parikh, S., Schorry, E.K. & Von Stein, D. (2007). The immature spine in type-1 neurofibromatosis. J Bone Joint Surg Am Vol. 89, Suppl. 1, pp. 123–142

DeBella, K., Poskitt, K., Szudek, J. & Friedman, J.M. (2000a). Use of "unidentified bright objects" on MRI for diagnosis of neurofibromatosis 1 in children. Neurology Vol. 54, No. 8, pp. 1646 -1651

DeBella, K., Szudek, J. & Friedman, J.M. (2000b). Use of the national institutes of health criteria for diagnosis of neurofibromatosis 1 in children. Pediatrics. Vol. 105, No. 3, Pt. 1, pp. 608–614

Duman, O., Ozdem, S., Turkkahraman, D., Olgac, N.D., Gungor, F. & Haspolat, S. (2008). Bone metabolism markers and bone mineral density in children with neurofibromatosis type-1. Brain & Development. Vol. 30, No. 9, pp. 584–588

Durrani, A.A., Crawford, A.H., Chouhdry, S.N., Saifuddin, A. & Morley, T.R. (2000). Modulation of spinal deformities in patients with neurofibromatosis type 1. Spine (Phila Pa 1976). Vol. 25, No. 1, pp. 69-75.

Elefteriou F., Benson, M.D., Sowa, H., Starbuck, M., Liu, X., Ron, D., Parada, L.F. & Karsenty, G. (2006). ATF4 mediation ofNF1 functions in osteoblast reveals a nutritional basis for congenital skeletal dysplasiae. Cell Metab Vol. 4, No. 6, pp. 441-451

Elefteriou, F., Kolanczyk, M., Schindeler, A., Viskochil, D.H., Hock, J.M., Schorry, E.K., Crawford, A.H., Friedman, J.M., Little, D., Peltonen, J., Carey, J.C., Feldman, D., Yu X., Armstrong, L., Birch, P., Kendler, D.L., Mundlos, S., Yang, F.C., Agiostratidou, G., Hunter-Schaedle K. & Stevenson D.A. (2009). Skeletal abnormalities in neurofibromatosis type 1: approaches to therapeutic options. Am J Med Genet A. Vol. 149A, No. 10, pp. 2327-38

Ferner, R.E., Huson, S.M., Thomas, N., Moss, C., Willshaw, H., Evans, D.G., Upadhyaya, M., Towers, R., Gleeson, M., Steiger, C. & Kirby A. (2007). Guidelines for the diagnosis and management of individuals with neurofibromatosis 1 (NF1). J Med Genet Vol. 44, No. 2, pp. 81- 88

Friedman, J.M., Gutmann, D.H., MacCollin, M. & Riccardi, V.M. (Eds.)(1999). Neurofibromatosis: phenotype, natural history, and pathogenesis. Johns Hopkins University Press, ISBN: 080186285X, Baltimore MD

Friedman JM & Birch PH. Type 1 neurofibromatosis: a descriptive analysis of the disorder in 1,728 patients. Am J Med Genet. 1997 May 16;70(2):138-43

Greenwood, R.S., Tupler, L.A., Whitt, J.K., Buu, A., Dombeck, C.B., Harp, A.G., Payne, M.E., Eastwood, J.D., Krishnan, K.R. & MacFall J.R. (2005). Brain morphometry, T2-weighted hyperintensities, and IQ in children with neurofibromatosis type 1. Arch Neurol. Vol. 62, No. 12, pp. 1904–1908

Gutmann, D.H., Aylsworth, A., Carey, J.C., Korf, B., Marks, J., Pyeritz, R.E., Rubenstein, A., Viskochil, D. (1997). The diagnostic evaluation and multidisciplinary management of neurofibromatosis 1 and neurofibromatosis 2, JAMA. Vol. 278, No. 1, pp. 51-57.

Illes, T., Halmai, V., de Jonge, T. & Dubousset, J. (2001). Decreased bone mineral density in neurofibromatosis-1 patients with spinal deformities. Osteoporos Int. Vol. 12, No. 10, pp. 823–827

Jacquemin, C., Bosley, T.M., Liu, D., Svedberg, H. & Buhaliqa, A. (2002). Reassessment of sphenoid dysplasia associated with neurofibromatosis type 1. Am J Neuroradiol. Vol. 23, No. 4, pp. 644–648

Jacquemin, C., Bosley, T.M. & Svedberg, H. (2003). Orbit deformities in craniofacial neurofibromatosis type 1. Am J Neuroradiol. Vol. 24, No. 8, pp. 1678–1682

Jett, K. & Friedman, J.M. (2010). Clinical and genetic aspects of neurofibromatosis 1. Genet Med. Vol. 12, No 1, pp. 1-11

Jouhilahti, E.M., Peltonen, S., Heape, A.M. & Peltonen, J. (2011). The pathoetiology of neurofibromatosis 1. Am J Pathol. Vol. 178, No. 5, pp. 1932-9

Karwacki, M.W. & Wozniak, W. (2006). Neurofibromatosis--an inborn genetic disorder with susceptibility to neoplasia. Med Wieku Rozwoj. Vol. 10, No. 3, Pt. 2, pp. 923-48

Khong, P.L., Goh, W.H., Wong, V.C., Fung, C.W. & Ooi, G.C. (2003). MR imaging of spinal tumors in children with neurofibromatosis 1. Am J Roentgenol. Vol 180, No. 2, pp. 413-417.

Kolanczyk, M., Kossler, N., Kuhnisch, J., Lavitas, L., Stricker, S., Wilkening, U., Manjubala, I., Fratzl, P., Sporle, R., Herrmann, B.G., Parada, L., Kornak, U. & Mundlos S. (2007). Multiple roles for neurofibromin in skeletal development and growth. Hum Mol Genet. Vol. 16, No. 8, pp. 874-886

Kolanczyk, M., Kuehnisch, J., Kossler, N., Osswald, M., Stumpp, S., Thurisch, B., Kornak, U. & Mundlos, S. (2008). Modelling neurofibromatosis type 1 tibial dysplasia and its treatment with lovastatin. BMC Med. No. 6, p. 21.

Konishi, K., Nakamura, M., Yamakawa, H., Suzuki, H., Saruta, T., Hanaoka, H. & Davatchi, F. (1991). Hypophosphatemic osteomalacia in von Recklinghausen neurofibromatosis. Am J Med Sci. Vol. 301, No. 5, pp. 322-328

Kuorilehto, T., Nissinen, M., Koivunen, J., Benson, M.D. & Peltonen, J. (2004). NF1 tumor suppressor protein and mRNA in skeletal tissues of developing and adult normal mouse and NF1-deficient embryos. J Bone Miner Res. Vol. 19, No. 6, pp. 983-9

Lammert, M., Friedman, J.M., Roth, H.J., Friedrich, R.E., Kluwe, L., Atkins, D., Schooler, T., Mautner, V.F. (2006). Vitamin D deficiency associated with number of neurofibromas in neurofibromatosis 1. J Med Genet. Vol. 43, No. 10, pp. 810-3

Lammert, M., Friedrich, R.E., Friedman, J.M., Mautner, V.F., Tucker T. (2007). Early primary tooth eruption in neurofibromatosis 1 individuals. Eur J Oral Sci. Vol. 115, No. 5, pp. 425-426

Larizza, L., Gervasini, C., Natacci, F. & Riva, P. (2009). Developmental abnormalities and cancer predisposition in neurofibromatosis type 1. Curr Mol Med. Vol. 9, No. 5, pp. 634-53

Lee, H.C. & Cho, D.Y. (2006). Assessment of sacrum scalloping in neurofibromatosis type 1 caused by a giant cell lesion of the sacrum. Surg Neurol Vol. 65, No. 2, pp. 194-198 (discussion p 198)

Mensink, K.A., Ketterling, R.P., Flynn, H.C., Knudson, R.A., Lindor, N.M., Heese, B.A., Spinner, R.J. & Babovic-Vuksanovic, D. (2006). Connective tissue dysplasia in five new patients with NF1 microdeletions: further expansion of phenotype and review of the literature. J Med Genet. Vol. 43, No. 2, p. e8

Neurofibromatosis. Conference statement. National Institutes of Health Consensus Development Conference. (1988). Arch Neurol. Vol. 45, No. 5, pp. 575-8

Ramachandran, M., Tsirikos, A.I., Lee, J. & Saifuddin, A. (2004). Whole-spine magnetic resonance imaging in patients with neurofibromatosis type 1 and spinal deformity. J Spinal Disord Tech. Vol. 17, No. 6, pp. 483-491

Radtke, H.B., Sebold, C.D., Allison, C., Haidle, J.L. & Schneider, G. (2007). Neurofibromatosis type 1 in genetic counseling practice: recommendations of the National Society of Genetic Counselors. J Genet Couns. Vol. 16, No. 4, pp. 387-407

Riccardi, V.M. (2010). Neurofibromatosis type 1 is a disorder of dysplasia: the importance of distinguishing features, consequences, and complications. Birth Defects Res A Clin Mol Teratol. Vol. 88, No.1, pp. 9-14

Schindeler, A., Ramachandran, M., Godfrey, C., Morse, A., McDonald, M., Mikulec, K. & Little, D.G. (2008). Modeling bone morphogenetic protein and bisphosphonate combination therapy in wild-type and Nf1 haploinsufficient mice. J Orthop Res. Vol. 26, No. 1, pp. 65-74

Schindeler, A., Birke, O., Yu, N.Y., Morse, A., Ruys, A., Baldock, P.A. & Little, D.G. (2011). Distal tibial fracture repair in a neurofibromatosis type 1-deficient mouse treated with recombinant bone morphogenetic protein and a bisphosphonate. J Bone Joint Surg Br. Vol. 93, No. 8, pp. 1134-9

Schonauer, C., Tessitore, E., Frascadore, L., Parlato, C. & Moraci, A. (2000). Lumbosacral dural ectasia in type 1 neurofibromatosis. Report of two cases. J Neurosurg Sci Vol. 44, No. 3, pp. 165-168 (and discussion p. 169)

Seitz, S., Schnabel, C., Busse B., Schmidt, H.U., Beil, F.T., Friedrich, R.E., Schinke, T., Mautner, V.F. & Amling, M. (2010). High bone turnover and accumulation of osteoid in patients with neurofibromatosis 1. Osteoporos Int. Vol. 21, No. 1, pp. 119-27

Stevenson, D.A., Moyer-Mileur, L.J., Carey, J.C., Quick, J.L., Hoff, C.J. & Viskochil, D.H. (2005). Case-control study of the muscular compartments and osseous strength in neurofibromatosis type 1 using peripheral quantitative computed tomography. J Musculoskelet Neuronal Interact. Vol. 5, No. 2, pp. 145-9

Stevenson, D.A., Moyer-Mileur, L.J., Murray, M., Slater, H., Sheng, X., Carey, J.C., Dube, B. & Viskochil, D.H. (2007). Bone mineral density in children and adolescents with neurofibromatosis type 1. J Pediatr. Vol. 150, No. 1, pp. 83-88

Stevenson, D.A., Schwarz, E.L., Viskochil, D.H., Moyer-Mileur, L.J., Murray, M., Firth S.D., D'Astous, J.L., Carey, J.C. & Pasquali, M. (2008). Evidence of increased bone resorption in neurofibromatosis type 1 using urinary pyridinium crosslink analysis. Pediatr Res. Vol. 63, No. , pp. 697-701

Szudek, J., Birch, P. & Friedman, J.M. (2000). Growth in North American white children with neurofibromatosis 1 (NF1). J Med Genet Vol. 37, No. 12, pp. 933-938

Tashjian A.H. Jr. & Gagel R.F. (2006). Teriparatide [human PTH(1-34)]: 2.5 years of experience on the use and safety of the drug for the treatment of osteoporosis. J Bone Miner Res. Vol. 21, No. 3, pp. 354-65

Tubbs, R.S. & Oakes, W.J. (2002). Dural ectasia in neurofibromatosis. Pediatr Neurosurg. Vol. 37, No. 6, pp. 331-332

Tucker, T., Birch, P., Savoy, D.M. & Friedman, J.M. (2007). Increased dental caries in people with neurofibromatosis 1. Clin Genet. Vol. 72, No. 6, pp. 524-7

Upadhyaya, M. (2011). Genetic basis of tumorigenesis in NF1 malignant peripheral nerve sheath tumors. Front Biosci. Vol. 16 (Jan. 1, 2011), pp. 937-51

Upadhyaya, M., Huson S.M., Davies, M., Thomas, N., Chuzhanova, N., Giovannini, S., Evans, D.G., Howard, E., Kerr, B., Griffiths, S., Consoli C., Side, L., Adams, D., Pierpont., M., Hachen, R., Barnicoat, A., Li, H., Wallace, P., Van Biervliet, J.P., Stevenson, D., Viskochil, D., Baralle, D., Haan, E., Riccardi, V., Turnpenny P., Lazaro, C. & Messiaen, L. (2007). An absence of cutaneous neurofibromas associated with a 3-bp inframe deletion in exon 17 of the NF1 gene (c. 2970-2972 delAAT): evidence of a clinically significant NF1 genotype-phenotype correlation. Am J Hum Genet. Vol. 80, No. 1, pp. 140 –151.

Virdis, R., Street, M.E., Bandello, M.A., Tripodi, C., Donadio, A., Villani, A.R., Cagozzi, L., Garavelli, L. & Bernasconi, S. (2003). Growth and pubertal disorders in neurofibromatosis type 1. J Pediatr Endocrinol Metab. Vol. 16, Suppl. 2, pp. 289–292

Visnapuu, V., Peltonen, S., Ellila, T., Kerosuo, E., Vaananen, K., Happonen, R.P. & Peltonen, J. (2007). Periapical cemental dysplasia is common in women with NF1. Eur J Med Genet. Vol. 50, No. 4, pp. 274–280

Vitale, M.G., Guha A. & Skaggs D.L. (2002). Orthopaedic manifestations of neurofibromatosis in children: an update. Clin Orthop Relat Res. No. 401, pp. 107-18

Walker, L., Thompson, D., Easton, D., Ponder, B., Ponder, M., Frayling, I. & Baralle, D. (2006). A prospective study of neurofibromatosis type 1 cancer incidence in the UK. Br J Cancer. Vol. 95, No. 2, pp. 233-8

Wang, Z. & Liu, Y. (2010). Research update and recent developments in the management of scoliosis in neurofibromatosis type 1. Orthopedics. Vol. 33, No. 5, pp. 335-41

Weixi, W., Nyman, J.S., Moss H., E., Gutierrez G., Mundy G.R., Xiangli Y. & Elefteriou F. (2010) Local Low-Dose Lovastatin Delivery Improves the Bone-Healing Defect Caused by Loss of Function in Osteoblasts. Journal of Bone and Mineral Research. Vol. 25, No 7, pp. 1658-1667

Williams, V.C., Lucas, J., Babcock, M.A., Gutmann., DH, Korf, B. & Maria, B.L. (2009). Neurofibromatosis type 1 revisited. Pediatrics; Vol. 123, No. 1, pp. 124 –133

Wozniak, W. & Karwacki, M.W. (2008). Is "watchful waiting" superior to surgery in children with neurofibromatosis type 1 presenting with extracranial and extramedullary tumor mass at diagnosis? Childs Nerv Syst. Vol. 24, No. 12, pp. 1431-6

Writing Group for the ISCD Position Development Conference: Diagnosis of osteoporosis in men, premenopausal women, and children. (2004). J Clin Densitom. Vol. 7, No. 1, pp. 17–26

Yang, F.C., Chen, S., Clegg, T., Li, X., Morgan, T., Estwick, S.A., Yuan, J., Khalaf, W., Burgin, S., Travers, J., Parada, L.F., Ingram, D.A., Clapp, D.W. (2006). Nf1+/- mast cells induce neurofibroma like phenotypes through secreted TGF-beta signaling. Hum Mol Genet. Vol. 15, No. 16, pp. 2421–2437

Yu, X., Chen, S., Potter, O.L., Murthy, S.M., Li, J., Pulcini, J.M., Ohashi, N., Winata, T., Everett, E.T., Ingram, D., Clapp, W.D. & Hock, J.M. (2005). Neurofibromin and its inactivation of Ras are prerequisites for osteoblast functioning. Bone. Vol. 36, No. , pp. 793–802

5

Post-Transplantation Bone Disease

Federico G. Hawkins, Sonsoles Guadalix,
Raquel Sanchez and Guillermo Martínez
Metabolic Unit, Endocrine Service, University Hospital 12 de Octubre,
Faculty of Medicine University Complutense, Madrid,
Spain

1. Introduction

Solid organ or stem cell transplantation is a well established procedure in the treatment of end-stage diseases (renal disease, chronic liver failure, end-stage pulmonary disease, heart failure). Improved outcome for these patients has allowed us to study some of the complications. One of these is metabolic bone disease, which can hinder their long-term survival and quality of life. In this chapter we have review our current understanding of the pathophysiology of bone loss before and after solid organ transplantation, and review recommendations for the prevention and treatment of osteoporosis in patients accepted into organ transplantation programs. There are a number of risk factors contributing to bone loss in these patients: hypogonadism, vitamin D deficiency, malabsorption, low body weight, physical inactivity, excessive use of tobacco or alcohol and immunosuppressive therapy. Management of pretransplant risk factors has improved, resulting in better bone mineral density (BMD) levels before transplantation (Guichelaar et al., 2006). After transplantation, rapid and marked bone loss is observed in the first 3-6 months. The speed of the bone loss suggests that corticosteroids are heavily involved. Greater bone loss at vertebral and hip sites and high rates of incident fragility fractures have been reported (Leidig-Bruckner et al., 2001).

2. Pathogenetic factors

Many factors contribute to the pathogenesis of osteoporosis after organ transplantation. These include bone disease preceding transplantation, immunosuppressive medications, nutritional and lifestyle factors, and derangements of the parathyroid-calcium-vitamin D and the pituitary gonadal axes (Table 1). However, specific pathophysiological features can also be found in different forms of end-stage diseases.

2.1 Pre-existing bone disease
2.1.1 Kidney disease
End-stage renal disease (ESRD) is associated with a form of bone disease that is generically referred as "renal osteodystrophy". Many mechanisms are involved in its pathophysiology including calcitriol deficiency, hypocalcemia, hyperphosphatemia, secondary hyperparathyroidism, metabolic acidosis, and aluminum overload. Kidney transplantation will improve many aspects of renal osteodystrophy, but parathyroid hyperplasia may not regress even when normal kidney function returns.

General Risk factors
Vitamin D Deficiency and secondary Hyperparathyroidism
Hypogonadism
Inactivity / Immobilization
Poor Nutrition
Low body weight
End Stage Renal Disease
Secondary hyperparathyroidism
Adinamic bone disease
Osteomalacia
Mixed Uremic disease
Metabolic Acidosis
Long term hemodyalysis
Medications: loop diuretics, heparin and warfarin.
Diabetic nephropathy
β-microglobulin amyloidosis
End-Stage Lung disease
Smoking
Chronic use of glucocorticoids
Hypercapnia
Hypoxia
Pancreatic insufficiency (cystic fibrosis).
Failure to attain peak bone mass (in patients who have cystic fibrosis).
Heart failure
Mild renal insufficiency
Medication: loop diuretics, heparin and warfarin.
Failure to attain peak bone mass (in patients with congenital heart disease).
End-Stage Liver Disease
Alcohol abuse
Cholestatic liver disease
Bone marrow transplant recipients
Chronic use of glucocorticoids
Chemotherapy
Growth hormone deficiency (in children)

Table 1. Risk Factors contributing to bone fragility before transplantation

There are several histological subtypes of renal osteodystrophy. The most common is osteitis fibrosa, characterized by increased bone turnover and typically associated with high serum PTH levels (secondary hyperparathyroidism). Osteomalacia is the least common type, with low bone formation and accumulation of unmineralized osteoid. A mixed disease of both, combining increased resorption and increased osteoid, can also exist. Adynamic bone disease is characterized by low bone formation without evidence of fibrosis.

Compared to the general population ESRD patients are 4.4 fold more likely to have a hip fracture and the prevalence of vertebral fracture is 21% higher (Alem et al., 2000). Some of the risk factors for fractures in general population are also seen in patients with renal osteodystrophy: older age, female gender, or low body weight. Specific risk factors in end-stage renal patients are duration of dialysis and peripheral vascular disease (Sethman-Breen et al., 2000).Although BMD in patients with renal osteodystrophy tends to be lower in cortical sites (forearm and hip) than cancellous sites (spine), there is not a clear relationship between the different histological types of renal osteodystrophy and bone density (Gerakis et al., 2000). Furthermore, BMD does not consistently predict fractures after kidney transplantation (Grotz et al., 1994). It is important to note that measurement of bone mineral density (BMD) and WHO criteria cannot be used to diagnose osteoporosis in patients with ESRD. This is because any of the several possible histological forms of renal bone disease may all be associated with low, normal or even elevated BMD.

2.1.2 Lung disease

Patients who are candidates for lung transplantation are highly likely to have osteoporosis before surgery. A retrospective study in patients with diffuse parenchymal lung disease referred for lung transplantation revealed that 30% and 49% of patients had lumbar or femoral osteoporosis respectively (Shane et al., 1996). Other authors found osteoporosis in 50% of the patients at lumbar spine and 61% at femoral neck (Tschopp et al., 2002). Several risk factors such as hypoxemia, malnutrition, vitamin D deficiency, smoking, decreased immobility and low body weight are involved. Cystic fibrosis is associated with additional risk factors such as hypogonadism, inflammatory bone-resorbing cytokines and pancreatic insufficiency that may impair the absorption of calcium and Vitamin D. In addition, most of the patients who undergo lung transplantation have experienced prior glucocorticoid therapy (Tschopp et al., 2002).

2.1.3 Cardiac disease

Osteoporosis and osteopenia are common in patients with severe congestive heart failure (CHF). Lumbar spine osteopenia has been found in 43% of patients, and spine osteoporosis (T-score $\leq$ -2.5 or Z-score $\leq$-2.0) in 12-40% of patients. Biochemical markers of bone turnover suggest the presence of increased bone resorption. Involved factors that contribute to bone loss include low serum 25-OH vitamin D, hypogonadism, immobilization and loop diuretic use. Long-term therapy with heparin has been associated with bone loss and vertebral fractures. However, in CHF oral anticoagulants (warfarin) usually are used chronically instead of heparin. Warfarin blocks vitamin K-dependent gamma-carboxylation of osteocalcin and impairs its binding with calcium. Secondary hyperparathyroidism may occur due to impaired renal function and abnormal vitamin D metabolism. Hypogonadotropic hypogonadism appears to be very common in males with CHF. Up to

30% of males with CHF evaluated before transplantation have low levels of testosterone, and this proportion could further increase after cardiac transplantation (Cohen et al., 2003). We have found that trabecular bone loss was related to pretransplantation time of waiting. Also bone resorption markers were increased at this stage reflecting a high bone turnover (Garcia Delgado et al., 2000).

2.1.4 Liver disease

Osteoporosis and osteopenia are frequent complications of chronic liver disease. Its prevalence is high in patients waiting for liver transplant, especially in cholestatic liver disease. In the most important series, densitometric osteoporosis has been described between 31% to 44% (Lopez et al., 1993, Newton et al., 2001, Solerio et al., 2003;Ninkovic et al., 2001; Guichelaar et al.., 2006).

A low bone turnover state has been found in biochemical measurements and histomorphometric analysis (Diamond et al., 1989). Osteocalcin levels are low and correlate with bone formation rate on bone biopsies, and show increases after successful transplantation. However, some reports describe increases in parameters reflecting bone resorption (osteoclast number and bone resorption surface) (Cuthbert et al., 1984).

Reduced bone formation has been related to several toxic factors that could inhibit osteoblast function as excessive alcohol intake or hyperbilirrubinemia. Also a lower IGF-1 sinthesis, that has a direct trophic action upon the osteoblast could be involved. Glucocorticoid used simultaneously reduces bone formation and increases bone resorption. Vitamin D metabolism plays a pivotal role. Patients with end-stage liver disease frequently have low serum levels of 25(OH) vitamin D, since 25-hydroxylation of colecalciferol occurs at the hepatocyte. Fat malabsorption also decreases 25 (OH) vitamin D. In addition, increased vitamin D catabolism, reduced levels of vitamin D-binding protein (DBP), or reduced sunlight exposure can further decrease vitamin D serum levels. However, true osteomalacia is rare in cirrhotic patients (Table 2). Typically, successful liver transplantation reverses most of these factors. Hypogonadism frequently associated in these patients, could be partially responsible for the increased bone resorption.

Reducing bone formation:
-Ethanol excess
-Iron overload (hemochromatosis)
-Hyperbilirrubinemia
-Glucocorticoid use
-Decreased IGF-1
-Decreased 25 (OH) vitamin D_3
Increasing bone formation:
-Hypogonadism
-Glucocorticoid use

Table 2. Involved factors in hepatic osteodystrophy.

In the past two decades significant changes have occurred in the management of chronic liver disease, the waiting time for transplantation and immunosuppressive therapy. Recently an improvement in lumbar spine BMD T-scores pretransplant from -2.5 before 1990 to -1.7 after 1996 has been described (Guichelaar et al., 2006). This data can help to clarify the etiology of bone loss: the severity of liver disease has not changed, the duration of disease before transplantation has been extended and patients can reach older ages. However, nutritional status has improved and bilirubin values decreased. These factors may have contributed to increase BMD before transplantation.

2.1.5 Bone marrow
Bone marrow transplant (BMT) recipients have many known risk factors for developing bone loss: Failure to attain peak bone mass in children and adolescents, hypogonadism, inactivity and induction and consolidation regimens with high dose of chemotherapy, glucocorticoids and irradiation that may damage bone marrow stromal cells and colony-forming unit fibroblast , reducing osteoblastic differentiation. A study in patients before BMT (after chemotherapy) show osteopenia in 24% and osteoporosis in only 4% (Schulte et al., 2000).

2.2 Related to transplantation: Immunossupressor drugs and other factors
2.2.1 Glucocorticoids
Early bone loss has been observed in all solid organ transplants in the first 3 to 6 months, increasing the incidence of osteoporosis and osteopenia (Rodino et al., 1998; Leidig-Bruckner et al., 2001; Eastell et al., 1991). Bone loss primarily affects the spine and proximal femur. Some authors found greater impairment at this level (Keogh et al., 1999; Ninkovic et al., 2002). In patients who already have osteopenia or osteoporosis, this subsequent bone loss can result in a higher number of fractures (Eastell et al.., 1991; Leidig-Bruckner et al., 2001). Traditionally, it has been assumed that high doses of glucocorticoids required for immunosuppression play a major role in this loss. High doses (≥ 1 mg/kg/day) are commonly prescribed immediately after transplantation, with gradual dose reduction over several weeks or months. Total GCs exposure depends on the transplanted organ, number of rejection episodes, and different immunosupressive regimens.

The natural history of post-transplantation osteoporosis suggests that there are two main phases: the early one and the late one. The factors affecting the skeleton differ between this two phases.

The mechanisms associated with bone loss due to glucocorticoid treatment in the first phase are (Table 3):

1) An increase in bone resorption as a result of increased urinary calcium, decrease in intestinal calcium absorption, secondary hyperparathyroidism and hypogonadotropic hypogonadism; 2) Activation of osteoclastogenesis caused by increase of RANKL and decrease of osteoprotegerin (OPG). 3) Corticosteroid treatment decrease the proliferation and function of osteoblasts (by inhibiting the gene expression of osteocalcin, collagen type 1 and IGF-I) and induces its apoptosis (Canalis et al., 2002). **(Fig 1)**

In addition to their direct effects on bone tissue, glucocorticoids can induce severe myopathy, impairing balance and mobility, decreasing weight-bearing activity and increasing fall risk and fractures.

Increase in bone resorption as a result of increased urinary calcium.
Decrease in intestinal calcium absorption.
Secondary hyperparathyroidism.
Hypogonadotropic hypogonadism.
Activation of osteoclastogenesis caused by increase of RANKL and decrease of osteoprotegerine (OPG) levels.
Decrease in proliferation and function of osteoblasts (by inhibiting the gene expression of osteocalcin, collagen type 1 and IGF-I).
Decrease anabolic effects of TGF-beta.
Induces Osteoblast apoptosis.

Table 3. Effects of high doses of glucocorticoids in bone loss.

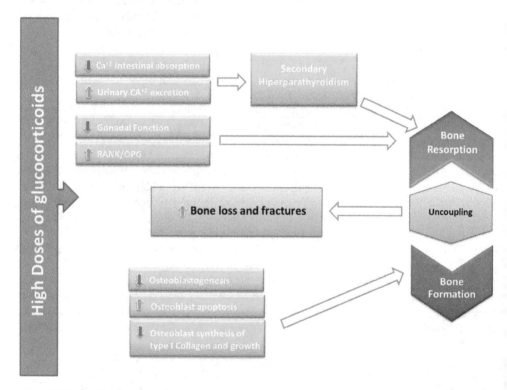

Fig. 1. Effect of high doses of glucocorticoids in bone loss

Effect of glucocorticoids in the WNT pathway: The Wnt pathway and the Bone Morphogenetic Protein (BMP) seem to be involved in the pathogenesis of glucocorticoid-induced osteoporosis, suppressing osteoblast differentiation and activity. BMP and Wnt pathway are regulated by several mechanisms: one of them are proteins that act as extracellular antagonists of BMP (Noggin, Chordin, Twisted gastrulation, Grelin, Sclerostin,

Follistatin and Dan), while others act as Wnt antagonist: Frizzled-related protein (sFRP), Dickkopf (Dkk) and Cerberus. Glucocorticoids can affect these signaling pathways, but the exact mechanisms are not been clarified. Recent studies suggest that glucocorticoids induce an alteration in osteoblast function by increasing Wnt antagonists with the subsequent suppression of this pathway. Recent reseach has shown that dexametasone, increases follistatin and DAN (BMP antagonists), sFRP-1(Wnt antagonist) and axin-2 (inhibitor of Wnt signal) . Simultaneously, alendronate and PTH (1-34), which have demostrated to be effective in the treatment of steroid osteoporosis, were able to antagonize the increase in this proteins induced by dexamethasone (Hayashi et al., 2008).

The potential impact of glucocorticoid dose as a determinant of bone loss is supported by the absence of bone loss at the lumbar spine and proximal femur in renal transplant patients treated with low doses of steroids and tacrolimus (Goffin et al., 2001). We have previously reported that steroid withdrawal in patients who have undergone a successful liver transplant accelerates the recovery of lumbar spine bone density without adverse effects on graft tolerance (Martínez Díaz-Guerra et al., 2002).

Moreover, higher rates of fracture occurring after cardiac (Shane et al., 1996) and lung (Shane et al., 1999) transplantation, in which higher doses of steroids are use, would be consistent with their role in the pathogenesis of post transplant osteoporosis.

The late phase observed in the postrasplant period takes place when the glucocorticoid doses are usually tapered below 5 mg per day. Then, osteoblast function recovers and consequently, an increase in bone formation and recoupling of bone remodeling activity is observed. During this later phase, rates of bone loss slow and there may even be some recovery, particularly in cancellous bone (Kulak et al., 2006). It is also found that despite an initial decrease in post transplant BMD, biopsies in the iliac crest showed improvement in histomorphometric parameters 4 months later (Guichelaar et al., 2003).

In conclusion, current evidence suggests that bone loss after transplantation is caused by an initial increase in bone turnover and resorption, plus a decrease in bone formation. Later, increases in bone formation could overcome resorption. These changes would be consistent with the rapid decrease in BMD observed in the first months after transplantation and recovery to baseline values, as most of studies show.

2.2.2 Other immunosuppressive drugs

The effect of these drugs in humans is difficult to study because they are used in conditions that by themselves affect bone remodeling, and they are rarely used in monotherapy so, the potential deleterious effect of one single agent could not be ascertained.

The role of calcineurin inhibitors in post-transplant bone loss is unknown. Tacrolimus is a calcineurin inhibitor that suppresses T cell activation and the production and release of IL-2 and other cytokines. It induces severe trabecular bone loss in rats, but this effect appears to be less severe in humans (Epstein, 1996). Cyclosporin A (CyA), another calcineurin inhibitor, also appears to have adverse effects in mouse models, inducing high turnover and reducing bone mass. Some studies in humans suggest a similar effect in patients with liver (Giannini et al., 2000), and cardiac (Thiebaud et al., 1996) transplantation. In a research of 360 patients with liver transplantation due to chronic cholestatic liver disease, the post transplant bone gain was lower, and the number of fractures was higher in patients treated with CyA than in those receiving tacrolimus (Guichelaar et al., 2007). Other authors have found greater fracture incidence in patiens receiving CyA treatment than in those treated with tacrolimus (Monegal et al., 2001).

In other liver transplanted recipients study, although bone mass losses were similar in patients on CyA regimen than in those on tacrolimus, histomorphometric changes after transplantation were different between groups. Patients treated with tacrolimus had an improvement in trabecular bone architecture compared with patients receiving CyA (Guichelaar et al., 2004). These findings suggest that patients treated with tacrolimus may have faster recovery of bone metabolism after the initial phase of bone loss compared with those treated with CyA.

A study comparing CsA monotherapy versus prednisone and azathioprine regimen in renal transplant recipients did not found any differences in bone loss or bone histomorphometric parameters (Cueto-Manzano et al., 2003). Furthermore, a major side-effect of CsA therapy is dose-related nephrotoxicity, often leading to secondary hyperparathyroidism, which may also adversely affect bone health.

Other immunosupresive agents such as Mycophenolate mofetil (104), rapamycin or azathioprine have shown no effects on bone in murine models (Maalouf et al., 2005).

3. Bone loss and fractures after transplantation

The majority of longitudinal studies show a decrease in bone mineral density at the lumbar spine and hip that occurs in the first year after solid organ transplantation. The amount of bone loss ranges between 3% and 10%, particularly in the first 3-6 months. Rapid bone loss and major involvement of lumbar spine (trabecular bone tissue) are findings probably related to the large doses of glucocorticoids used immediately after transplantation. Rates of lumbar spine bone loss slow thereafter, with stabilization by 6–12 months and even some recovery after liver, lung, and heart transplantation. However, most studies do not document recovery of bone mass at the hip. BMD changes after renal transplantation are different since continued bone loss after the rapid initial bone loss may be observed. Prevalence of densitometric osteoporosis is quite variable depending on type of organ transplantation and time elapsed since transplantation (Hawkins et al., 1994).

With regard to fractures, a high incidence of them (between 20% and 40% in most studies) has been documented. In heart and liver transplant recipients, the incidence of new fractures parallels the timing of the most rapid bone loss, with most fractures occurring within the first year after transplantation (Eastell R, 1991; Henderson et al., 1995; Shane et al., 1996; Ramsey-Goldman et al., 1999).

Fractures usually affect the spine and ribs in liver, cardiac, or lung recipients, whereas long bones are more easily fractured in renal transplant recipients. However, fracture incidence may have decreased in the last years. This is probably related to the wide implementation of immunosuppressive regimens that use lower doses of glucocorticoids and for a shorter period of time. Indeed, bone loss and fractures remain unacceptably high in several recent studies.

Risk factors for fractures after transplantation include older age, prevalent fractures before transplantation, postmenopausal status, and lower body mass index. Additional risk factors in renal transplant recipients include the presence of diabetes mellitus and prolonged dialysis. The predictive roles of pretransplantation BMD and cumulative glucocorticoid dose are controversial. Associations between these risk factors and bone loss or fractures are not consistent across studies. Even patients with normal pre-transplant BMD may suffer fracture after transplantation. Therefore, it is usually not possible with current clinical tools to predict whether individual transplant recipients will fracture after transplantation.

In a nested case-control study of transplant recipients (kidney, liver, lung, heart), multivariate analysis showed that post-transplant fracture rate was highest among those with a history of hyperthyroidism, pretransplant diabetes, fracture, or corticosteroid use, and among those currently exposed to antidepressants, narcotics, sirolimus, and loop diuretics (Shane et al., 2009 uptodate). Use of bisphosphonates or calcitonin was also a predictor of fracture, likely indicating the presence of pre-transplant osteoporosis.

In some studies, the rate of post-transplant fracture is decreasing, in part due to increased recognition of the problem, which has resulted in changes in immunosuppressive regimens (reduction in dose and duration of glucocorticoids) and earlier identification and treatment for osteoporosis (Shane et al., 2004; Compston et al., 2003)

3.1 Kidney transplantation

Rates of bone loss are greatest in the first 3-18 months and range from 4-9% at the spine and 5-8% at the hip.

After renal transplantation fractures affect appendicular sites (hips, long bones, ankles, feet) more commonly than axial sites (spine and ribs). The majority of fractures occur within the first 3 years. Fracture prevalence varies from 7-11% in nondiabetic renal transplant recipients, but is considerably higher in patient transplanted because of diabetic nephropathy and in those who receive kidney-pancreas transplants. (Nowacka-Cieciura et al., 2006)

With regard to the difference in the prevalence of fracture in end stage renal disease patients referred to kidney transplant or those who continued dialysis, a large study realized with 101,039 patients with end stage renal disease demonstrated that kidney transplantation was associated with a 34% greater risk of hip fracture than continued dialysis (Nisbeth et al., 1994).

3.2 Lung transplantation

During the first year after lung transplantation, rates of bone loss at the lumbar spine and femoral neck range from 2 to 5%. In another study conducted with 70 patients awaiting lung transplantation the prevalence of vertebral fractures was 29% in patients with chronic obstructive pulmonary disease and 25% in patients with cystic fibrosis (Shane et al., 1996). Fracture rates are also high during the first year after lung transplantation, ranging from 18 to 37%.

3.3 Cardiac transplantation

The most rapid rate of bone loss occurs in the first year. Spinal BMD declines by 6-10% during the first 6 months, whereas femoral neck BMD falls by 6-11% in the first year. The rate of bone loss slows after the first year and spine BMD may increase after the third year (Cohen et al., 2003). Densitometric osteoporosis at the lumbar spine and femoral neck has been reported in approximately 28% and 20% respectively of long term transplant patients (Chou et al., 2006).

Vertebral fracture incidence ranges from 20-36% during the first 1 to 3 years after cardiac transplantation. One prospective study shows that 36 percent of all patients and 54 percent of women sustained a fracture after this procedure, 85 percent of which occurred within the first six months (Shane et al., 1996). Women with the lowest pretransplant hip BMD were at highest risk of fracture. In men, pretransplant BMD did not differ between those who went on to fracture and those who did not.

3.4 Liver transplantation

Spine BMD declines by 2-24% during the first year in earlier studies, particularly during the first 3-6 months. Some authors report higher rates of bone loss and fracture in patients who have alcoholic cirrhosis, primary biliary cirrhosis, and primary sclerosing cholangitis (Lopez 1992). Rates of bone loss have been lower in more recent studies. In the second year after transplantation, lumbar BMD recovered or even exceeded baseline levels (Guichelaar et al., 2006). Although early studies showed a predominance of post-transplant bone loss and fractures in the lumbar spine (Compston et al., 2003), more recent studies reported higher bone loss at the hip (Keogh et al., 1999; Ninkovic et al., 2002; Crawford et al., 2006). It seems that there are differences in the natural evolution of lumbar and femoral BMD, with greater loss of femoral bone that persists after the first year after transplantation. As an example, after 3 years, BMD at the femoral neck improved, but still remained below baseline levels (Monegal A, 2001). Other studies found a decrease in BMD at the femoral neck at 6 and 12 months, even despite treatment with bisphosphonates, suggesting a lesser effect of these drugs at cortical bone (Keogh et al., 1999), (Ninkovic et al., 2002), (Monegal et al., 2009).

Fracture rates after liver transplantation are highest in the first 6-12 months. Range from 24 to 65% and the ribs and spine are the most common sites. Women with primary biliary cirrhosis and the most severe preexisting bone disease appear to be at greatest risk. In a study of 37 patients receiving liver transplantation between 1993 and 1995, an incidence of 27% of vertebral fractures in the first three months after transplantation was found (Ninkovic et al., 2000). A subsequent study of the same group, done between 1995 and 1998, showed that this incidence was only 5%. Between both studies there was a considerable reduction in the dose and duration of glucocorticoid treatment, although the use of cyclosporine and tacrolimus barely changed (Ninkovic et al., 2002).

3.5 Bone marrow transplantation

The pattern of bone loss after bone marrow transplantation (BMT) is different from other forms of osteoporosis, being more persistent and severe in cortical bones, such as femoral neck than in trabecular bones, such as lumbar spine (Hatutman et al., 2011)). Bone marrow transplant (BMT) recipients have many known risk factors for developing decreased bone mineral density after transplantation. The pathogenesis of bone disease following BMT differs from others form of post-transplantation osteoporosis; recipients are usually younger and the time from the diagnosis to the BMT does not exceed 2 years; history of prolonged bed rest is uncommon. Immunosuppressive drugs are used in relatively low doses and for short periods of time (Ebeling et al., 1999). Glucocorticoid use is restricted to the treatment of graft-versus- host disease (GVHD).

Lumbar spine BMD declines by 2-9% and femoral neck BMD falls 6-11% during the first year following transplantation. Lumbar spine BMD begins to recover after 12 months, returning to baseline levels at 48 months. The extent of recovery at the femoral neck is less (Schulte et al., 2004). The presence of chronic GVHD is another factor associated with higher risk of osteoporosis in these patients. Avascular necrosis develops in 10-20% of allogenic

BMT patients; its development may be facilitated by a deficit in bone marrow stromal stem cell regeneration and low osteoblast number.

4. PTH. 25-OH-D. Bone remodeling in postransplantation bone disease

4.1 PTH

Elevated PTH levels have an adverse effect on bone health increasing turnover and decreasing bone mass, especially in cortical bone.

Some studies reflect a slight increase in PTH levels in the first month after transplantation. It could be related to vitamin D deficiency, calcium malabsorption or decreased tubular reabsorption of calcium, consequence of steroid treatment (Compston et al., 1996). PTH levels may remain elevated in the long-term due to chronic renal failure induced by cyclosporin (Floreani A, 2001; Crosbie et al., 1999).

4.2 25-OH vitamin D

Inadequate levels of vitamin D have been described in patients with end-stage liver diseases prior to liver transplantation, and this may play a role in the aetiology of lower mineralization after transplantation. Our group found that 91% of liver transplanted patients had insufficient serum levels of 25(OH)D at transplantation time. After adequate supplementation, serum 25(OH)D levels increased from 3 months onwards (Guadalix et al., 2011). A positive correlation between serum 25(OH)D levels at 3 months and BMD increase at 6 months was found suggesting that this vitamin has a positive effect on mineralization (Crosbie et al., 1999). In our study serum 25(OH)D levels showed positive correlation with the percentage change in total hip and femoral neck BMD at 12 months of treatment (Guadalix et al., 2011). These results suggest that vitamin D could have a main role in bone loss prevention after liver transplantation.

4.3 Bone remodeling in postransplantation bone disease

Bone turnover markers can provide information about the mechanisms of bone loss in post-transplant period.Our group has previously reported an increase in bone turnover markers such as osteocalcin after liver transplantation (Valero et al., 1995; Hawkins et al., 1994). No significant changes in urinary hydroxyproline, one and two years after transplant were found; however urinary excretion of NTX (amino-terminal telopeptide of collagen type I) showed a significant decrease after two years compared with baseline values(Giannini et al., 2000), while other found that values of deoxypyridinoline doubled compared to baseline, two months after transplantation (Crosbie et al., 1999). We also found that β-CTX decreased as from 3 months both in patients on bisphosphonate treatment as in patients receiving only calcium plus vitamin D, reflecting a reduction of bone resorption after liver transplantation (Guadalix et al., 2011). Greater reductions in β-CTX may be obtained with intravenuous bisphosphonates. A significant decrease in urinary deoxypyridinoline in heart transplant recipienters after intravenous pamidronate traeatment (Shane et al., 1998) and in β-CTX levels 6 months after liver transplanted in 13 patients treated with intravenous zoledrónico acid (Misof et al., 2008) was found. Other investigators found an early increase (one and 3 months after heart transplantation) in resorption markers hydroxyproline, pyridonoline and desoxypyridinoline and a decreased in osteocalcin, recovering all baseline values at 6 months (Shane et al., 1997). Several studies have investigated the OPG / RANKL in the post-transplant period. Results are not homogeneous. High levels of both, OPG and RANKL in the first 14 days after liver transplantation compared to the control group were found (Fabrega et al., 2006). In the other hand, serum OPG in 57 patients at 3 and 6 months after cardiac transplantation wa correlated with bone loss at the lumbar spine and femoral neck sites, after 6 months. Serum OPG alone accounted for 67% of the variance of lumbar spine bone density changes over the first 6 months post transplantation leading to the conclussion that serum OPG levels decline consistently in all patients following initiation of immunosuppressive therapy and are independently correlated with changes in bone density (Fahrleitner et al., 2003).In another study in patients with kidney transplant, levels of OPG and RANKL did not differ between healthy volunteers and transplant patients (Malyszko et al., 2003).

5. Gonadal status and postransplatation bone disease

Hypogonadotropic hypogonadism is frequently found both before and after transplantation and may play a role in the multifactorial pathogenesis of immunosuppression-induced bone loss. Sex-steroid deficiency in either sex results in an increase in bone turnover with an imbalance in bone formation and bone resorption. Few studies have assessed the status of gonadal function after transplantation and its relationship with bone mass. Many premenopausal women and men undergoing solid organ transplantation have temporary hypogonadism, most often related to the effects of glucocorticoids and chronic illnesses (Fleischer et al., 2008; Tauchmanovà et al., 2005). In some cases (i.e. chemotherapy and/or radiation therapy for hematopoietic stem cell transplantation), hypogonadism is permanent (Tauchmanovà et al., 2003). In men and women undergoing transplantation, testosterone and estrogen-progestin replacement, respectively, have been shown to slow bone loss (Isoniemi et al., 2001; Kananen et al., 2005). Hypogonadism is a common finding among patients with terminal liver disease, especially in males. Incidence was estimated up to 70% (Guichelaar et al., 2004). There are few studies about change in sex hormones after liver transplantation, some authors have reported an increase in free testosterone, although the recovery of normal levels has not been achieved in all patients (Floreani et al., 2001; Monegal et al., 2001). In a study of 10 liver transplant recipients followed for 12 months after transplantation, before transplantation, 90% of patients had a decrease in testosterone levels and reported decreased libido and erectile dysfunction .After transplant, total testosterone levels had doubled, and free testosterone increased tenfold. Patients reported early improvement in sexual function (6 to 8 weeks after transplantation). It was suggested that pretransplant abnormalities in gonadal function are mainly due to liver failure and are reversible in most patients (Madersbacher et al., 1996). In premenopausal women, normal menses usually resumes after liver transplantation (Mass et al., 1996).

Low levels of testosterone are quite common early after cardiac transplantation, and may be found in up to 50% of men (Guo et al., 1998). In addition, a significant relationship between low levels of serum testosterone and rates of femoral neck bone loss during the first 6 month after transplantation have been found by some authors (Shane et al., 1997). Fleischer et al., (2008) studied 108 male heart transplant patients. One month after transplantation, total testosterone levels were below normal in 63% of them while 33% had decreased levels of free testosterone. 15% of patients had elevated gonadotropin a month after transplantation, increasing to 29% at 6 months. These data suggest a suppression of the hypothalamic-pituitary-gonadal axis immediately after transplantation, with subsequent recovery. Authors attributed this to steroid therapy. Prednisone dose was found to be the main determinant of the values of total and free testosterone). No relationship was found between post-transplant bone loss and testosterone levels, probably because patients were treated with calcitriol or alendronate.

In most studies, testosterone levels return to normal by 6 to 12 months after transplantation (Sambrook et al., 1994) but up to 20% of patients receiving prednisone and cyclosporine A may persist with low serum total testosterone levels 3 years after cardiac transplantation (Stempfle et al., 1999).

Regarding the role of other immunosuppressive agents on gonadal function cyclosporine A decreases testosterone by affecting both the hypothalamic-pituitary- gonadal axis (Sikka et al., 1988) and by direct inhibition of testicular synthesis of testosterone in murine models (Seethalakshmi et al., 1990). However, cyclosporine did not seem to affect testosterone levels in humans (Fleisher et al., 2008; Samojlik et al., 1992).

Some authors recommend hormonal treatment in post transplant osteoporosis in men and premenopausal women with hypogonadism, if there are no contraindications (Shane et al., 2009 up-to-date). Androgen replacement therapy has shown skeletal benefit (increase in BMD) only in men with hypogonadism. It has been demonstrated in an uncontrolled study of postmenopausal liver transplantation recipients, that the use of transdermal estradiol was effective in increasing BMD of lumbar spine and femoral neck over a period of two years (Isoniemi et al., 2001).

6. Prevention and treatment of osteoporosis

6.1 General measures before transplantation

The same measures used to prevent osteoporosis in the general population apply to transplant recipients, regardless of the pretransplant BMD measurement. It is recomended that all candidates for organ transplantation follow a throughfully evaluation in order to identificate and correct risk factors and to implement measures to improve bone health (Table 4).

Before Transplantation	After transplantation
- Measurement lumbar spine and hip BMD. If BMD is low, it should be evaluated secondary causes of osteoporosis. - Patients with kidney failure should be avaluated and treated for renal osteodystrophy. - Perform spine radiograph to detect prevalent fractures. - Recommend appropriate intake of calcium (1000-mg/day) and vitamin D (800 IU). - Patients with osteoporosis should be evaluated and treated according to general guidelines.	- Consider initiating preventive therapy in most patient (even those with normal BMD): calcium, vitamin D and antiresorptive agents. - Perform annual BMD measurement. - Perform annual Spine Radiograph. - Annual measurement of bone turnover markers.

Table 4. General recommendations for prevention and treatment of osteoporosis

Lifestyle factors, such as immobilization, smoking, and alcohol abuse, should be avoided. Concomitant use of medications that can negatively impact skeletal health should be minimized whenever possible. Hypogonadism should be sought and corrected, particularly in males, where symptoms are easily confounded with those of preexisting chronic disease or adverse effects of concomitant medication. All patients should receive the recommended daily allowance for calcium (1000-15000 mg/day) and vitamin D (800 IU/day). Higher vitamin D doses should be given if the patient is vitamin D deficient (serum 25-hydroxyvitamin D level >20 ng/ml [50 nmol/L]). Although calcium and vitamin D do not prevent transplantation-related bone loss, randomized trials assessing antiresorptive therapy, such as bisphosphonates, have been carried out in the setting of concomitant calcium and vitamin D repletion.

Prevention of early bone loss after transplantion have been reported with specific resistance training programs (Mitchell et al., 2003). Regular weight-bearing exercise (30 minutes, three times per week) has proved also to be beneficial for the prevention and treatment of osteoporosis. Because of the high prevalence of osteopenia and osteoporosis in patients awaiting transplantation and the morbidity caused by osteoporosis after transplantation, it is recommended that candidates for organ transplantation undergo measurements of BMD of the hip and spine, preferably at the time of acceptance to the waiting list. Low BMD before transplantation has been pointed out as a risk factor for fractures after transplantation. In addition, spine radiographs should be performed to detect prevalent fractures .Patients who have a history of fracture or have osteoporosis on DXA (T-score ≤ -2.5) before transplantation should be evaluated for secondary causes. When a secondary cause (i.e. hypogonadism) is identified, appropriate treatment is recommended prior to transplant. In addition to the treatment (when possible) of secondary causes, some patients may benefit from additional osteoporosis therapy, such as bisphosphonates, while awaiting transplant. Patients with osteopenia should be considered for prevention (calcium, vitamin D and/or antirresorptives) evaluating risk factors. Alternatively, patients with normal BMD can defer medical therapy until immediately after transplantation. For patients with end-stage renal disease, an evaluation and treatment for renal osteodystrophy according to accepted guidelines is highly recommended.

6.2 Therapeutic measures of post-transplantion bone loss

Several drugs have been studied for the treatment of osteoporosis after transplantation. Many of these studies were done with small number of patients, were not randomized or not compared with control group. Also, patients were not selected based on T-score or risk factor (beyond the transplant). There is no consensus on candidates for the treatment or the drug of choice.Given the accelerated bone loss that occurs immediately after transplantation many experts recommend preventive treatment for all patients receiving solid organ transplantation, regardless of pretransplant BMD (Maalouf NM, 2005; Cohen et al., 2006). This approach is based on observational data that show an overlap in BMD values between the pre-transplant patients with posttransplant fracture and those without fractures (Leidig-Bruckner et al., 2001; Shane et al., 1996). The lack of reliable clinical predictors to identify individual patients who will experience osteoporotic fractures renders all transplant recipients candidates for preventive therapy. Treatment should be started immediately after transplantation.

Since lumbar BMD starts to recover in many patients at 12 months after transplantation, long-term treatment may be unnecessary (Cohen et al., 2006). Duration of treatment depends on patient characteristics, such as time of steroid therapy withdrawal, presence of other risk factors for low bone mineral density and fractures as well as information provided by the measurement of BMD.

Another approach to the management of transplanted patients is to apply similar guidelines as those used for the prevention of glucocorticoid-induced osteoporosis. There are several guidelines for the prevention of glucocorticoid-induced osteoporosis. Collectively, they suggest preventive therapy for patients with clinical risk factors for osteoporosis and fracture (age ≥65 years, previous fragility fracture) or in patients without other risk factors if BMD T-score is below -1.0 or -1.5 (Shane E, 2009).

6.2.1 Bisphosphonates

These potent antiresorptive agents are an obvious option in preventing the rapid bone loss, that occurs mainly in the early phase after transplantation. Bisphosphonates are considered the medical therapy of choice for the prevention of transplantation-related bone loss. Although there are conflicting data both oral and intravenous bisphosphonates appear to be effective in these patients.

Below shows some of the results obtained with bisphosphonates treatment in different types of transplants.

In a study of 99 subjects receiving stem cell transplantation, patients were randomly assigned to receive calcium and vitamin D or calcium and vitamin D plus pamidronate (60 mg intravenously six times over the first post-transplant year). Treatment with pamidronate prevented spine bone loss (0 percent in pamidronate group versus -2.9 percent in calcium group), and reduce hip bone loss (-5.5 percent and -7.8 percent in the pamidronate and calcium-vitamin D groups, respectively) (Kananen et al., 2005).

In a trial of 62 adults undergoing liver transplantation, patients were randomly assigned to receive infusions of zoledronic acid (4 mg) or placebo within seven days of transplantation. BMD was measured 3, 6, 9, and 12 months later. Zoledronic acid group lost significantly less bone at the hip at all time points (Crawford BA, 2006). In the spine, the zoledronic acid group lost less bone at three months, but the difference between the two groups was no longer significant at 12 months because of improvements between 3 and 12 months in the placebo group. Zoledronic acid sometimes caused postinfusion hypocalcemia and temporary secondary hyperparathyroidism.

Oral bisphosphonates are also effective in preventing bone loss after transplantation (Shane et al., 2004; Atamaz et al., 2006). As an example, in a trial of 98 subjects receiving a liver transplant, subjects randomly assigned to alendronate (70 mg weekly) versus no alendronate had significant increases in lumbar spine (5.1and 8.9 percent) and femoral neck (4.3 and 8.7 percent) BMD at 12 and 24 months, respectively, compared with the control group (Atamaz et al., 2006). All subjects received calcium (1000 mg daily) and calcitriol (0.5 mcg daily).

Our group studied the effect of risedronate in liver transplant patient. The main findings of our study are that liver transplanted patients with low bone mineral density who receive either Risendronate combined with calcium and vitamin D3 or vitamin D3 and calcium alone showed a significant increase in spine BMD at 12 months compared to baseline values. In addition, risedronate patients showed a significant increase in intertrochanteric BMD, but we were not able to find any significant differences between groups. Hence, these results suggest that weekly risedronate after liver transplantation combined with 1000 mg/day of calcium and 800 IU/day of vitamin D are not superior to the administration of calcium and vitamin D alone (Guadalix S, 2011). Significant improvement in BMD at the lumbar spine was also observed 12 months after liver transploant in the control group. This response may be related to the administration of calcium and vitamin D3 itself, but also to improvement in general health, mobility, muscle mass, and nutrition as a consequence of better liver function.

A recent meta-analysis in 364 liver transplant patients from 6 randomized controlled trials have found that bisphosphonate therapy improved lumbar spine BMD by 0.03 g/cm^2 (95% CI 0.01-0.05 g/cm^2, p=0.02) at 12 months post-liver transplantation compared to the control group. However, a statistically significant change in femoral neck BMD could not be demonstrated in this meta-analysis. Data on fractures could not be analyzed (Kasturi et al., 2010). In a study of 34 lung transplant recipients (with cystic fibrosis antecedents), pamidronate therapy versus calcium and vitamin D showed a significant increase in bone mass at 2 years in lumbar spine and total femur. There was no difference in fracture incidence (Aris et al., 2000).

In patients after allogenic stem cell transplantation pamidronate reduced bone loss at the spine, femoral neck and hip by 5.6, 7.7 and 4.9% respectively after 12 month of treatment. However, at 24 month, only differences at BMD of total hip remained statistically significant between study groups (Grigg et al., 2006). Other study in 12 patients treated with zoledronic acid show that 12 month after infusion, total hip BMD increased in 75% of the patients and femoral neck BMD increased in 11 of 12 patients. Spinal BMD only increase in four (D'Souza et al., 2006).

Based upon the above trials, we suggest bisphosphonates as first choice for prevention of transplantation-related bone loss. There are few data to support the use of one bisphosphonate over another. Many of the trials used intravenous bisphosphonates due to ease of administration, especially in post-transplant patients who are required to take many oral medications. There are no trials comparing oral to intravenous bisphosphonates in the immediate post-transplant setting. The decision should be based upon individual patient preferences and abilities. The safety and efficacy of bisphosphonates for prevention of transplantation-related bone loss in patients with chronic kidney disease has not been carefully evaluated, and in general, there is limited data on the level of renal impairment at which bisphosphonate use should be avoided and whether this level is the same for iv bisphosphonates. In the majority of trials, individuals with serum creatinine concentrations above the upper limits of normal were excluded from participation. Despite these concerns, however, it is usually recommend their use after renal transplantation, at least during the first year when rates of bone loss are most rapid.

6.3 Other therapies

Replacement doses of calcium and vitamin D (400-1000 IU/day) do not prevent clinically significant bone loss after transplantation, but active metabolites of vitamin D could reduce post-transplantation bone loss, probably by reversing glucocorticoid-induced decreases in intestinal calcium absorption.

6.3.1 Calcidiol (25-hydroxivitamin D) and alfacalcidol (1α-hydroxivitamin D)

In renal transplant recipients calcidiol (40 μgr/day) prevents spine and femoral bone loss and is associated with a significant decrease in vertebral deformities (Talalaj et al., 1996). Consistently with these findings, our group have found that in patients randomized immediately after cardiac transplantation to 32000 IU/week of oral calcidiol for 18 months, lumbar spine BMD increased ~5%, whereas those who received cyclical etidronate or nasal calcitonin, showed decreases in spine BMD (Garcia-Delgado et al., 1997). Also, alfacalcidol therapy has been associated with an increase in BMD or prevention of additional bone loss in renal (El-Agroudy et al., 2003) and cardiac recipients (Van Cleemput et al., 1996).

6.3.2 Calcitriol
Calcitriol may suppress bone resorption indirectly by facilitating intestinal calcium absorption and suppressing PTH secretion. Studies of calcitriol alone and those that compare calcitriol and bisphosphonates suggest that calcitriol may also prevent early post-transplant bone loss, particularly at the proximal femur. Positive effects on BMD have been found with higher doses of calcitriol (> 0.50 μgr/day) in heart, lung or renal transplantation, whereas lower doses (0.25 μgr/day) are relatively ineffective. Use of calcitriol requires close monitoring of serum and 24 hour urine calcium, because it is associated with hypercalcemia and hypercalciuria in >50% patients.In a study of 65 patients undergoing cardiac or single lung transplantation, patients were randomly allocated to receive placebo or calcitriol (0.5-0.75 microg/day), the latter for either 12 months or 24 months. Bone loss at the proximal femur was significantly reduced or prevented by treatment with calcitriol for 2 years compared with treatment with calcium alone (Sambrook et al., 2000).
Other randomized study compared the efficacy of 6 months treatment with either calcitriol (0.5 microg/day) or two cycles of etidronate plus calcium in preventing bone loss in 41 patients undergoing cardiac or lung transplantation. Compared with an untreated reference group, both therapies offered significant protection at 6 months in lumbar spine and etidronate provided significant protective carryover after therapy had been discontinued (Henderson et al., 2001).Although calcitriol appears to be effective in preventing bone loss after transplantation (Sambrook et al., 2000; Shane E, 2004) it should not be selected as first-line treatment because of their limited effectiveness and narrow therapeutic window.

6.3.3 Calcitonin
Although calcitonin is effective in preventing bone loss in postmenopausal women, it has not been shown to be superior to calcium in transplant recipients (Välimäki et al., 1999). In one trial, the combination of continuos oral calcitriol (0.5 microg/day) and nasal salmon calcitonin (200 U/day) for the first 3 months was inferior to intravenous pamidronate (0.5 mg/kg body weight) every third month in attenuating bone loss three months after cardiac transplant but similar at 18 months in 26 cardiac transplant recipients (Bianda et al., 2000).

6.3.4 Recombinant parathyroid hormone (PTH)
PTH 1-34 (teriparatide) has been shown to improve BMD in patients with glucocorticoid-induced osteoporosis, but there are few studies evaluating PTH for the prevention of post-transplant osteoporosis. It a small trial 24 kidney recipients patients were treated with 20 μg of teriparatide/daily/6 months, it was shown that femoral neck BMD was stable compared to the placebo group. Lumbar spine BDM and radial BMD, histomorphometric bone volume and bone matrix mineralization status remained unchanged in both groups. (Cejka et al., 2008). Recombinant parathyroid hormone (PTH) has not been well studied in this population. Patients who have received total body irradiation during hematopoietic stem cell transplantation or who have primary or secondary elevations in PTH are not candidates for recombinant PTH therapy.

6.3.5 New therapies

Promising new agents for transplantation osteoporosis include new potent anticatabolic drugs such as human antibodies to receptor activator of nuclear factor kb-ligand (RANKL) (denosumab), and catepsin k inhibitors.

6.4 Monitoring

There is no consensus on the optimal strategy for monitoring patients on therapy. Patients on antiresorptive therapy are measured BMD every year after transplantation. Patients with normal BMD can be follow up with DXA every two years, depending also of other risk factors . In patients who require continuous treatment with glucocorticoids (prednisone ≥ 5 mg / day), BMD measurement is recommended annually. An effort should be made to find the lowest prednisone dose compatible with graft survival.

7. Summary and conclusions

Although bone loss and fractures after transplantation seem to be lower than those reported years ago, they remain being a main long term postransplant complication. An effective approach should incorporate pre-transplant measures to detect and to treat preexisting bone diseases. Oral or intravenous bisphosphonates, in conjunction with calcium and vitamin D, are effective in preventing post-transplantation bone loss when started shortly after grafting. The optimal dose, timing, and frequency, particularly of intravenous bisphosphonate administration, remain to be determined. At present, most controlled trials lack sufficient statistical power to demonstrate efficacy for fracture prevention, so treatment regimens are based on results of effects on the surrogate end-points, bone densitometry, and bone turnover markers. More studies are required to determine the best agent and route of administration to prevent this common complication of organ transplantation. The future challenge is to achieve adequate immunosuppression without corticosteroids, with drugs not damaging bone. This approach, together with improved bone health before the transplant would be an effective strategy to reduce post-transplant osteoporosis.

8. Acknowledgement

The authors received funding from Fundación Mutua Madrileña (n° 2005-072) and from Asociacion para la investigacion de Osteoporosis y Enfermedades Endocrinas.

9. References

Alem AM, Sherrard DJ, Gillen DL, Weiss NS, Beresford SA, Heckbert SR, Wong C, Stehman-Breen C. 2000. Increased risk of hip fracture among patients with end-stage renal disease.,*Kidney Int.* 58:396–399.

Atamaz F, Hepguler S, Akyildiz M, Karasu Z, Kilic M. 2006, Effects of alendronate on bone mineral density and bone metabolic markers in patients with liver transplantation. *Osteoporos Int* 17:942.

Aris RM. 2000 Efficacy of pamidronate for osteoporosis in patients with cystic fibrosis following lung transplantation. *Am J Respir Crit Care Med.* Sep;162(3 Pt 1):941-6.

Braith RW, Magyari PM, Fulton MN, Lisor CF, Vogel SE, Hill JA, Aranda JM Jr. 2006. Comparison of calcitonin versus calcitonin + resistance exercise as prophylaxis for osteoporosis in heart transplant recipients. *Transplantation.* Apr 27;81(8):1191-5.

Braith RW. 2007 Comparison of alendronate vs alendronate plus mechanical loading as prophylaxis for osteoporosis in lung transplant recipients: a pilot study. *J Heart Lung Transplant.* Feb;26(2):132-7.

Bianda T, Linka A, Junga G, Brunner H, Steinert H, Kiowski W, Schmid C, 2000Prevention of osteoporosis in heart transplant recipients: a comparison of calcitriol with calcitonin and pamidronate. *Calcif Tissue Int*; 67:116.

Canalis E, Delany AM. Mechanisms of glucocorticoid action in bone. 2002 *Ann N Y Acad Sci.* Jun;966:73-81.

Cejka D, Benesch T, Krestan C, Roschger P, Klaushofer K, Pietschmann P, Haas M. 2008 Effect of teriparatide on early bone loss after kidney transplantation, *Am J Transplant* 1864-70

Chou NK, Su IC, Kuo HL, Chen YH, Yang RS, Wang SS. 2006 Bone mineral density in long term Chinese heart transplant recipients: a cross-sectional study. *Transplant Prc*;38(7): 2141-2144

Cohen A, Shane E. 2003 Osteoporosis after solid organ and bone marrow transplantation. *Osteoporos Int.* Aug;14(8):617-30.

Cohen A, Ebeling, P, Sprague, S, and Shane, E. 2006. Transplantation Osteoporosis. *Primer on the Metabolic Bone Diseases and Disorders of Mineral Metabolism*, sixth edition. American Society of Bone and Mineral Research 56:302.

Cohen A, Addesso V, McMahon DJ, Staron RB, Namerow P, Maybaum S, Mancini D, Shane E. 2006 Discontinuing antiresorptive therapy one year after cardiac transplantation: effect on bone density and bone turnover. *Transplantation.* Mar 15;81(5):686-91.

Compston JE, Greer S, Skingle SJ, Stirling DM, Price C, Friend PJ, Alexander G 1996 Early increase in plasma parathyroid hormone levels following liver transplantation. *J Hepatol.* Nov;25(5):715-8.

Compston JE. 2003Osteoporosis after liver transplantation. Liver. *Transpl.* Apr;9(4):321-30.

Crawford BA, Kam C, Pavlovic J, Byth K, Handelsman DJ, Angus PW, McCaughan GW. 2006 Zoledronic acid prevents bone loss after liver transplantation: a randomized, double-blind, placebo-controlled trial. *Ann Intern Med.* Feb 21;144(4):239-48.

Crosbie OM, Freaney R, McKenna MJ, Curry MP, Hegarty JE. 1999 Predicting bone loss following orthotopic liver transplantation. *Gut*;44(3):430-4.

Cuthbert JA, Pak CY, Zerwekh JE, Glass KD, Combes B. 1984 Bone disease in primary biliary cirrhosis: increased bone resoprtion and turnover in the asence of osteoporosis or osteomalacia. *Hepatology*; 4:1-8

Cueto-Manzano AM, Konel S, Crowley V, France MW, Freemont AJ, Adams JE, Mawer B, Gokal R, Hutchison AJ. 2003 Bone histopathology and densitometry comparison between cyclosporine as monotherapy and prednisolone plus azathioprine dual immunosuppression in renal transplant patients. *Transplantation*; 75:2053-2058.

Diamond TH, Stiel D, Lunzer M, McDowall D, Eckstein RP, Posen S. 1989 Hepatic osteodystrophy:state and dynamic bone histomorphometry and serum bone GLA protein in 80 patients with chronic liver disease. *Gastroenterology*; 96; 213-221

D`Souza AB, Grigg AP, Szer J, Ebeling PR. 2006 Zoledronic acid prevents bone loss after allogenic haemopoietic stem cell transplantation. *Int Med J*; 36:600.

Eastell R, Dickson ER, Hodgson SF, Wiesner RH, Porayko MK, Wahner HW1991. Rates of vertebral bone loss before and after liver transplantation in women with primary biliary cirrhosis. *Hepatology.* 1991 Aug;14(2):296-300.

Ebeling PR, Thomas DM, Erbas B, Hopper JL, Szer J, Grigg AP. 1999Mechanisms of bone loss following allogeneic and autologous hemopoietic stem cell transplantation.*J Bone Miner Res*. Mar;14(3):342-50.

El-Agroudy AE, El-Husseini AA, El-Sayed M, Ghoneim MA. 2003 Preventing bone loss in renal transplant recipients with vitamin D. *J Am Soc Nephrol*;14:2975-2979.

Epstein S. 1996 Post-transplantation bone disease: the role of immunosuppressive agents and the skeleton. *J Bone Miner Res*. Jan;11(1):1-7.

Fabrega E, Orive A, Garcia-Unzueta M, Amado JA, Casafont F, Pons-Romero F. . 2006 Osteoprotegerin and receptor activator of nuclear factor-kappaB ligand system in the early post-operative period of liver transplantation. *Clin Transplant* May-Jun;20(3):383-8.

Fahrleitner A, Prenner G, Kniepeiss D, Iberer F, Tscheliessnigg KH, Piswanger-Sölkner C, Obermayer-Pietsch B, Leb G, Dobnig H. 2003 Serum osteoprotegerin is a major determinant of bone density development and prevalent vertebral fracture status following cardiac transplantation. *Bone* Jan;32(1):96-106.

Floreani A, Mega A, Tizian L, Burra P, Boccagni P, Baldo V, Fagiuoli S, Naccarato R, Luisetto G. 2001 Bone metabolism and gonad function in male patients undergoing liver transplantation: a two-year longitudinal study. *Osteoporos Int*.;12(9):749-54.

Fleischer J, McMahon DJ, Hembree W, Addesso V, Longcope C, Shane E. S 2008 Serum testosterone levels after cardiac transplantation. Transplantation. Mar 27;85(6):834-9.

Garcia-Delgado I, Prieto S, Gil-Fraguas L, Robles E, Rufilanchas JJ, Hawkins F. 1997;Calcitonin, etidronate, and calcidiol treatment in bone loss after cardiac transplantation. *Calcif Tissue Int* 60:155-159.

Garcia-Delgado I, Gil-Fraguas L, Robles E, Martinez G, Hawkins F. 2000;Clinical factors associated with bone mass loss previous to cardiac transplantation. *Med Clin (Barc)* 114: 761-4

Gerakis A, Hadjidakis D, Kokkinakis E, Apostolou T, Raptis S, Billis A. 2000. Correlation of bone mineral density with the histological findings of renal osteodystrophy in patients on hemodialysis. *J Nephrol*;13:437-443.

Giannini S, Nobile M, Ciuffreda M, Iemmolo RM, Dalle Carbonare L, Minicuci N. Long-term persistence of low bone density in orthotopic liver transplantation. *Osteoporos Int.* 2000;11:417-24.ç

Goffin E, Devogelaer JP, Depresseux G, Squifflet JP, Pirson Y. . 2001 Osteoporosis after organ transplantation. LancetMay 19;357:1623.

Grotz WH, Mundinger FA, Gugel B, Exner V, Kirste G, Schollmeyer PJ 1994 Bone fracture and osteodensitometry with dual x-ray absorptiometry in kidney transplant recipients. *Transplantation*;58:912-915.

Guadalix S, Martínez-Díaz-Guerra G, Lora D, Vargas C, Gómez-Juaristi M, Cobaleda B, Moreno E, Hawkins F. . 2011 Effect of early risedronate treatment on bone mineral density and bone turnover markers after liver transplantation: a prospective single-center study. *Transpl Int*;24(7):657-665.

Guichelaar MM, Malinchoc M, Sibonga JD, Clarke BL, Hay JE. . 2003 Bone histomorphometric changes after liver transplantation for chronic cholestatic liver disease. *J Bone Miner Res* .Dec;18(12):2190-9.

Guichelaar MM, Malinchoc M, Sibonga J, Clarke BL, Hay JE. 2004 Immunosuppressive and postoperative effects of orthotopic liver transplantation on bone metabolism. *Liver Transpl.* May;10(5):638-47.

Guichelaar MM, Kendall R, Malinchoc M, Hay JE. 2006 Bone mineral density before and after OLT: long-term follow-up and predictive factors. *Liver Transpl*;12(9):1390-402.

Guichelaar MM, Schmoll J, Malinchoc M, Hay JE. 2007 Fractures and avascular necrosis before and after orthotopic liver transplantation: long-term follow-up and predictive factors. *Hepatology.* Oct;46(4):1198-207.

Grigg AP, Shuttleworth P, Reynolds J, Schwarer AP, Szer J, Bradstock K, Hui C, Herrmann R, Ebeling PR. 2006 Pamidronate reduces bone loss after allogenic stem cell transplantation. *JCEM* 91(10):3835-3843.

Guo CY, Jonson A, Locke TJ, Esatell R. 1998 Mechanisms of bone loss after cardiac transplantation. *Bone;* 22:267-271.

Hautmann AH, Elad S, Lawitschka A, Greinix H, Bertz H, Halter J, Faraci M, Christian Hofbauer L, Lee S, Wolff D, Holler E. 2011 Metabolic bone disease in patients after allogenic hematopoietic stem cell transplantation: Report from the Consensus Conference on Clinical Practice in chronic graft-versus-host disease. *Transplant International Transpl Int.* Sep;24(9):867-879. t).

Hawkins FG, Leon M, Lopez MB, Valero MA, Larrodera L, Garcia-Garcia I, Loinaz C, Moreno Gonzalez E.. 1994 Bone loss and turnover in patients with liver transplantation. *Hepatogastroenterology*;41(2):158-61.

Hayashi K, Yamaguchi T, Yano S, Kanazawa I, Yamauchi M, Yamamoto M, Sugimoto T. 2009 BMP/Wnt antagonists are upregulated by dexamethasone in osteoblasts and reversed by alendronate and PTH: Potential therapeutic targets for glucocorticoid-induced osteoporosis. *Biochem Biophys Res Commun.* Feb 6;379(2):261-6. Epub 2008 Dec 25

Henderson NK, Sambrook PN, Kelly PJ, Macdonald P, Keogh AM, Spratt P, Eisman JA. 1995. Bone mineral loss and recovery after cardiac transplantation. *Lancet.* Sep 30;346(8979):905

Henderson K. 2001 Protective effect of short-tem calcitriol or cyclical etidronate on bone loss after cardiac or lung transplantation. *J Bone Miner Res* Mar;16(3):565-71.

Isoniemi H, Appelberg J, Nilsson CG, Mäkelä P, Risteli J, Höckerstedt K. 2001 Transdermal oestrogen therapy protects postmenopausal liver transplant women from osteoporosis. A 2-year follow-up study. *J Hepatol.* Feb;34(2):299-305.

Kasturi KS, Chennareddygari S, Mummadi RR. 2010 Effect of bisphosphonates on bone mineral density in liver transplant patients: a meta-analysis and systematic review of randomized controlled trials. *Transpl Int*;23(2):200-7.

Kananen K, Volin L, Laitinen K, Alfthan H, Ruutu T, Välimäki MJ. 2005 Prevention of bone loss after allogeneic stem cell transplantation by calcium, vitamin D, and sex hormone replacement with or without pamidronate. *J Clin Endocrinol Metab*; 90:3877.

Keogh JB, Tsalamandris C, Sewell RB, Jones RM, Angus PW, Nyulasi IB, Seeman. 1999 Bone loss at the proximal femur and reduced lean mass following liver transplantation: a longitudinal study. *Nutrition.* Sep;15(9):661-4.

Kulak CAM, Shane E. Transplantation osteoporosis: biochemical correlates of pathogenesis and treatment. In: Seibel MJ, Robbins SP, Bilezikian JP (eds). Dynamics of bone and cartilage metabolism, 2 nd edition. San Diego: Academic Press, 2006. Pp 515-26.

Leidig-Bruckner G, Hosch S, Dodidou P, Ritschel D, Conradt C, Klose C, Otto G, Lange R, Theilmann L, Zimmerman R, Pritsch M, Ziegler R.. 2001.Frequency and predictors of osteoporotic fractures after cardiac or liver transplantation: a follow-up study. Lancet;357(9253):342-7.

Lopez MN, Gonzalez Pinto I, Hawkins F, Valero MA, Leon M, Loinaz G, Garcia I, Gomez R, Moreno E 1992. Effect of liver transplantation and immunosuppressive treatment on bone mineral density. Transplantation Proceedings; 24:3044-46

Maalouf NM, Shane E. 2005 Osteoporosis after solid organ transplantation. J Clin Endocrinol Metab. Apr;90(4):2456-65.

Madersbacher S, Ludvik G, Stulnig T, Grunberger T, Maier U. 1996 The impact of liver transplantation on endocrine status in men. Clin Endocrinol (Oxf). Apr;44(4):461-6.

Malyszko J, Malyszko JS, Wolczynski S, Mysliwiec M. 2003 Osteoprotegerin and its correlations with new markers of bone formation and bone resorption in kidney transplant recipients. Transplant Proc. Sep;35(6):2227-9.

Mass K, Quint EH, Punch MR, Merino RM. 1996 Gynecological and reproductive function after liver transplantation. Transplantation 62:476-479.

Martínez Díaz-Guerra G, Gómez R, Jódar E, Loinaz C, Moreno E, Hawkins F. 2002. Long-term follow-up of bone mass after orthotopic liver transplantation: effect of steroid withdrawal from the immunosuppressive regimen. Osteoporos Int 13(2):147-50.

Mitchell MJ, Baz MA, Fulton MN, Lisor CF, Braith RW. 2003 Resistance training prevents vertebral osteoporosis in lung transplant recipients. Transplantation. Aug 15;76(3):557-62.

Misof BM, Bodingbauer M, Roschger P, Wekerle T, Pakrah B, Haas M, Kainz A, Oberbauer R, Mühlbacher F, Klaushofer K. 2008 Short-term effects of high-dose zoledronic acid treatment on bone mineralization density distribution after orthotopic liver transplantation. Calcif Tissue Int;83(3):167-75.

Monegal A, Navasa M, Guañabens N, Peris P, Pons F, Martinez de Osaba MJ, Ordi J, Rimola A, Rodés J, Muñoz-Gómez 2001. Bone disease after liver transplantation: a long-term prospective study of bone mass changes, hormonal status and histomorphometric characteristics. Osteoporos Int.;12(6):484-92.

Monegal A, Navasa M, Guañabens N, Peris P, Pons F, Martínez de Osaba MJ, Rimola A, Rodés J, Muñoz-Gómez J. 2001 Bone mass and mineral metabolism in liver transplant patients treated with FK506 or cyclosporine A. Calcif Tissue IntFeb;68(2):83-6.

Monegal A, Guañabens N, Suárez MJ, Suárez F, Clemente G, García-González M, De la Mata M, Serrano T, Casafont F, Tome S, Barrios C, Navasa M. 2009 Pamidronate in the prevention of bone loss after liver transplantation: a randomized controlled trial. Transpl Int. Feb;22(2):198-206.

Newton J, Francis R, Prince M, James O, Bassendine M, Rawlings D, Jones D. 2001 Osteoporosis in primary biliary cirrhosis revisited. Gut. Aug;49(2):282-7.

Ninkovic M, Skingle SJ, Bearcroft PW, Bishop N, Alexander GJ, Compston JE. 2000 Incidence of vertebral fractures in the first three months after orthotopic liver transplantation. Eur J Gastroenterol Hepatol. Aug;12(8):931-5.

Ninkovic M, Love SA, Tom B, Alexander GJ, Compston JE. 2001 High prevalence of osteoporosis in patients with chronic liver disease prior to liver transplantation. Calcif Tissue Int. Dec;69(6):321-6.

Ninkovic M, Love S, Tom BD, Bearcroft PW, Alexander GJ, Compston JE. 2002 Lack of effect of intravenous pamidronate on fracture incidence and bone mineral density after orthotopic liver transplantation. *J Hepatol.* Jul;37(1):93-100.

Nisbeth U, Lindh E, Ljunghall S, Backman U, Fellström B. 1994 Fracture frequency after kidney transplantation. *Transplant Proc.* Jun;26(3):1764

Nowacka-Cieciura E, Cieciura T, Baczkowska T, Kozińska-Przybył O, Tronina O, Chudziński W, Pacholczyk M, Durlik M. 2006 Bisphosphonates are effective prophylactic of early bone loss after renal transplantation. *Transplant Proc.* Jan-Feb;38(1):165-7

Ramsey-Goldman R, Dunn JE, Dunlop DD, Stuart FP, Abecassis MM, Kaufman DB, Langman CB, Salinger MH, Sprague SM 1999. Increased risk of fracture in patients receiving solid organ transplants. *J Bone Miner Res* 14:456.

Rodino MA, Shane E. 1998 Osteoporosis after organ transplantation. *Am J Med.* May;104(5):459-69.

Sambrook P . 2000 Effect of calcitriol on bone loss after cardiac or lung transplantation. *J Bone Miner Res.* Sep;15(9):1818-24.

Samojlik E, Kirschner MA, Ribot S, Szmal E. 1992 Changes in the hypothalamic-pituitary-gonadal axis in men after cadaver kidney transplantation and cyclosporine therapy. *J Androl.* Jul-Aug;13(4):332-6.

Schulte C, Beelen DW, Schaefer UW, Mann K. 2000 Bone loss in long-term survivors after transplantation of hematopoietic stem cells: a prospective study. *Osteopor Int;* 11:344-353.

Schulte CM, Beelen DW. 2004 Bone loss following hematopoietic stem cell transplantation: a long-term follow-up. *Blood.* May 15;103(10):3635-43.

Seethalakshmi L, Flores C, Carboni AA, Bala R, Diamond DA, Menon M. 1990 Cyclosporine: its effects on testicular function and fertility in the prepubertal rat. *J Androl.* Jan-Feb;11(1):17-24.

Shane E, Rivas M, Staron RB, Silverberg SJ, Seibel MJ, Kuiper J, Mancini D, Addesso V, Michler RE, 1996 Factor-Litvak P. Fracture after cardiac transplantation: a prospective longitudinal study. *J Clin Endocrinol Metab.* May;81(5):1740-6.

Shane E, Silverberg SJ, Donovan D, Papadopoulos A, Staron RB, Addesso V, Jorgesen B, McGregor C, Schulman L . 1996 Osteoporosis in lung transplantation candidates with end-stage pulmonary disease. *Am J Med.* Sep;101(3):262-9.

Shane E, Rivas M, McMahon DJ, Staron RB, Silverberg SJ, Seibel MJ, Mancini D, Michler RE, Aaronson K, Addesso V, Lo SH. 1997 Bone loss and turnover after cardiac transplantation. *J Clin Endocrinol Metab.* May;82(5):1497-506.

Shane E, Rodino MA, McMahon DJ, Addesso V, Staron RB, Seibel MJ, Mancini D, Michler RE, Lo SH.. 1998; Prevention of bone loss after heart transplantation with antiresorptive therapy: a pilot study. *J Heart Lung Transplant* 17(11):1089-96.

Shane E, Papadopoulos A, Staron RB, Addesso V, Donovan D, McGregor C, et al. Bone loss and fracture after lung transplantation. Transplantation. 1999 Jul 27;68(2):220-7.

Shane E, Addesso V, Namerow PB, McMahon DJ, Lo SH, Staron RB, Zucker M, Pardi S, Maybaum S, Mancini D. 2004 Alendronate versus calcitriol for the prevention of bone loss after cardiac transplantation. *N Engl J Med.* Feb 19;350(8):767-76

Shane E. Osteoporosis after solid organ or stem cell transplantation. UpToDate. Basow, DS (Ed), UpToDate, Waltham, MA.ed; 2009.

Sikka SC, Bhasin S, Coy DC, Koyle MA, Swerdloff RS, Rajfer J. 1988 Effects of cyclosporine on the hypothalamic-pituitary-gonadal axis in the male rat: mechanism of action. *Endocrinology.* Aug;123(2):1069-74.

Solerio E, Isaia G, Innarella R, Di Stefano M, Farina M, Borghesio E, Framarin L, Rizzetto M, Rosina F. 2003 Osteoporosis: still a typical complication of primary biliary cirrhosis? *Dig Liver Dis.* May;35(5):339-46.

Stehman-Breen CO, Sherrard DJ, Alem AM, Gillen DL, Heckbert SR, Wong CS, Ball A, Weiss NS 2000 Risk factors for hip fracture among patients with end-stage renal disease. *Kidney Int;*58: 2200–2205.

Talalaj M, Gradowska L, Marcinowska-Suchowierska E, Durlik M, Gaciong Z, Lao M. Efficiency of preventive treatment of glucocorticoid-induced osteoporosis with 25-hydroxyvitamin D3 and calcium in kidney transplant patients. Transplant Proc 1996;28:3485–7.

Tauchmanovà L, Selleri C, De Rosa G, Esposito M, Orio F Jr, Palomba S, Bifulco G, Nappi C, Lombardi G, Rotoli B, Colao A 2003 . Gonadal status in reproductive age women after haematopoietic stem cell transplantation for haematological malignancies. *Hum Reprod* 18:1410.

Tauchmanovà L, Selleri C, De Rosa G, Esposito M, Di Somma C, Orio F, Palomba S, Lombardi G, Rotoli B, Colao A. 2005 Endocrine disorders during the first year after autologous stem-cell transplant. *Am J Med;* 118:664.

Thiebaud D, Krieg MA, Gillard-Berguer D, Jacquet AF, Goy JJ, Burckhardt P. 1996 Cyclosporine induces high bone turnover and may contribute to bone loss after heart transplantation. *Eur J Clin Invest.* Jul;26(7):549-55.

Tschopp O, Boehler A, Speich R, Weder W, Seifert B, Russi EW, Schmid C. 2002.Osteoporosis before lung transplantation: association with low body mass index, but not with underlying disease. *Am J Transplant.* Feb;2(2):167-72.

Van Cleemput J, Daenen W, Geusens P, Dequeker P, Van De Werf F, Van Haecke J. Prevention of bone loss in cardiac transplant recipients. A comparison of biphosphonates and vitamin D. Transplantation 1996;61:1495–9.

Valero MA, Loinaz C, Larrodera L, Leon M, Moreno E, Hawkins F. 1995Calcitonin and bisphosphonates treatment in bone loss after liver transplantation. *Calcif Tissue Int;*57(1):15-9.

Välimäki MJ, Kinnunen K, Tähtelä R, Löyttyniemi E, Laitinen K, Mäkelä P, Keto P, Nieminen M. 1999.A prospective study of bone loss and turnover after cardiac transplantation: effect of calcium supplementation with or without calcitonin. *Osteoporos Int.* 10(2):128-36.

Välimäki MJ, Kinnunen K, Volin L, Tähtelä R, Löyttyniemi E, Laitinen K, Mäkelä P, Keto P, Ruutu T. 1999; A prospective study of bone loss and turnover after allogeneic bone marrow transplantation: effect of calcium supplementation with or without calcitonin. *Bone Marrow Transplant* 23:355.

Vedi S, Ninkovic M, Garrahan NJ, Alexander GJ, Compston JE. 2002 Effects of a single infusion of pamidronate prior to liver transplantation: a bone histomorphometric study. *Transpl Int;* 15(6):290-5.

6

The Phytoestrogens, Calcitonin and Thyroid Hormones: Effects on Bone Tissue

Branko Filipović and Branka Šošić-Jurjević
University of Belgrade, Institute for Biological Research"Siniša Stanković"
Serbia

1. Introduction

The skeleton is a metabolically active organ that undergoes remodeling throughout life. This involves a complex process by which old bone is continuously replaced by new tissue. Bone remodeling refers to the sequential, coupled actions of osteoclasts and osteoblasts. In conditions of sex hormone deficiency during advancing age, after the menopause or andropause, the rate of remodeling increases and bone formation is reduced relative to resorption. These alterations can cause microarchitectural deterioration of bone tissues, which increases bone loss as a predisposition to the occurrence of osteoporosis (Rehman et al., 2005). However, in contrast to postmenopausal osteoporosis in women, age-related bone loss in men is less well defined.

Numerous studies attest to the importance of estrogen in bone remodeling, evident from the finding that hormone replacement therapy (HRT) administered in a dose-dependent manner effectively prevented bone loss in postmenopausal women (Lindsay et al., 1976, 1984). However, in addition to protective effects on bone, HRT is associated with an increased risk for breast, endometrial, ovarian or prostate cancers (Davison & Davis, 2003; Loughlin & Richie, 1997; Nelson et al., 2002). Therefore, it is important to examine alternative approaches for prevention and treatment of osteoporosis without side effects. It is well known that the incidence of osteoporosis-related fractures is significantly lower in Southern and Eastern Asian women than in Western women (Tham et al., 1998). One possible reason for this difference is a high intake of phytoestrogen-rich plants, which Asian people eat more often than Western people (Ho et al., 2003). As a result, over the past decade a number of clinical trials for prevention of bone loss have assessed the effectiveness of plant derived non-steroidal phytoestrogens found in a wide variety of foods, most notably soybean. Isoflavones, which include daidzein and genistein are a class of phytoestrogens that act like estrogens. Since these compounds bind to estrogen receptors (ERs) and have estrogen-like activity (Branca, 2003), they have attracted much attention because of their potential benefit in the prevention and treatment of osteoporosis.

In addition to the phytoestrogen-mediated protective mechanisms against bone loss, recent evidence suggests that daidzein may also act on rat bone tissue through enhancement of thyroid C cell activity (Filipović et al., 2010). Namely, thyroid C cells produce the hormone, calcitonin (CT), which lowers plasma calcium concentration by suppressing osteoclast activity. Synthesis of CT and its release from C cells were decreased in conditions of gonadal hormone deficiency (Filipović et al., 2003, 2007; Isaia et al., 1989; Lu et al., 2000; Sakai et al., 2000). Due to its osteoprotective properties, CT is widely applied in the therapy of osteoporosis.

It is known that parathyroid hormone (PTH) is a major factor involved in the systemic regulation of bone resorption. Phytoestrogens may affect the parathyroid gland and reduce PTH secretion (Wong et al., 2002), suggesting that one way in which these compounds inhibit bone loss may be through reducing PTH levels.

Thyroid hormones are essential for normal bone maturation *in utero* and during early life. In adults an excess of thyroid hormones in the body affects the remodeling system in cortical and trabecular bone and may contribute to the development of osteoporosis (Kung, 1994). Receptors for these hormones are present in bone cells and they may directly increase bone resorption (Abu et al., 1997; Rizzoli et al., 1986). Additionally, thyroid-stimulating hormone (TSH), which stimulates the release of thyroid hormones, positively influences bone remodeling. Therefore, demonstrating both anabolic and antiresorptive effects, TSH may represent a promising candidate for the treatment of osteoporosis (Sendak et al., 2007).

In this chapter we will describe the known effects of phytoestrogens on bone. In addition to the direct action of these plant compounds, special attention will be paid to their influence on thyroid C and follicular cells, as producers of CT and thyroid hormones, using the latest data in the literature and our own results. These hormones, together with PTH may be involved in the indirect effects of phytoestrogens on bone tissue.

2. Bone cells and bone remodeling

Bone is a dynamic organ that undergoes remodeling throughout life. This process results from the separate action of bone forming cells called osteoblasts and bone resorbing cells called osteoclasts. Osteoblasts are responsible for the production of bone matrix constituents and are found in clusters on bone surfaces (Fig 1). They originate from multipotent mesenchymal stem cells, which have the capacity to differentiate into osteoblasts or other cells, such as adipocytes, chondrocytes, myoblasts and fibroblasts (Bianco et al., 2001). A mature osteoblast that is trapped in the bone matrix and remains isolated in lacunae becomes an osteocyte. (Fig.1). Bone formation involves production and maturation of the osteoid matrix, followed by mineralization of the matrix. Osteoblasts produce growth factors, such as insulin-like growth factor (IGF), platelet-derived growth factor (PDGF), basic fibroblast growth factor (bFGF), transforming growth factor-β (TGF- β) and bone morphometric protein (BMP) (Canalis et al., 1993, 1993a; Chen et al., 2004; Globus et al., 1989; Rydzel et al., 1994). These factors regulate osteoblast activity in an autocrine and paracrine manner.

Osteoclasts are large multinucleate cells responsible for bone resorption. They are derived from hematopoetic cells of the mononuclear lineage (Teitelbaum, 2000) (Fig.1). Osteoclasts have an abundant Golgi complex, mitochondria and transport vesicles loaded with lysosomal enzymes, such as tartrate-resistant acid phosphatase (TRAP) and cathepsin K. These enzymes are secreted via the specialized (ruffler border) plasma membrane of osteoclasts into the bone-resorbing compartment (Väänänen et al., 2000). The process of osteoclast attachment to the bone is complex and involves binding of integrins expressed in osteoclasts with specific amino acid sequences within proteins at the surface of the bone matrix and cytoskeleton activation (Davies et al., 1989; Reinholt et al., 1990). Dynamic structures, called podozomes allow movement of osteoclasts across the bone surface. Bone resorption occurs due to acidification and proteolysis of the bone matrix. As a result of this resorptive activity in contact with the surface of calcified bone, osteoclasts create resorptive lacunae. Osteoclast function is regulated both by locally acting cytokines and by systemic hormones.

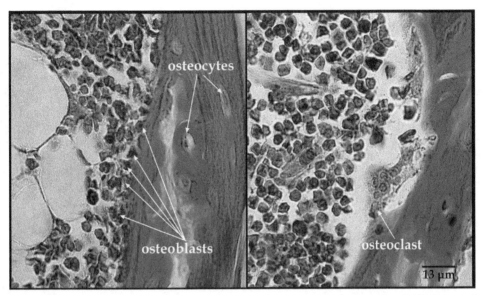

Fig. 1. Bone cells – osteoblasts, osteocytes and osteoclasts; unpublished image of Filipović et al.

In homeostatic equilibrium, bone resorption and formation are balanced. It appears that osteoclasts and osteoblasts closely collaborate in the remodeling process in what is called a "Basic Multicellular Unit", or BMU. This indicates that a coupling mechanism must exist between formation and resorption (Frost, 1964), although its nature is not known. Organization of the BMU in cortical and trabecular bone differs. Between 2% and 5% of cortical bone is remodeled each year. The remodeling process in trabecular bone is mainly a surface event. Due to the much larger surface to volume ratio, it is more actively remodeled than cortical bone, with remodeling rates that can be up to 10 times higher (Lee & Einhorn, 2001).

The remodeling cycle consists of three consecutive phases: resorption, reversal and formation. Resorption begins with the migration of partially differentiated preosteoclasts, which form multinucleated osteoclasts on the bone surface. During the reversal phase, mononuclear cells prepare the resorption lacunae for bone formation and provide signals for osteoblast differentiation and migration (Eriksen et al., 1990). Bone formation starts with activation of preosteoblasts to differentiate into osteoblasts. They secrete bone-matrix proteins to form the organic matrix, which is later mineralized. During this period, osteoblasts completely replace the resorbed bone by new tissue. After this phase, the surface is covered with flattened lining cells and a prolonged resting period ensues until a new remodeling cycle is initiated. Duration of the resorption phase is about 2 weeks, the reversal phase lasts for up to 4 or 5 weeks, while the formation phase can continue for 4 months.

At each remodeling site, bone resorption is coupled with bone formation, locally released growth factors and cytokines acting as mediators of this process (Canalis et al., 1988; Mundy, 1995). The decrease of bone mass, which may be due to different causes, is a consequence of an imbalance between the amount of mineral and matrix removed and that subsequently incorporated into each resorption cavity (Kanis et al., 1990).

3. Phytoestrogens in bone protection

Phytoestrogens are structurally and functionally similar to estrogens and their estrogenic activity may occur through ERs. There are three main classes of phytoestrogens: isoflavonoids, coumestans and lignans (Fig. 2). Due to their estrogenic and anti-estrogenic activity, they are termed - natural selective ER modulators (SERMs). Therefore, soybean isoflavones have received great attention as alternatives to HRT for the prevention of postmenopausal osteoporosis. Genistein and daidzein, the main isoflavones in soybean, may protect against osteoporosis, because they can affect both types of bone cells.

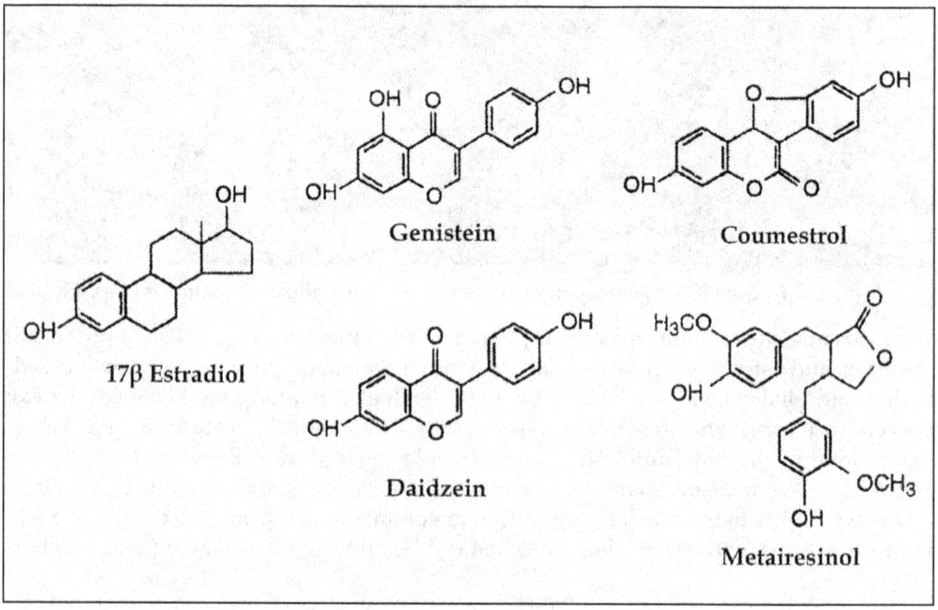

Fig. 2. Structure of 17β estradiol, isoflavones (genistein and daidzein), coumestan (coumestrol) and lignans (metairesinol); Filipović et al.

Isoflavones can stimulate the proliferation and differentiation of osteoblasts. Thus, the presence of genistein or daidzein led to a significant increase in protein synthesis, alkaline phosphatase activity, and DNA content in cultures of osteoblastic MC3T3-E1 cells (Sugimoto & Yamaguchi, 2000, 2000a; Yamaguchi & Sugimoto, 2000).

In addition to a stimulating effect on bone formation, these plant compounds may also suppress osteoclastic bone resorption in vitro. Thus, genistein was found to induce apoptosis of osteoclasts isolated from rat femoral tissues. Daidzein also decreased the number of these bone resorbing cells in rats (Gao & Yamaguchi, 1999) and their development in cultures of porcine bone marrow (Rassi et al., 2002). Osteoclast activity is regulated by phosphorylation of cell membrane constituents, involving tyrosine kinases. As a naturally tyrosine kinase inhibitor, genistein was found to suppress avian osteoclastic activity through inhibition of tyrosine kinase (Blair et al., 1996). Genistein also caused a significant increase in tyrosine phosphatase activity, which is a negative regulator of osteoclastogenesis and osteoclast-resorbing activity in mutant mice (Aoki et al., 1999; Gao &Yamaguchi, 2000) (Fig 3).

While investigations in vitro give clues about the effects of isoflavones on individual bone cells, studies in vivo provide knowledge about their influence in intact systems. Aged gonadectomized female and male rodents are suitable animal models for studying osteoporosis (Comelekoglu et al., 2007; Filipović et al., 2007; Pantelić et al., 2010; Vanderschueren et al., 1992.) Using them it has been demonstrated that isoflavones can prevent bone loss in female rats and mice after ovariectomy (Ovx) (Blum et al., 2003; Erlandsson et al., 2005; Fonseca & Ward, 2004; Ishimi et al., 1999; Lee et al., 2004; Om & Shim, 2007; Ren et al., 2007; Wu et al., 2004). The bone-preventing effects of isoflavones were also confirmed in male orchidectomized (Orx) rats and mice (Filipović et al., 2010; Ishimi et al., 2002; Khalil et al., 2005; Soung et al., 2006; Wu et al., 2003). On the contrary, some studies showed that isoflavones had minimal or no effects on bone loss in animal models (Bahr et al., 2005; Nakai et al., 2005; Picherit et al., 2001). Moreover, in the monkey, a nonhuman primate, dietary isoflavones do not effectively prevent ovariectomy-induced bone loss (Register et al., 2003). However, others suggested that soy phytoestrogens were protective against loss of bone volume (Ham et al., 2004).

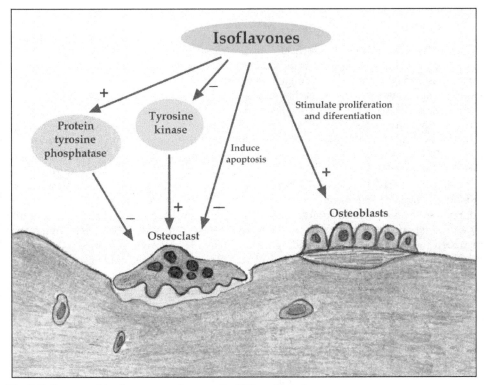

Fig. 3. Influence of isoflavones on bone cells; Filipović et al.

During recent years, numerous human studies have evaluated the effect of soy protein-containing isoflavones or pure isoflavones on bone mass. However, the results of these observational and dietary interventional investigations have been variable and conflicting. In general, isoflavone supplementation studies indicate a beneficial effect on bone mass (Huang et al., 2006; Lydeking-Olsen et al., 2004; Newton et al., 2006), no effect (Anderson et al., 2002; Arjmandi et al., 2005; Brink et al., 2008; Wu et al., 2006) or a possible negative effect in terms of increased circulating concentrations of biochemical markers associated with bone resorption (Geppert et al., 2004; Wanger et al., 2000).

The large heterogeneity of these results may be due to study design, differences regarding hormonal status of the subjects, together with the duration, type and dose of isoflavone supplementation. In addition, bone sparing benefits may depend on the extent of conversion of isoflavones to metabolites. Thus, equol binds with greater affinity to ERs than daidzein from which it is derived (Setchell et al., 2002). Equol production is dependent on the intestinal microflora and there are large interindividual differences in this metabolism. Some people produce more equol than others. Also, production of this metabolite may at least partially explain why the beneficial effects of isoflavones observed in laboratory rodents, which consistently produce high levels of equol, have not been easily recapitulated in humans, where this is not the case. Generally, the relative importance of phytoestrogens in human health must be resolved and longer-term studies are needed to determine their effects on human bone tissue.

4. Phytoestrogens – Mechanisms of action in bone

Although the mechanisms by which soy phytoestrogens may alter bone remodeling are still not completely known, Atmaca et al. (2008) state that they act on both osteoblasts and osteoclasts through genomic and nongenomic pathways.

Due to their low molecular weight these plant compounds can pass through cell membranes and interact with receptors and enzymes (Adlercreutz et al., 1998). Phytoestrogens possess estrogenic activity and act as natural SERMs. This suggests that their effect on bone can be achieved by binding to ERs. Both α and β subtypes of ERs have been identified in bone (Arts et al., 1997; Onoe et al., 1997). The protective effect of phytoestrogens is probably achieved mainly through binding to ER-β, the expression of which is increased during bone mineralization (Arts et al., 1997; Kuiper et al., 1998). In addition to ERs, phytoestrogens can bind to androgenic receptors and act as phytoandrogens (Chen & Chang, 2007).

Both genistein and daidzein stimulate osteoblast proliferation, differentiation and activation by an ER-dependent mechanism (De Wilde et al., 2004; Pan et al., 2005). These isoflavones regulated the synthesis of core binding factor-1 (Cbfa-1) and bone morphogenic protein-2 (BMP-2), which is involved in the differentiation of osteoblasts (De Wilde et al., 2004; Jia et al., 2003; Pan et al., 2005). Genistein and daidzein activate peroxisome proliferator activator receptors (PPARs). The balance between PPAR and ER activation may govern the balance between adipogenesis and osteoblastogenesis (Dang et al., 2003, 2004).

Osteoclasts express the receptor activator of nuclear factor kappa B (RANK) (Hsu et al., 1999), while the receptor activator of nuclear factor kappa B ligand (RANK-L) and osteoprotegerin (OPG) is expressed by osteoblasts (Udagawa et al., 1999). Binding of RANKL to RANK stimulates osteoclastogenesis, whereas binding of RANK-L to OPG prevents RANK-L – RANK binding and indirectly inhibits osteoclastogenesis (Fuller et al., 1998; Theoleyre et al., 2004). The relative levels this triad of proteins are important for controlling osteoclastogenesis. It was shown that isoflavones may increase the activity of osteoblasts by stimulating the secretion of OPG and RANK-L (De Wilde et al., 2004; Yamagishi et al., 2001) (Fig. 4).

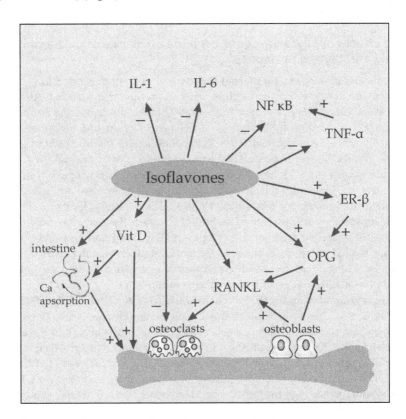

Fig. 4. Mechanisms of isoflavone action in bone; Filipović et al.

Proinflammatory cytokines, such as interleukin (IL)-1, IL-6, and tumor necrosis factor α (TNF-α), stimulate osteoclastogenesis and bone resorption. These effects can be achieved by both RANK-L dependent and RANK-L-independent mechanisms (Collin-Osbody et al., 2001; Katagiri et al., 2002). Isoflavones have been shown to inhibit IL-6 synthesis by MC3T3-E1/4 osteoblast-like cells in vitro (Chen et al., 2003; Suh et al., 2003) and to reduce serum IL-1β and TNF-α concentrations in Ovx rats (Li, 2003). Also, a soy supplemented diet may inhibit serum concentrations of proinflammatory cytokines in postmenopausal women (Huang et al., 2005).

In addition to osteoclastogenesis, isoflavones appear to influence osteoclast activity through inhibition of inward rectifier K+channels in osteoclasts. This leads to membrane depolarization, intracellular influx of Ca2+ and inhibition of bone resorption (Okamoto et al., 2001). One beneficial effect of isoflavones on bone is increased intestinal calcium absorption (Fig. 4). However, it is not known whether the mechanism(s) by which isoflavones influence calcium absorption include interactions with intestinal ER and/or vitamin D receptor-mediated calcium transport or not (Arjmandi et al., 2002).

Nongenomic effects do not involve ERs. These effects of phytoestrogens include inhibition of tyrosine kinase which directly modulate osteoclastic acid secretion (Blair et al., 1996; Williams et al., 1998) or topoisomerase I and II, which helps to regulate cell differentiation and the cell replication cycle (Okura et al., 1998; Yamagishi et al., 2001).

5. Indirect effects of phytoestrogens on bone – The role of calcitonin, parathyroid and thyroid hormones

5.1 Effects of phytoestrogens on thyroid C cells and calcitonin production

Thyroid C cells are dispersed neuroendocrine cells that produce many bioregulatory peptides, among which CT is considered the most important. This calcium regulating hormone lowers plasma calcium concentration by inhibiting osteoclast activity. In addition to sex steroids, a voluminous literature has accumulated for therapeutic use of CT in treating osteoporosis. Thus, C cells may also be very important in the pathogenesis of osteoporosis.

The C cells are mostly located in the middle of the thyroid lobes and appear in clusters or as solitary cells between follicular cells and the capillary wall. They have a round, elliptical or polygonal shape and never face the follicular lumen. The nucleus is located in the center of the cell. The most salient ultrastructural feature of C cells is the numerous round secretory granules that fill extensive areas of the cytoplasm. The Golgi complex and endoplasmic reticulum are well developed. There is a moderate number of mitochondria, which are mostly round to elongate in shape and not uniformly distributed. Lysosomes are large and contain acid phosphatase and other lysosomal enzymes (Fig. 5).

CT suppresses the number and motility of osteoclasts (Gao & Yamaguchi, 1999; Zaidi et al., 1990) and induces a change in their contractile elements (Hunter et al., 1989). Also, CT increases osteoblast proliferation by acting on components of the insulin-like growth factor system (Farley et al., 2000) and enhancing alkaline phosphatase activity, which is associated with increased synthesis and deposition of bone matrix collagen (Farley et al., 1988, 1992; Ito et al., 1987). The action of CT bone formation is at least in part, mediated via CT receptors located on osteoblasts, through the cAMP second messenger system (Farley et al., 1992; Villa et al., 2003).

It was shown that gonadal hormone deficiency affects thyroid C cell activity. Thus, synthesis of CT and its release from rat C cells were decreased after Ovx due to lack of estrogens (Filipović et al., 2002, 2003; Sakai et al. 2000). Also, the decline in testosterone level induced by Orx altered thyroid C cell structure and reduced the synthesis and release of CT (Filipović et al., 2007; Lu et al., 2000). The same effects were noticed after Orx or the natural menopause in women (Isaia et al. 1989). On the other hand, estrogen treatment was found to have a stimulatory effect on CT secretory activity of C cells in Ovx rats (Grauer et al., 1993; Filipović et al., 2003), Orx rats (Filipović et al., 2010a) and women (Isaia et al., 1992). In addition to estrogen, chronic calcium administration after Ovx increased the release of CT from C cells without affecting CT synthesis, suggesting that estrogen plays an important role in CT synthesis (Filipović et al., 2005). On the other hand, CT administration, which may be useful for treatment of osteoporosis, negatively affected rat thyroid C cells by a negative feedback mechanism (Sekulić et al., 2005).

Among the few studies concerning the potential effects of phytoestrogens on CT production, the influence of ipriflavone, a derivative of isoflavone, on CT synthesis and secretion was investigated. Administration of ipriflavone to intact rats had a gender-related effect on serum CT, which increased in females, but no significant change was seen in male rats (Watanabe et al., 1992). With regard to the inhibitory effect of testosterone on the synthesis of some enzymes it is possible that testosterone inhibited ipriflavone-stimulated CT synthesis (Weiner & Dias, 1990).

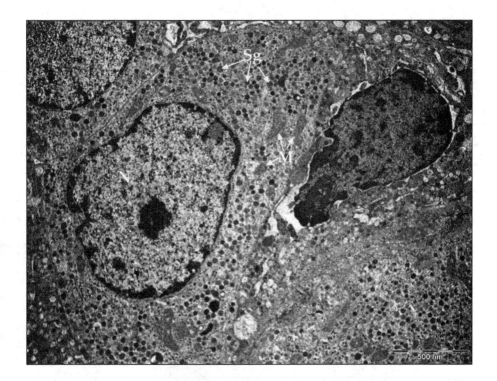

Fig. 5. Ultrastructure of a thyroid C cell; nucleus (N), mitochondria (M), secretory granules (Sg); unpublished image of Filipović et al.

Recently the first experimental data suggesting that daidzein affects thyroid C cells and stimulates CT secretory activity in Orx middle-aged rats were presented (Filipović et al., 2010). The androgen deficiency after Orx strongly affected thyroid C cell structure and reduced the synthesis and release of CT. Daidzein treatment decreased immunoreactivity for CT, significantly increased C cell volume (Fig. 6) and slightly raised serum CT concentration.

Daidzein administration also decreased bone turnover, prevented loss of cancellous bone and the plate-like structure was recovered after trabecular bone destruction caused by Orx (Fig. 7). Based on these results, the authors suggested that, besides direct action on the skeleton, daidzein may affect bone structure indirectly through enhancement of thyroid C cell activity (Filipović et al., 2010).

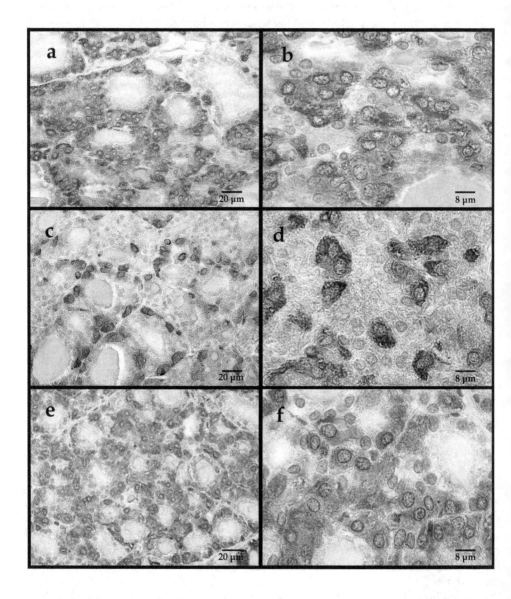

Fig. 6. Calcitonin producing thyroid C cells in control (a, b), orchidectomized (c, d) and orchidectomized rats treated with daidzein (e, f); immuno-staining for calcitonin; unpublished image of Filipović et al.

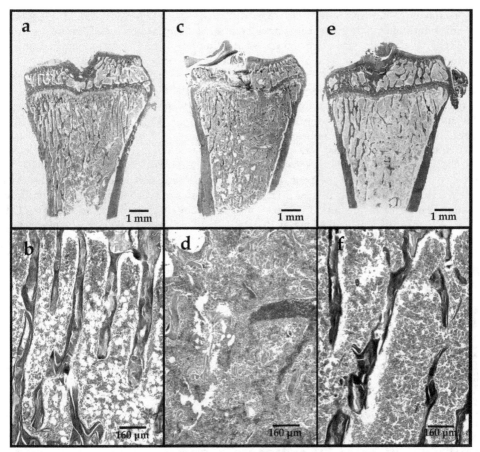

Fig. 7. Trabecular microarchitecture of the proximal tibial metaphysis in control (a, b), orchidectomized (c, d) and orchidectomized rats treated with daidzein (e, f); azan staining method; unpublished image of Filipović et al.

5.2 Effects of phytoestrogens on parathyroid hormone production

Parathyroid glands are constituted of chief, clear and oxyphilous cells. The chief cells synthesize and secrete PTH and are arranged in rather dense cords or nests around abundant capillaries. These cells are oval or polygonal in shape. The nucleus is irregularly shaped, with a few spots of chromatin located in the margin, and the nuclear membrane is infolded. The plasma membrane shows interdigitations. Mitochondria are dispersed throughout the cytoplasm. The cisternae of the rough-surfaced endoplasmic reticulum are arranged in parallel arrays or randomly distributed in the cytoplasm. The Golgi complexes are well developed. Storage granules are filled with finely particulate electron-dense material (Fig. 8).

PTH plays an important role in calcium homeostasis and has a critical role in bone turnover. It antagonizes CT produced by thyroid C cells and acts directly on bone and kidney to increase Ca influx into the blood circulation. This hormone increases the tubular reabsorption of calcium and induces increased conversion of 25(OH)-D to 1,25(OH)2-D, which enhances intestinal calcium absorption and increases skeletal calcium mobilization.

PTH has a biphasic effect on bone, as it stimulates bone formation when given intermittently, whereas continuous infusion reduces bone mass (Kim et al., 2003). Treatment with PTH significantly increases ALP activity, which suggests that this hormone modulates SaOS-2 osteoblastic cell differentiation and has an anabolic effect on bone. However, increases in RANKL mRNA and decreased OPG mRNA expression in SaOS-2 cells due to PTH indicates induction of bone resorption (Chen & Wong, 2006).

Elevated PTH secretion contributes to the greater bone resorption in osteoporosis which is related to estrogen deficiency. Estrogen therapy prevented the increase in PTH levels associated with the menopause (Khosla et al., 1997). Similarly, phytoestrogens behave as estrogen and may prevent the bone loss caused by estrogen deficiency in female animals and women through reduction of PTH levels. It was shown that phytoestrogens from medical plants can lower serum PTH levels in aged menopausal monkeys (Trisomboon et al. 2004). Also, postmenopausal women with habitually high intakes of dietary isoflavones had significantly lower levels of serum PTH and higher BMD (Mei et al., 2001). These plant compounds bind to ERs in the kidney, gastrointestinal tract and bone and improve calcium absorption resulting in a secondary decrease in the PTH level. Moreover, phytoestrogens may directly reduce PTH secretion from the parathyroid gland (Wong et al., 2002).

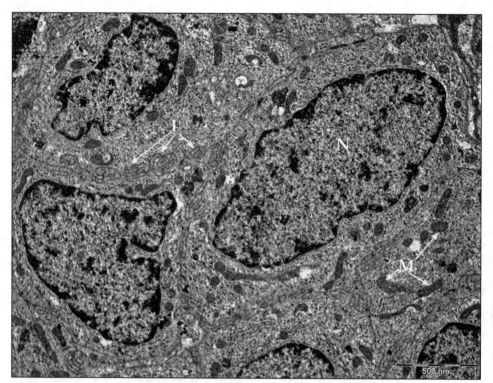

Fig. 8. Ultrastructure of parathyroid chief cells; nucleus (N), mitochondria (M), interdigitations of the plasma membrane (I); unpublished image of Pantelić et al.

Mimicking the effect of estrogen, phytoestrogens can modulate the action of PTH on bone. Thus, one study in vitro showed that pre-treatment of SaOS-2 osteoblastic cells with genistein enhanced PTH-induced ALP activity and attenuated PTH up regulation of RANKL mRNA expression and PTH down regulation of OPG mRNA expression (Chen & Wong, 2006).

5.3 Effects of phytoestrogens on thyroid glands and thyroid hormones production

Hypothalamic–pituitary–thyroid axis (HPT) plays a key role in skeletal development, attainment of peak bone mass and regulation of adult bone turnover (Gogakos et al., 2010; Roef et al., 2011). Additionally, thyroid disorders are associated with alterations in bone metabolism (Lakatos, 2003).

Soy-food, soy-based infant formula, as well as dietary supplements containing purified soybean isoflavones, genistein and daidzein, are increasingly consumed in typical "Western" diet in the recent years. Commonly cited reasons for using soy infant formula are to feed infants who are allergic to dairy products or are intolerant of lactose, galactose, or cow-milk protein (Tuohy, 2003). In elderly, reason is potential health benefit of soybean isoflavones in protection of age-related diseases, including osteoporosis (Setchell, 1998).

Structurally, soybean isoflavones genistein and daidzein are polyphenolic compounds, similar to estradiol-17β and bind with a weaker potency to both types of ERs, with higher affinity for ERβ (Kuiper et al., 1998). Despite the numerous beneficial effects of soy isoflavones, epidemiological and experimental data also exist showing an adverse effect on human health, namely on reproductive and thyroid axis. The association between high soy isoflavones intake and goitrogenesis, as well as protective effect of adequate iodine intake, was reported both in humans (Chorazy et al.1995; Van Wyk et al., 1959) and in different animal models (Ikeda et al., 2000; Kimura et al., 1976; McCarrison, 1933).

Therefore, besides the direct beneficial effect of soybean phytoestrogens on bone tissue, isoflavones may also act indirectly, through endocrine disruption and interference with HPT axis. Most researchers who examined osteoprotective potential of isoflavones did not include in their research examining of the thyroid status. We will address that aspect in this subchapter.

5.3.1 Phytoestrogens, thyroid hormones and skeletal development

Normal thyroid function in childhood is essential for development of endochondral and intramembranous bone, for normal linear growth, as well as for establishing peak bone mass. Hypothyroidism in children causes growth arrest, delayed bone maturation, and epiphyseal dysgenesis, while T_4 replacement results in rapid catch-up growth (Basset & Williams, 2003). Exposure to soybean isoflavones during development may alter thyroid hormone concentrations and disturb feedback regulation of HPT axis, and these effects can be more serious than in the adults.

Soy infant formula is fed to infants as a replacement for human milk, or as an alternative to cow milk formula. Genistein is the predominant isoflavone found in soy infant formula (58-67%), followed by daidzein (29-34%) and glycitein (5-8%) and infants fed soy infant formula have higher daily intakes of genistein and other isoflavones than other populations (Patisaul & Jefferson, 2010). The question of whether or not soy infant formula is safe has been widely debated for more than a decade, and early epidemiological studies demonstrated that infants fed adapted soy formula without iodine supply were hypothyroid (Van Wyk et al., 1959). This effect was eliminated by supplementing commercial soy infant formulas with iodine, or by switching to cow milk (Chorazy et al., 1995). Today, soy formula is regularly supplied with iodine and a more recent study demonstrated no significant changes in the serum level of bone alkaline phosphatase, osteocalcin, intact PTH, and the urinary levels of the markers of bone metabolism in children (mean age of 37 months) fed with soy formula (Giampietro et al., 2004). However, infants with congenital hypothyroidism fed with iodine supplemented diet still need higher doses of L-thyroxine (Jabbar et al., 1997). This finding is of particular importance, keeping in mind that the consequence of congenital and juvenile acquired hypothyroidism is retardation of skeletal development and that the effects of T_4 replacement (achievement of predicted adult height) strongly depend on the duration of untreated hypothyroidism (Rivkees et al., 1988).

Soybean isoflavones may functionally disrupt the thyroid hormone (TH) system by influencing different steps such as synthesis, transport, action and metabolism of TH. Genistein and daidzein inhibit the activity of thyroid peroxidase (TPO), the key enzyme in the synthesis of thyroid hormones, both in vitro and in vivo (Chang & Doerge, 2000; Divi et al., 1997; Doerge & Chang, 2002). Besides the inhibitory effects of isoflavones on TPO, iodine deficiency is important risk factor for thyroid dysfunction and goiter development, both in humans and in rats. An adequate iodine supply is a way to prevent goitrogenic effects of soy bean isoflavones, especially in the high-risk group of patients with congenital hypothyroidism.

Besides the serum concentrations of TH, biological activity of T_3 on bone tissue is determined by the membrane transporters of TH, local expression and activity of deiodinase enzymes and receptors for TSH and TH. Polymorphisms in above mentioned genes are associated with important chronic skeletal diseases, including osteoporosis and osteoarthritis (Andersen et al., 2002, 2003; Peeters et al., 2006).

Entry of T_3 and T_4 into target cells is determined by the active uptake of free hormones by specific cell membrane transporters: monocarboxylate transporter-8 (MCT8), MCT10 and organic acid transporter protein-1c1 (OATP1c1) (van der Deure et al., 2010). MCT8 is expressed in growth plate chondrocytes, bone forming osteoblasts and bone resorbing osteoclasts at all stages of cell differentiation, and its expression is regulated by thyroid status (Capelo et al., 2009), although its functional importance is still unclear. It seems that OATP1c1 is not expressed in the mouse skeleton (Capelo et al., 2009), but there are still no data regarding expression of MCT10. Tyrosine kinase inhibitors sunitinib and imatinib inhibit MCT8 – mediated iodothyroinine transport (Schweizer et al., 2010), but there are still no data regarding possible effects of genistein, which is a potent thyrosine kinase inhibitor as well, on cellular transport of TH.

Deiodinase (Dio) enzymes determine the intracellular levels of bioactive T3 and thus cell-specific gene expression. Expression of deiodinases is tissue specific: Dio 1 enzyme is not expressed in bone, while Dio 2 plays an important role in local regulation of thyroid hormone signaling during fetal bone development. In the adult skeleton Dio 2 activity is restricted to osteoblasts (Williams et al., 2008). Dio 2 expression and activity are inhibited by high concentrations of substrate (T_4) and thus are maximal in hypothyroidism and suppressed in thyrotoxicosis. Locally regulated activity of Dio 2 in osteoblasts maintains intra-cellular T_3 concentrations constant over the euthyroid range and preserves optimal bone mineralization. Inactivating deiodinase type 3 (Dio 3) is expressed in the skeleton, although the highest levels of enzyme activity occur in growth plate chondrocytes prior to weaning (Yen, 2001). Genistein inhibit both Dio 1 and Dio 2 activity in vitro (Mori et al., 1996), but the physiological importance of this mechanism is still unclear.

Based on analyses of rare monogenic diseases and the results of animal studies, it was proposed that T_3 play a key role in bone development, while TSH is not required for normal skeletal development (Bassett et al., 2008). T_3 enters the nucleus and binds to its nuclear receptors (TR). There are three functional TRs: TRα1, TRβ1 and TRβ2, encoded by the THRA and THRB genes. These receptors act as hormone inducible transcription factors that regulate expression of T_3-responsive target genes (Yen, 2001). Both TRα1 and TRβ1 isoforms are expressed in bone and TRα1 levels are at least 10-fold greater than TRβ1. These findings support the opinion that TRα1 is the principal mediator of T_3 action in bone (Bassett & Williams, 2009; O'Shea et al., 2003).

In vitro experiments demonstrated that effects of T_3 in osteoblastic cell lines and primary osteoblast cultures depend on species, cell type, anatomic origin, differentiation phase and duration of the treatment. T_3 was reported to increase expression of osteocalcin, osteopontin, type I collagen, alkaline phosphatase, IGF-I and its regulatory binding proteins IGF1BP-2 and -4 (Milne et al., 2001; Pereira et al., 1999; Varga et al., 2004). Therefore, T_3 may exert its stimulatory effect on osteoblasts via complex pathways involving many growth factors and cytokines.

5.3.2 Phytoestrogens, thyroid hormones and osteoporosis prevention

Similar to osteoporosis, thyroid diseases are much more common in elderly women than in men and is associated with significant morbidity if left untreated (Schindler 2003; Suchartwatnachai et al., 2002). Still, this fact does not imply a causal relationship between the two diseases and many patients may independently develop both. Hypothyroidism occurs in 10% of females and 2% of males in patients older than 60 years. The prevalence of hyperthyroidism in the elderly is approximately 2% (Maugeri et al., 1996), though other authors reported that 10 to 15% of elderly patients were hyperthyroid (Kennedy & Caro, 1996). Thyrotoxicosis increase risk in developing secondary osteoporosis (Amashukeli et al., 2010; Lakatos, 2003).

Thyroid hormones play a significant role in maintaining adult bone homeostasis. Results of clinical and experimental studies are consistent and demonstrate that hypothyroid state slows down bone turnover and affect overall gain in bone mass and mineralization. By contrast, bone resorption and formation are accelerated in hyperthyroidism, while the remodeling cycle is shortened (Davies et al., 2005). Increased bone turnover and osteoporosis in thyrotoxicosis are attributed to the thyroid hormone excess and are not a consequence of deficient TSH receptor (TSHR) signaling. However, TSH may play a direct role in regulation of bone turnover, since TSH receptor was identified in osteoblasts. The experiment with ovariectomized rats, which were treated with low doses of TSH (insufficient to alter serum T_3, T_4 or TSH levels), demonstrated that TSH treatment prevented bone loss and increased bone mass (Sampath et al., 2007; Sun et al., 2008). Although the TSHR is expressed in osteoblasts, current data from in vitro studies are contradictory and suggest that TSH may enhance, inhibit or have no effect on osteoblast differentiation and function (Bassett et al., 2008).

Prevention and treatment of osteoporosis involve Ca and vitamin D supplementation, as well as different drug therapy approaches, which include bisphosphonate, salmon CT and estrogen or androgen replacement therapy for menopausal women and andropausal men, respectively. In addition, in recent years, numerous discussions on safety and benefit of synthetic steroids (both estrogens and androgens) favor the trend towards consumption of "green" natural "phytosteroids" or "phyto-selective modulator of ERs". That is why nutritional supplements and concentrated extracts containing purified soybean phyto-SERMs genistein and daidzein are increasingly used as alternative therapy for osteoporosis and other age-related diseases in both sexes (Ramos, 2007; Setchell, 1998; Tham et al., 1998). However, all these treatments may affect thyroid function as well.

Not so many researchers have tried to link effects of supplementation or drug treatment on bone metabolism with modulation of thyroid hormone levels. Rodents are considered useful models for thyroid studies, even though significant differences between rodent and human thyroid physiology have been reported (Choksi et al., 2003; Poirier et al., 1999). Rat thyrocytes are characterized by abundant granular endoplasmic reticulum, well developed Golgi, prominent lysosomes, luminal (apical) microvilli, small mitochondria, and round nuclei with homogeneous chromatin (Fig. 9).

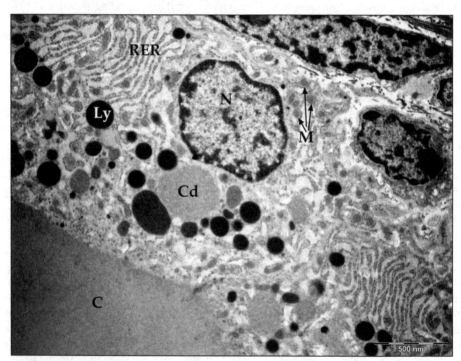

Fig. 9. Ultrastructure of thyroid follicular cell; nucleus (N), mitochondria (M), rough endoplasmatic reticulum (RER), lysosomes (Ly), colloidal droplets (Cd), colloid (C); unpublished image of Šošić-Jurjević et al.

In our laboratory we demonstrated that chronic Ca administration to middle-aged female rats significantly decreased the volume density of the thyroid follicular epithelium, epithelium's height and the index of activation rate, which are morphometric parameters of TH synthetic and secretory potential of thyrocytes (Šošić -Jurjević et al., 2002). Consistent with histomorphometric changes, reduced serum levels of total T_4 and T_3 were detected (Šošić -Jurjević et al., 2006). At the same time, we determined significant decrease of serum osteocalcin and urinary Ca, as biochemical parameters of reduced bone turnover after Ca treatment (unpublished data). In vitro studies with FTRL-5 cells demonstrated that Ca did not affect the morphology of these cells, but when administered together with TSH, it acted directly, by reducing the thyrotropin stimulatory effect (Gaberscek et al., 1998). Isoform VI of adenilyl cyclase, the enzyme crucial for TSH-induced activation of thyroid follicular cells, was found negatively modulated by Ca in human and dog thyroids (Vanvooren et al., 2000). Doses of Ca were chosen to mimic human exposure to high doses of Ca in treatment of osteoporosis. We can speculate that slowing down of thyroid hormone synthesis may be an indirect mechanism, which lead to decreased bone turnover detected after Ca treatment under our experimental conditions.

Sex steroids, estrogen and testosterone, play an important role in bone physiology and pathology. Endogenous estrogens are regularly produced in bone via aromatase enzyme activity, and exert their effects through ER, which are also detected in male bones (Carani et al., 1997; Grumbach & Auchus, 1999; Korach, 1994). Bone cells are sensitive to both estrogens and androgens, and aromatase inhibition causes similar degree of osteoporosis in male animals as orchidectomy (Vanderschueren et al., 1998).

There is a close relationship between sex steroids and thyroid function. Epidemiological studies suggest that the use of estrogens may contribute to the pathogenesis of thyroid tumors (Ron et al., 1987). Experimental studies on rodents demonstrated numerous sex-related differences in thyroid function and, in general, adult male rodents have higher levels of TSH than females associated with lower T_4 and higher plasma levels of T_3 (Capen, 1997). The results related to treatment effects of sex steroids on different set points of thyroid function are inconsistent and depend on experimental conditions: type of experimental animal, animal's age and applied dose (Chen & Wallfish, 1978; Henderson et al., 1982; Sekulić et al., 2007). Our previous results demonstrated an inhibitory effect of pharmacologic doses of estradiol (previously used in human studies for treatment of osteoporosis) on thyroid follicular cells in ovariectomized young adult and ovarium-intact young and middle-aged rats, (Sekulić et al., 2006; Šošić -Jurjević et al., 2005, 2006a), as well as after treatments of orchidectomized 16-month-old rat males with 10 times lesser dose of estradiol dipropionate (Sekulić et al., 2010). We choose the dose of estradiol in the experiment which was previously reported to prevent bone loss in males (Fitts et al., 2001; Vanderput et al., 2001). Consistent with literature data, we also detected decreased serum osteocalcin levels, accompanied by decreased urinary Ca concentration in Orx rats treated with EDP (unpublished data). Contrary to effects of estradiol, testosterone treatment of castrated middle-aged males moderately increased serum TSH and total T_4 levels (Sekulić et al., 2010), but similarly to estradiol treatment, decreased both serum osteocalcin levels and urinary Ca concentration (unpublished data). Therefore, it seems that the direct effect of sex steroids on bone tissue is more relevant for the net result of replacement therapy on bone protection then the indirect effect, mediated through modulation of thyroid function.

Direct negative effect of isoflavones on thyroid hormone synthesis, by significant blocking of TPO activity (more than 60%), has been well described. Genistein and daidzein were demonstrated to block both TPO-catalyzed reactions: iodination of thyrosine residues of Tg, and T_4 formation by coupling reactions, but this effect was eliminated by iodine (Chang & Doerge, 2000; Divi et al., 1997; Doerge & Chang 2002). Despite significant inactivation of this enzyme, serum thyroid hormone levels were unaffected by isoflavone treatments in young adult rats of both sexes. The authors supposed that soy could cause goiter, but only in animals or humans consuming diets marginally adequate in iodine, or who were predisposed to develop goiter. Most other authors, who performed their studies on young adult animals of both sexes, also reported that soy or isoflavones alone, in the absence of other goitrogenic stimulus, did not affect thyroid weights, histopathology and the serum levels of TSH and thyroid hormones (Chang & Doerge, 2000; Schmutzler et al., 2004). The thyroid function becomes impaired with aging in rodents, and the number of thyroid dysfunction increase in elderly population (Donda & Lemarchand-Béraud, 1989; Reymond et al., 1992). We were the first who demonstrated that therapeutic doses of both genistein and daidzein induce hypertrophy of Tg-immunopositive follicular epithelium and colloid depletion (Fig. 10), and reduce the level of serum thyroid hormones, accompanied by

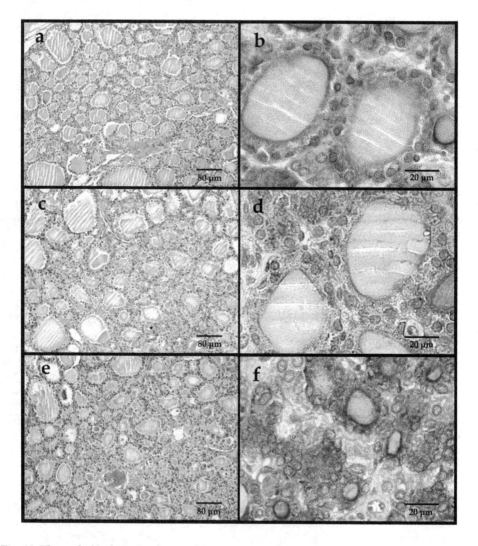

Fig. 10. Thyroid gland tissue of control (a, b), orchidectomized (c, d) and orchidectomized rats treated with daidzein (e, f); hematoxylin-eosin and immuno-staining for thyroglobulin; unpublished image of Šošić-Jurjević et al.

increased serum TSH, in orchidectomized (Orx) middle-aged male rats fed a iodine-sufficient soy-free diet (Šošić -Jurjević et al., 2010). Our research team obtained that both genistein and daidzein increased bone mass following orchidectomy of middle-aged males (Filipovic et al., 2010 and unpublished data). Therefore, decreased serum level of TH might contribute to the detected increase in trabecular bone mass, and decrease in bone turnover in aged male orchidectomized rat model.

6. Conclusion

Phytoestrogens have the potential to maintain bone health. Owing to their properties, these plant-derived non-steroidal compounds have a potential beneficial role in delaying or preventing osteoporosis. Therefore, they have attracted much attention as alternatives to HRT. As SERM, phytoestrogens may generate a bone protective effect via stimulation of osteoblastic bone formation and inhibition of osteoclastic bone resorption. Proposed molecular mechanisms are based on their ER-mediated effects. In addition to direct action, phytoestrogens can affect bone structure indirectly, by stimulating or inhibiting the synthesis of certain hormones, i.e. through increased synthesis of CT from thyroid C cells, as well as reduction of PTH and thyroid hormone levels.

7. Acknowledgment

This work was supported by the Ministry of Education and Science of the Republic of Serbia, Grant No. 173009. The authors express their gratitude to the late Dr Dana Brunner for her guidance and contribution, to Mrs. Anna Nikolić and Mr. Kristijan Jurjević for assistance with English manuscript preparation.

8. References

Abu, EO., Bord, S., Horner, A., Chatterjee, VK. & Compston, JE. (1997). The expression of thyroid hormone receptors in human bone. *Bone*, Vol. 21, pp. 137-142

Adlercreutz, H. (1998). Evolution, nutrition, intestinal microflora, and prevention of cancer: a hypothesis. *Proc Soc Exp Biol Med*, Vol. 217, pp. 241–246

Amashukeli, M., Giorgadze, E., Tsagareli, M., Nozadze, N. & Jeiranashvili, N. (2010). The impact of thyroid diseases on bone metabolism and fracture risk. *Georgian Med News*, Vol. 184-185, pp. 34-39

Andersen, S., Bruun, NH., Pedersen, KM. & Laurberg, P. (2003). Biologic variation is important for interpretation of thyroid function tests. *Thyroid*, Vol. 13, pp. 1069-1078

Andersen, S., Pedersen, KM., Bruun, NH. & Laurberg, P. (2002). Narrow individual variations in serum T(4) and T(3) in normal subjects: a clue to the understanding of subclinical thyroid disease. *J Clin Endocrinol Metab*, Vol. 87, pp. 1068-1072

Anderson, JJ., Chen, X., Boass, A., Symons, M., Kohlmeier, M., Renner, JB. & Garner, SC. (2002). Soy isoflavones: no effects on bone mineral content and bone mineral density in healthy, menstruating young adult women after one year. *J Am Coll Nutr*, Vol. 21, pp. 388–393

Aoki, K., Didomenico, E., Sims, NA., Mukhopadhyay, K., Neff, L., Houghton, A., Amling, M., Levy, JB., Horne, WC. & Baron, R. (1999). The tyrosine phosphatase SHP-1 is a negative regulator of osteoclastogenesis and osteoclast resorbing activity: Increased resorption and osteopenia in mev/mev mutant mice. Bone, Vol. 25, pp. 261-267

Arjmandi, BH., Khalil, DA. & Hollis, BW. (2002). Soy protein: its effects on intestinal calcium transport, serum vitamin D, and insulin-like growth factor-I in ovariectomized rats. Calcif Tissue Int, Vol. 70, pp. 483-487

Arjmandi, BH., Lucas, EA., Khalil, DA., Devareddy, L., Smith, BJ., McDonald, J., Arquitt, AB., Payton, ME. & Mason, C. (2005). One year soy protein supplementation has positive effects on bone formation markers but not bone density in postmenopausal women. Nutr J, Vol. 4, pp. 8

Arts, J., Kuiper, GG., Janssen, JM., Gustafsson, JA., Lowik, CW., Pols, HA. & van Leeuwen, JP. (1997). Differential expression of estrogen receptors alpha and beta mRNA during differentiation of human osteoblast SV-HFO cells. Endocrinology, Vol. 138, pp. 5067- 5070

Atmaca, A., Kleerekoper, M., Bayraktar, M. & Kucuk, O. (2008). Soy isoflavones in the management of postmenopausal osteoporosis. Menopause, Vol. 15, pp. 748–757

Bahr, JM., Nakai, M., Rivera, A., Walsh, J., Evans, GL., Lotinun, S., Turner, RT., Black, M. & Jeffery, EH. (2005). Dietary soy protein and isoflavones: minimal effects on bone and no effect on the reproductive tract of sexually mature ovariectomized Sprague-Dawley rats. Menopause, Vol. 12, pp. 165-173

Bassett, JH. & Williams, GR. (2003). The molecular actions of thyroid hormone in bone.Trends Endocrinol Metab, Vol. 14, pp. 356-164

Bassett, JH., Williams, AJ., Murphy, E., Boyde, A., Howell, PG., Swinhoe. R., Archanco, M., Flamant , F., Samarut, J., Costagliola, S., Vassart, G., Weiss, RE., Refetoff, S. & Williams, GR. (2008). A lack of thyroid hormones rather than excess thyrotropin causes abnormal skeletal development in hypothyroidism. Mol Endocrinol, Vol. 22, pp. 501-512

Bassett, JH. & Williams, GR. (2009). The skeletal phenotypes of TRalpha and TRbeta mutant mice. J Mol Endocrinol, Vol. 42, pp. 269-282

Bianco, P., Riminucci, M., Gronthos, S. & Robey, PG. (2001). Bone marrow stromal stem cells: nature, biology, and potential applications. Stem Cells, Vol. 19, pp. 180-192

Blair, HC., Jordan, SE., Peterson, TG. & Barnes, S. (1996). Variable effects of tyrosine kinase inhibitors on avian osteoclastic activity and reduction of bone loss in ovariectomized rats. J Cell Biochem, Vol. 61, pp. 629-637

Blum, SC., Heaton, SN., Bowman, BM., Hegsted, M. & Miller, SC. (2003). Dietary soy protein maintains some indices of bone mineral density and bone formation in ovariectomized rats. J Nutr, Vol. 133, pp. 1244-1249

Branca, F. (2003). Dietary phyto-oestrogens and bone health. Proc Nutr Soc, Vol. 62, pp. 877–887

Brink, E., Coxam, V., Robins, S., Wahala, K., Cassidy, A. & Branca, F. (2008). Long-term consumption of isoflavone-enriched foods does not affect bone mineral density, bone metabolism, or hormonal status in early postmenopausal women: a randomized, double-blind, placebo controlled study. Am J Clin Nutr, Vol. 87, pp. 761–770

Canalis, E., McCarthy, T. & Centrella, M. (1988). Growth factors and the regulation of bone remodeling. J Clin Invest, Vol. 81, pp. 277-281

Canalis, E., Pash, J. & Varghese, S. (1993). Skeletal growth factors. *Crit Rev Eukaryot Gene Expr*, Vol. 3, pp. 155-166

Canalis, E., Pash, J., Gabbitas, B., Rydziel, S. & Varghese, S. (1993a). Growth factors regulate the synthesis of insulin-like growth factor-I in bone cell cultures. *Endocrinology*, Vol. 133, pp. 33-38

Capelo, LP., Beber, EH., Fonseca, TL. & Gouveia, CH. (2009). The monocarboxylate transporter 8 and L-type amino acid transporters 1 and 2 are expressed in mouse skeletons and in osteoblastic MC3T3-E1 cells. *Thyroid*, Vol. 19, pp. 171-178

Capen, C. (1997). Mehanicistic data and risk assesment of selected toxic end points of the thyroid gland. *Toxicologic Pathology*, Vol. 25, pp. 39-48

Carani, C., Qin, K., Simoni, M., Faustini-Fustini, M., Serpente, S., Boyd, J., Korach, KS. & Simpson, ER. (1997). Effect of testosterone and estradiol in a man with aromatase deficiency. *N Engl J Med*, Vol. 337, pp. 91-95

Chang, HC. & Doerge, DR. (2000). Dietary genistein inactivates rat thyroid peroxidase in vivo without an apparent hypothyroid effect. *Toxicol Appl Pharmacol*, Vol. 168, pp. 244-252

Chen, D., Zhao, M. & Mundy, GR. (2004). Bone morphogenetic proteins. *Growth Factors*, Vol. 22, 233-241

Chen, HJ. & Walfish, PG. (1978). Effects of estradiol benzoate on thyroid-pituitary function in female rats. *Endocrinology*, Vol. 103, pp. 1023-1030

Chen, JJ. & Chang, HC. (2007). By modulating androgen receptor coactivators, daidzein may act as a phytoandrogen. *Prostate*, Vol. 67, pp. 457-462

Chen, WF. & Wong, MS. (2006). Genistein modulates the effects of parathyroid hormone in human osteoblastic SaOS-2 cells. *Br J Nutr*, Vol. 95, pp. 1039-1047

Chen, XW., Garner, SC., Quarles, LD. & Anderson, JJB. (2003). Effects of genistein on expression cell of bone markers during MC3T3-E1 osteoblastic differentiation. *J Nutr Biochem*, Vol. 14, pp. 342–349

Choksi, NY., Jahnke, GD., St Hilaire, C. & Shelby, M. (2003). Role of thyroid hormones in human and laboratory animal reproductive health. Birth Defects *Res B Dev Reprod Toxicol*, Vol. 68, pp. 479-491

Chorazy, PA., Himelhoch, S., Hopwood, NJ., Greger, NG. & Postellon, DC. (1995). Persistent hypothyroidism in an infant receiving a soy formula: case report and review of the literature. *Pediatrics*, Vol. 96, pp. 148-150

Collin-Osdoby, P., Rothe, L., Anderson, F., Nelson, M., Maloney, W. & Osdoby, P. (2001). Receptor activator of NF-kappa B and osteoprotegerin expression by human microvascular endothelial cells, regulation by inflammatory cytokines, and role in human osteoclastogenesis. *J Biol Chem*, Vol. 276, pp. 20659– 20672

Comelekoglu, U., Bagis, S., Yalin, S., Ogenler, O., Yildiz, A., Sahin, NO., Oguz, I. & Hatungil, R. (2007). Biomechanical evaluation in osteoporosis: ovariectomized rat model. *Clin Rheumatol*, Vol. 26, pp. 380-384

Dang, ZC., Audinot, V., Papapoulos, SE., Boutin, JA. & Lowik, C. (2003). Peroxisome proliferator-activated receptor gamma (PPAR gamma) as a molecular target for the soy phytoestrogen genistein. *J Biol Chem*, Vol. 278, pp. 962–967

Dang, ZC. & Lowik, C. (2004). The balance between concurrent activation of ERs and PPARs determines daidzein-induced osteogenesis and adipogenesis. *J Bone Miner Res*, Vol. 19, pp. 853–861

Davies, J., Warwick, J., Totty, N., Philp, R., Helfrich, M. & Horton, M. (1989). The osteoclast functional antigen, implicated in the regulation of bone resorption, is biochemically related to the vitronectin receptor. *J Cell Biol*, Vol. 109, pp. 1817-1826

Davies, TF, Ando, T., Lin, RY., Tomer, Y. & Latif, R. (2005). Thyrotropin receptor-associated diseases: from adenomata to Graves disease. *J Clin Invest*, Vol. 115, pp. 1972-1983

Davison, S. & Davis, SR. (2003). Hormone replacement therapy: current controversies. *Clin Endocrinology*, Vol. 58, pp. 249–261

DeWilde, A., Lieberherr, M., Colin, C. & Pointillart, A. (2004). A low dose of daidzein acts as an ER beta-selective agonist in trabecular osteoblasts of young female piglets. *J Cell Physiol*, Vol. 200, pp. 253–262

Divi, RL., Chang, HC. & Doerge, DR. (1997). Anti-thyroid isoflavones from soybean: isolation, characterization, and mechanisms of action. *Biochem Pharmacol*, Vol. 54, pp. 1087-1096

Doerge, DR. & Chang, HC. (2002). Inactivation of thyroid peroxidase by soy isoflavones, in vitro and in vivo. *J Chromatogr B Analyt Technol Biomed Life Sc*, Vol. 777, pp. 269-279

Donda, A. & Lemarchand-Béraud, T. (1989). Aging alters the activity of 5'-deiodinase in the adenohypophysis, thyroid gland, and liver of the male rat. *Endocrinology*. Vol. 124, pp. 1305-1309

Eriksen, EF., Hodgson, SF., Eastell, R., Cedel, SL., O'Fallon, WM. & Riggs, BL. (1990). Cancellous bone remodeling in type I (postmenopausal) osteoporosis: quantitative assessment of rates of formation, resorption, and bone loss at tissue and cellular levels. *J Bone Miner Res*, Vol. 5, pp. 311-319

Erlandsson, MC., Islander, U., Moverare, S., Ohlsson, C. & Carlsten, H. (2005). Estrogenic agonism and antagonism of the soy isoflavone genistein in uterus, bone and lymphopoiesis in mice. *APMIS*, Vol. 113, pp. 317-323

Farley, JR., Tarbaux, NM., Hall, SL., Linkhart, TA. & Baylink, DJ. (1988). The anti-bone-resorptive agent calcitonin also acts in vitro to directly increase bone formation and bone cell proliferation. *Endocrinology*, Vol. 123, pp. 159-167

Farley, JR., Hall, SL., Herring, S. & Tarbaux, NM. (1992). Two biochemical indices of mouse bone formation are increased, in vivo, in response to calcitonin. *Calcif Tissue Int*, Vol. 50, pp. 67–73

Farley, J., Dimai, HP., Stilt-Coffing, B., Farley, P., Pham, T. & Mohan, S. (2000). Calcitonin increases the concentration of insulin-like growth factors in serum-free cultures of human osteoblast-line cells. *Calcif Tissue Int*, Vol. 67, pp. 247–254

Filipović, B., Šošić -Jurjević, B., Manojlović-Stojanoski, M., Nestorović, N., Milošević, V. & Sekulić, M. (2002). The effect of ovariectomy on thyroid C cells of adult rats. *Yugoslov Med Biohem*, Vol. 21, pp. 345-350

Filipović, B., Šošić -Jurjević, B., Nestorović, N., Manojlović Stojanoski, M., Kostić N., Milošević, V. & Sekulić M. (2003). The thyroid C cells of ovariectomized rats treated with estradiol. *Histochem Cell Biol*, Vol. 120, pp. 409-414

Filipović, B., Šošić -Jurjević, B., Manojlović Stojanoski, M., Nestorović, N., Milošević V. & Sekulić M. (2005). The effect of chronic calcium treatment on thyroid C cells in ovariectomized rats. *Life Sci*, Vol. 77, pp. 121-129

Filipović, B., Šošić -Jurjević, B., Ajdžanović, V., Trifunović, S., Manojlović Stojanoski, M., Ristić, N., Nestorović, N., Milošević, V. & Sekulić M. (2007) The effect of orchidectomy on thyroid C cells and bone histomorphometry in middle-aged rats. *Histochem Cell Biol*, Vol. 128, pp. 153–159

Filipović, B., Šošić -Jurjević, B., Ajdzanović, V., Brkić, D., Manojlović-Stojanoski, M., Milosević, V. & Sekulić M. (2010). Daidzein administration positively affects thyroid C cells and bone structure in orchidectomized middle-aged rats. *Osteoporos Int*, Vol. 21, pp. 1609-1616

Filipović B., Šošić -Jurjević B., Ajdžanović V., Pantelić J., Nestorović N. & Sekulić M. Estardiol effects the function of neuroendocrine C cells in orchidectomized middle-aged rat thyroid gland. (2010a). *The 7th International Congress of Neuroendocrinology*, p. 180, Rouen, France, July 11-15, 2010

Fitts, JM., Klein, RM. & Powers, CA. (2001). Estrogen and tamoxifen interplay with T(3) in male rats: pharmacologically distinct classes of estrogen responses affecting growth, bone, and lipid metabolism, and their relation to serum GH and IGF-I. *Endocrinology*, Vol. 142, pp. 4223-4235

Fonseca, D. & Ward, WE. (2004). Daidzein together with high calcium preserve bone mass and biomechanical strength at multiple sites in ovariectomized mice. *Bone*, Vol. 35, pp. 489-497

Frost, HM. (1964). Dynamics of bone remodeling. In: *Frost HM (ed) Bone Biodynamics. Littel, Brown, Boston*, pp 315-333

Fuller, K., Wong, B., Fox, S., Choi, Y. & Chambers, TJ. (1998). TRANCE is necessary and sufficient for osteoblast-mediated activation of bone resorption in osteoclasts. *J Exp Med*, Vol. 188, pp. 997– 1001

Gaberscek, S., Stiblar-Martincic, D. & Kalisnik, M. (1998). The influence of calcium on thyroid follicular cells FRTL-5 in vitro. *Folia Biol (Praha)*, Vol. 44, pp. 49-52

Gao, YH. & Yamaguchi, M. (1999). Suppressive effect of genistein on rat bone osteoclasts: apoptosis is induced through Ca2+ signaling. *Biol Pharm Bull*, Vol. 22, pp. 805–809

Gao, YH. & Yamaguchi, M. (2000) Suppressive effect of genistein on rat bone osteoclasts: involvement of protein kinase inhibition and protein tyrosine phosphatase activation. *Int J Mol Med*, Vol. 5, pp. 261-267

Geppert, J., Baier, S., Zehn, N., Gouni-Berthold, I., Berthold, HK., Reinsberg, J. & Stehle, P. (2004). Short-term effects of high soy supplementation on sex hormones, bone markers, and lipid parameters in young female adults. *Eur J Nutr*, Vol. 43, pp. 100–108

Giampietro, PG., Bruno, G., Furcolo, G., Casati, A., Brunetti, E., Spadoni, GL. & Galli, E. (2004). Soy protein formulas in children: no hormonal effects in long-term feeding. *J Pediatr Endocrinol Metab*, Vol. 17, pp. 191-196

Globus, RK., Plouet, J. & Gospodarowicz, D. (1989). Cultured bovine bone cells synthesize basic fibroblast growth factor and store it in their extracellular matrix. *Endocrinology*, Vol. 124, pp. 1539-1547

Gogakos, AI., Duncan Bassett, JH. & Williams, GR. (2010). Thyroid and bone. *Arch Biochem Biophys*, Vol. 503, pp. 129-136

Grauer, A., Klein, P., Naveh-Many, T., Silver, J., Ziegler, R. & Raue, F. (1993). Diminished calcitonin secretion after ovariectomy without apparent reduction in calcitonin content in the rat. *Horm Metab Res*, Vol. 25, pp. 389-390

Grumbach, MM. & Auchus, RJ. (1999). Estrogen: consequences and implications of human mutations in synthesis and action. *J Clin Endocrinol Metab*, Vol. 84, pp. 4677-4694

Ham, KD. & Carlson CS. (2004). Effects of estrogen replacement therapy on bone turnover in subchondral bone and epiphyseal metaphyseal cancellous bone of ovariectomized cynomolgus monkeys. *J Bone Miner Res*, Vol. 19, pp. 823-829

Henderson, KM., McNeilly, AS. & Swanston, IA. (1982). Gonadotrophin and steroid concentrations in bovine follicular fluid and their relationship to follicle size. *J Reprod Fertil*, Vol. 65, pp. 467-473

Ho, SC., Woo, J., Lam, S., Chen, YM., Sham, A. & Lau, J. (2003). Soy protein consumption and bone mass in early postmenopausal Chinese women. *Osteoporos Int*, Vol. 14, pp. 835-842

Hsu, HL., Lacey, DL., Dunstan, CR., Solovyev, I., Colombero, A., Timms, E., Tan, HL., Elliott, G., Kelley, MJ., Sarosi, I., Wang, L., Xia, XZ., Elliott, R., Chiu, L., Black, T., Scully, S., Capparelli, C., Morony, S., Shimamoto, G., Bass, MB. & Boyle, WJ. (1999). Tumor necrosis factor receptor family member RANK mediates osteoclast differentiation and activation induced by osteoprotegerin ligand. *Proc Nat Acad Sci*, Vol. 96, pp. 3540-3545

Huang, YF., Cao, SM., Nagamani, M., Anderson, KE., Grady, JJ. & Lu, LJW. (2005). Decreased circulating levels of tumor necrosis factor-alpha in postmenopausal women during consumption of soy-containing isoflavones. *J Clin Endocr Metab*, Vol. 90, pp. 3956-3962

Huang, HY., Yang, HP., Yang, HT., Yang, TC., Shieh, MJ. & Huang, SY. (2006). One-year soy isoflavone supplementation prevents early postmenopausal bone loss but without a dosedependent effect. *J Nutr Biochem*, Vol. 17, pp. 509-517

Hunter, SJ., Schraer, H. & Gay, CV. (1989). Characterization of the cytoskeleton of isolated chick osteoclasts: effect of calcitonin. *J Histochem Cytochem*, Vol. 37, pp. 1529-1537

Ikeda, T., Nishikawa, A., Imazawa, T., Kimura, S. & Hirose, M. (2000). Dramatic synergism between excess soybean intake and iodine deficiency on the development of rat thyroid hyperplasia. *Carcinogenesis*, Vol. 21, pp. 707-713

Isaia, GC., Campagnoli, C., Mussetta, M., Massobrio, M., Salamono, G., Gallio, M. & Molinatti, GM. (1989). Calcitonin and lumbar bone mineral content during oestrogen-progesterone administration in postmenopausal women. *Maturitas*, Vol. 11, pp. 287-294

Isaia, GC., Mussetta, M., Massobrio, M., Sciolla, A., Gallio, M. & Molinatti, GM. (1992). Influence of estrogens on calcitonin secretion. *J Endocrinol Invest*, Vol. 15, pp. 59-62

Ishimi, Y., Miyaura, C., Ohmura, M., Onoe, Y., Sato, T., Uchiyama, Y., Ito, M., Wang, X., Suda, T. & Ikegami, S. (1999). Selective effects of genistein, a soybean isoflavone, on B-lymphopoiesis and bone loss caused by estrogen deficiency. *Endocrinology*, Vol. 140, pp. 1893-1900

Ishimi, Y., Yoshida, M., Wakimoto, S., Wu, J., Chiba, H., Wang, X Takeda, K. & Miyaura C. (2002). Genistein, a soybean isoflavone, affects bone marrow lymphopoiesis and prevents bone loss in castrated male mice. *Bone*, Vol. 31, pp. 180-185

Ito, N., Yamazaki, H., Nakazaki, M., Miyahara, T., Kozuka, H. & Sudo, H. (1987). Response of osteoblastic clonal cell line (MC3T3-E1) to [Asu]eel calcitonin at a specific cell density or differentiation stage. *Calcif Tissue Int*, Vol. 40, pp. 200–205

Jabbar, MA., Larrea, J. & Shaw, RA. (1997). Abnormal thyroid function tests in infants with congenital hypothyroidism: the influence of soy-based formula. *J Am Coll Nutr*, Vol. 16, pp. 280-282

Jia, TL., Wang, HZ., Xie, LP., Wang, XY. & Zhang, RQ. (2003). Daidzein enhances osteoblast growth that may be mediated by increased bone morphogenetic protein (BMP) production. *Biochem Pharmacol*, Vol. 65, pp. 709–715

Kanis, JA., Aaron, JE., Evans, D., Thavarajah, M. & Beneton, M. (1990). Bone loss and age-related fractures. *Exp Gerontol*, Vol. 25, pp. 289-296

Katagiri, T. & Takahashi, N. (2002). Regulatory mechanisms of osteoblast and osteoclast differentiation. *Oral Dis*, Vol. 8, pp. 147– 159

Kennedy, JW. & Caro, JF. (1996). The ABC of managing hyperthyroidism in the older patient. *Geriatrics*, Vol. 51, pp. 22-32

Khalil, DA., Lucas, EA., Smith, BJ., Soung, DY., Devareddy, L., Juma, S., Akhter, MP., Recker, R. & Arjmandi, BH. (2005). Soy isoflavones may protect against orchidectomy-induced bone loss in aged male rats. *Calcif Tissue Int.* Vol. 76, pp. 56–62

Khosla, S., Atkinson, EJ., Melton, LJ III. & Riggs, BL. (1997). Effects of age and estrogen status on serum parathyroid hormone levels and biochemical markers of bone turnover in women: a populationbased study. *J Clin Endocrinol Metab*, Vol. 82, pp. 1522–1527

Kim, CH., Takai, E., Zhou, H., von Stechow, D., Müller, R., Dempster, DW. & Guo, XE. (2003). Trabecular bone response to mechanical and parathyroid hormone stimulation: the role of mechanical microenvironment. *J Bone Miner Res*, Vol. 18, pp. 2116-2125

Kimura, S., Suwa, J., Ito, M. (1976). Sato, H. Development of malignant goiter by defatted soybean with iodine-free diet in rats. *Gann*, Vol. 67, pp. 763-765

Korach, KS. (1994). Insights from the study of animals lacking functional estrogen receptor. *Science*, Vol. 266, pp. 1524-1527

Kuiper, GG., Lemmen, JG., Carlsson, B., Corton, JC., Safe, SH., van der Saag, PT., van der Burg, B. & Gustafsson, JA. (1998). Interaction of estrogenic chemicals and phytoestrogens with estrogen receptor beta. *Endocrinology*, Vol. 139, pp. 4252–4263

Kuiper, GG., Lemmen, JG., Carlsson, B., Corton, JC., Safe, SH., van der Saag, PT., van der Burg, B. & Gustafsson, JA. (1998). Interaction of estrogenic chemicals and phytoestrogens with estrogen receptor beta. *Endocrinology*, Vol. 139, pp. 4252–4263

Kung, AWC. (1994). The effect of thyroid hormone on bone metabolism and osteoporosis. *J Hong Kong Med Assoc*, Vol. 46, pp. 247-251

Lakatos, P. (2003). Thyroid hormones: beneficial or deleterious for bone? *Calcif Tissue Int*, Vol. 73, pp. 205-209

Lee, CA. & Einhorn, T. (2001). In: *Osteoporosis*, edited by Marcus, Feldman & Kelsey, pp. 3-20

Lee, YB., Lee, HJ., Kim, KS., Lee, JY., Nam, SY., Cheon, SH. & Sohn HS. (2004). Evaluation of the preventive effect of isoflavone extract on bone loss in ovariectomized rats. *Bioscience, Biotechnology and Biochemistry*, Vol. 68, pp. 1040-1045

Li, BB. & Yu, SF. (2003). Genistein prevents bone resorption diseases by inhibiting bone resorption and stimulating bone formation. *Biol Pharm Bull*, Vol. 26, pp. 780–786

Lindsay, R., Hart, DM., Aitken, JM., MacDonald, ED., Anderson, JB. & Clarke, AC. (1976). Long-term prevention of postmenopausal osteoporosis by oestrogen. *Lancet*, Vol. 1, pp. 1038–1041

Lindsay, R., Hart, DM. & Clark, DM. (1984). The minimum effective dose of estrogen for prevention of postmenopausal bone loss. *Obstet Gynecol*, Vol. 63, pp. 759–763

Loughlin, K. & Richie, J. (1997). Prostate cancer after exogenous testosterone treatment for impotence. *J Urology*, Vol. 157, pp.1845

Lu, CC., Tsai, SC., Chien, EJ., Tsai, CL. & Wang, PS. (2000). Age-related differences in the secretion of calcitonin in male rats. *Metabolism*, Vol. 49, pp. 253–258

Lydeking-Olsen, E., Beck-Jensen, JE., Setchell, KD. & Holm-Jensen, T. (2004). Soymilk or progesterone for prevention of bone loss: a 2 year randomized, placebo- ontrolled trial. *Eur J Nutr*. Vol. 43, pp. 246–257

Maugeri, D., Salvatore Russo, M., Carnazzo, G., Di Stefano, F., Catanzaro, S., Campagna, S., Romano, G., Franze, C., Motta, M., Panebianco, P. (1996). Altered laboratory thyroid parameters indicating hyperthyroidism in elderly subjects. *Arch Gerontol Geriatr*, Vol. 22, pp. 145-153

McCarrison, R. (1993). A Paper on FOOD AND GOITRE. *Br Med J*, Vol. 14, pp. 671-675

Mei, J., Yeung, SS. & Kung, AW. (2001). High dietary phytoestrogen intake is associated with higher bone mineral density in postmenopausal but not premenopausal women. *J Clin Endocrinol Metab*, Vol. 86, pp. 5217-5221

Milne, M., Quail, JM., Rosen, CJ. & Baran, DT. (2001). Insulin-like growth factor binding proteins in femoral and vertebral bone marrow stromal cells: expression and regulation by thyroid hormone and dexamethasone. *J Cell Biochem*, Vol. 81, pp. 229-240

Mori, K., Stone, S., Braverman, LE. & Devito, WJ. (1996). Involvement of tyrosine phosphorylation in the regulation of 5'-deiodinases in FRTL-5 rat thyroid cells and rat astrocytes. *Endocrinology*, Vol. 137, pp. 1313-1318

Mundy, GR. (1995). Local control of bone formation by osteoblasts. *Clin Orthop Relat Res*, Vol. 313, pp. 19-26

Nakai, M., Cook, L., Pyter, LM., Black, M., Sibona, J., Turner, RT., Jeffery, EH. & Bahr, JM. (2005). Dietary soy protein and isoflavones have no significant effect on bone and a potentially negative effect on the uterus of sexually mature intact Sprague-Dawley female rats. *Menopause*, Vol. 12, pp. 291-298

Nelson, HD., Humphrey, LL., Nygren, P., Teutsch, SM. & Allan, JD. (2002). Postmenopausal hormone replacement therapy: scientific review. *JAMA*, Vol. 288, pp. 872-881

Newton, KM., LaCroix, AZ., Levy, L., Li, SS., Qu, P., Potter, JD. & Lampe, JW. (2006) Soy protein and bone mineral density in older men and women: a randomized trial. *Maturitas*, Vol. 55, pp. 270–277

Okamoto, F., Okabe, K. & Kajiya, H. (2001). Genistein, a soybean isoflavone, inhibits inward rectifier K+ channels in rat osteoclasts. *Jap J Physiol*, Vol. 51, pp. 501–509

Okura, A., Arakawa, H., Oka, H., Yoshinari, T. & Monden, Y. (1998). Effect of genistein on topoisomerase activity and on the growth of [val 12] Ha-ras transformed NIH 3T3 cells. *Biochem Biophys Res Commun*, Vol. 157, pp. 183-189

Om, AS. & Shim, JY. (2007). Effect of daidzein, a soy isoflavone, on bone metabolism in Cd-treated ovariectomized rats. *Acta Biochim Pol*, Vol. 54, pp. 641-646

Onoe, Y., Miyaura, C., Ohta, H., Nozawa, S. & Suda, T. (1997). Expression of estrogen receptor in rat bone. *Endocrinology*, Vol. 138, pp. 4509-4512

O'Shea, PJ., Harvey, CB., Suzuki, H., Kaneshige, M., Kaneshige, K., Cheng, SY. & Williams, GR. (2003). A thyrotoxic skeletal phenotype of advanced bone formation in mice with resistance to thyroid hormone. *Mol Endocrinol*, Vol. 17, pp. 1410-1424

Pan, W., Quarles, LD., Song, LH., Yu, YH., Jiao, C., Tang, HB., Jiang, CH., Deng, HW., Li, YJ., Zhou, HH. & Xiao, ZS. (2005). Genistein stimulates the osteoblastic differentiation via NO/cGMP in bone marrow culture. *J Cell Biochem*, Vol. 94, pp. 307-316

Pantelić, J., Filipović, B., Šošić -Jurjević, B., Medigović, I. & Sekulić, M. (2010). Effects of testosterone and estradiol treatment on bone histomorphometry in orchidectomized middle-aged rats. *Proceedings of 4th Serbian Congress for Microscopy*, pp. 143-144, Belgrade, Serbia, October 11-12, 2010

Patisaul, HB. & Jefferson, W. (2010). The pros and cons of phytoestrogens. *Front Neuroendocrinol*, Vol. 31, pp. 400-419

Peeters, RP., van der Deure, WM. & Visser, TJ. (2006). Genetic variation in thyroid hormone pathway genes; polymorphisms in the TSH receptor and the iodothyronine deiodinases. *Eur J Endocrinol*, Vol. 155, pp. 655-662

Pereira, RC., Jorgetti, V. & Canalis, E. (1999). Triiodothyronine induces collagenase-3 and gelatinase B expression in murine osteoblasts. *Am J Physiol*, Vol. 77, pp. E496-E504

Picherit, C., Bennetau-Pelissero, C., Chanteranne, B., Lebecque, P., Davicco, MJ., Barlet, JP. & Coxam, V. (2001). Soybean isoflavones dose-dependently reduce bone turnover but do not reverse established osteopenia in adult ovariectomized rats. *J Nutr*, Vol. 131, pp. 723-728

Poirier, LA., Doerge, DR., Gaylor, DW, Miller, MA, Lorentzen, RJ., Casciano, DA., Kadlubar, FF. & Schwetz, BA. (1999). An FDA review of sulfamethazine toxicity. *Regul Toxicol Pharmacol*, Vol. 30 pp. 217-222

Ramos, S. (2007). Effects of dietary flavonoids on apoptotic pathways related to cancer chemoprevention. *J Nutr Biochem*, Vol. 18, pp. 427-442

Rassi, CM., Lieberherr, M., Chaumaz, G., Pointillart, A. & Cournot, G. (2002). Down-regulation of osteoclast differentiation by daidzein via caspase 3. *J Bone Miner Res*, Vol. 17, pp. 630-638

Register, TC., Jayo, MJ. & Anthony, MS. (2003). Soy phytoestrogens do not prevent bone loss in postmenopausal monkeys. *J Clin Endocrinol Metab*, Vol. 88, pp. 4362-4370

Rehman, HU. & Masson, EA. (2005). Neuroendocrinology of female aging. *Gender Medicine*, Vol. 2, pp. 41-56

Reinholt, FP., Hultenby, K., Oldberg, A. & Heinegård, D. (1990). Osteopontin--a possible anchor of osteoclasts to bone. *Proc Natl Acad Sci U S A*, Vol. 87, pp. 4473-4475

Ren, P., Ji, H., Shao, Q., Chen, X., Han, J. & Sun, Y. (2007).Protective effects of sodium daidzein sulfonate on trabecular bone in ovariectomized rats. *Pharmacology*, Vol. 79, pp. 129-136

Reymond, F., Dénéréaz, N. & Lemarchand-Béraud, T. (1992). Thyrotropin action is impaired in the thyroid gland of old rats. *Acta Endocrinol (Copenh)*, Vol. 126, pp. 55-63

Rivkees, SA., Bode, HH. & Crawford, JD. (1988). Long-term growth in juvenile acquired hypothyroidism: the failure to achieve normal adult stature. *N Engl J Med*, Vol. 318, pp. 599-602

Rizzoli, R., Poser, J. & Bürgi, U. (1986). Nuclear thyroid hormone receptors in cultured bone cells. *Metabolism*, Vol. 35, pp. 71-74

Roef, G., Lapauw, B., Goemaere, S., Zmierczak, H., Fiers, T., Kaufman, J.M. & Taes Y. (2011). Thyroid hormone status within the physiological range affects bone mass and density in healthy men at the age of peak bone mass. *Eur J Endocrinol*, Vol. 164, pp. 1027-1034

Ron, E., Kleinerman, RA., Boice, JDJr., LiVolsi, VA., Flannery, JT. & Fraumeni, JFJr. (1987). A population-based case-control study of thyroid cancer. *J Natl Cancer Inst*, Vol. 79, pp. 1-12

Rydziel, S., Shaikh, S. & Canalis, E. (1994). Platelet-derived growth factor-AA and -BB (PDGF-AA and -BB) enhance the synthesis of PDGF-AA in bone cell cultures. *Endocrinology*, Vol. 134, pp. 2541-2546

Sakai, K., Yamada, S. & Yamada, K. (2000). Effect of ovariectomy on parafollicular cells in the rat. *Okajimas Folia Anat Jpn*, Vol. 76, pp. 311–319

Sampath, TK., Simic, P., Sendak, R., Draca, N., Bowe, AE., O'Brien, S., Schiavi, SC., McPherson, JM. & Vukicevic, S. (2007). Thyroid-stimulating hormone restores bone volume, microarchitecture, and strength in aged ovariectomized rats. *J Bone Miner Res*, Vol. 22, pp. 849-859

Schindler, AE. (2003). Thyroid function and postmenopause. *Gynecol* Endocrinol, Vol. 17, pp. 79-85

Schmutzler, C., Hamann, I., Hofmann, PJ., Kovacs, G., Stemmler, L., Mentrup, B., Schomburg, L., Ambrugger, P., Grüters, A., Seidlova-Wuttke, D., Jarry, H., Wuttke, W. & Köhrle, J. (2004). Endocrine active compounds affect thyrotropin and thyroid hormone levels in serum as well as endpoints of thyroid hormone action in liver, heart and kidney. *Toxicology*, Vol. 205, pp. 95-102

Schweizer, U., Braun, D., Köhrle, J. & Hershman J. (2010). Tyrosine kinase inhibitors non – competitively inhibit MCT8-mediated iodothyronine transport. 14th International Thyroid Congress, Paris, 11-16 September, LB-12

Sekulić, M., Šošić -Jurjević, B., Filipović, B., Milošević, V., Nestorović, N. & Manojlović-Stojanoski, M. (2005). The effects of synthetic salmon calcitonin on thyroid C and follicular cells in adult female rats. *Folia Histochem Cytobiol*. Vol. 43, pp. 103-108

Sekulić, M., Šošić -Jurjević, B., Filipović, B., Manojlović-Stojanoski, M. & Milosević, V. (2006). Immunoreactive TSH cells in juvenile and peripubertal rats after estradiol and human chorionic gonadotropin treatment. *Acta Histochem*, Vol. 108, pp. 117-123

Sekulić, M., Šošić -Jurjević, B., Filipović, B., Nestorović, N., Negić, N., Stojanoski, MM. & Milosević, V. (2007). Effect of estradiol and progesterone on thyroid gland in pigs: a histochemical, stereological, and ultrastructural study. *Microsc Res Tech*, Vol. 70, pp. 44-49

Sekulić, M., Šošić -Jurjević, B., Filipović, B., Ajdzanović, V., Pantelić, J., Nestorović, N., Manojlović–Stojanoski, M. & Milosević V. (2010). Testosterone and estradiol differently affect thyroid structure and function i orchidectomized middle—aged rats. *14th International Thyroid Congress, Paris* p. 0302

Sendak, RA., Sampath, TK. & McPherson, JM. (2007). Newly reported roles of thyroid-stimulating hormone and follicle-stimulating hormone in bone remodelling. *Int Orthop*, Vol. 31, pp. 753-757

Setchell, KD. (1998). Phytoestrogens: the biochemistry, physiology, and implications for human health of soy isoflavones. *Am J Clin Nutr*, Vol. 68, pp. 1333S-1346S

Setchell, KDR., Brown, NM. & Lydeking-Olsen, E. (2002). The clinical importance of the metabolite equolVa clue to the effectiveness of soy and its isoflavones. *J Nutr*, Vol. 132, pp. 3577-3584

Šošić -Jurjević, B., Filipović, B., Nestorović, N., Lovren, M. & Sekulić, M. (2002), Effect of calcium on structural and morphometric features of thyroid gland tissue in middle-aged rat females. *Jug Med Biochem*, Vol. 21, pp. 261-267

Šošić -Jurjević, B., Filipović, B., Milosević, V., Nestorović, N., Manojlović-Stojanoski, M., Brkić, B. & Sekulić, M. (2005). Chronic estradiol exposure modulates thyroid structure and decreases T4 and T3 serum levels in middle-aged female rats. *Horm Res*, Vol. 63, pp. 48-54

Šošić -Jurjević, B., Filipović, B., Milosević, V., Nestorović, N., Negić, N. & Sekulić, M. (2006a). Effects of ovariectomy and chronic estradiol administration on pituitary-thyroid axis in adult rats. *Life Sci*, Vol. 79, pp. 890-897

Šošić -Jurjević, B., Filipović, B., Stojanoski-Manojlović, M. & Sekulić, M. (2006). Calcium administration decreases thyroid functioning in middle-aged female rats *Archives of Biological Sciences*, Vol. 58, pp. 31-32

Šošić -Jurjević, B., Filipović, B., Ajdzanović, V., Savin, S., Nestorović, N., Milosević, V. & Sekulić, M. (2010). Suppressive effects of genistein and daidzein on pituitary-thyroid axis in orchidectomized middle-aged rats. *Exp Biol Med (Maywood)*, Vol. 235, pp. 590-598

Soung, DY., Devareddy, L., Khalil, DA., Hooshmand, S., Patade, A., Lucas, EA. & Arjmandi, BH. (2006). Soy affects trabecular microarchitecture and favorably alters select bone-specific gene expressions in a male rat model of osteoporosis. *Calcif Tissue Int*, Vol. 78, pp. 385–391

Suchartwatnachai, C., Thepppisai, U. & Jirapinyo, M. (2002). Screening for hypothyroidism at a menopause clinic. *Int J Gynaecol Obstet*, Vol. 77, pp. 39-40

Sugimoto, E. & Yamaguchi, M. (2000). Anabolic effect of genistein in osteoblastic MC3T3-E1 cells. *Int J Mol Med*, Vol. 5, pp. 515-520

Sugimoto, E. & Yamaguchi, M. (2000a). Stimulatory effect of Daidzein in osteoblastic MC3T3-E1 cells. *Biochem Pharmacol*, Vol. 59, pp. 471-475

Suh, KS., Koh, G., Park, CY., Woo, JT., Kim, SW., Kim, JW., Park, IK. & Kim, YS. (2003). Soybean isoflavones inhibit tumor necrosis factor-alpha-induced apoptosis and the production of interleukin-6 and prostaglandin E-2 in osteoblastic cells. *Phytochemistry*, Vol. 63, pp. 209–215

Sun, L., Vukicevic, S., Baliram, R., Yang, G., Sendak, R., McPherson, J., Zhu, L.L., Iqbal, J., Latif, R., Natrajan, A., Arabi, A., Yamoah, K., Moonga, BS., Gabet, Y., Davies, TF., Bab, I., Abe, E., Sampath, K. & Zaidi, M. (2008). Intermittent recombinant TSH injections prevent ovariectomy-induced bone loss. *Proc Natl Acad Sci USA*, Vol. 105, pp. 4289-4294

Teitelbaum, SL. (2000). Bone resorption by osteoclasts. *Science*, Vol. 289, pp. 1504-1508

Tham, DM., Gardner, CD. & Haskell, WL. (1998). Clinical review 97: potential health benefits of dietary phytoestrogens: a review of the clinical, epidemiological, and mechanistic evidence. *J Clin Endocrinol Metab*, Vol. 83, pp. 2223–2235

Theoleyre, S., Wittrant, Y., Tat, SK., Fortun, Y., Redini, F. & Heymann, D. (2004). The molecular triad OPG/RANK/RANKL: involvement in the orchestration of pathophysiological bone remodeling. *Cytokine Growth Factor Rev*, Vol. 15, pp. 457–475

Trisomboon, H., Malaivijitnond, S., Suzuki, J., Hamada, Y., Watanabe, G. & Taya, K. (2004). Long-term treatment effects of Pueraria mirifica phytoestrogens on parathyroid hormone and calcium levels in aged menopausal cynomolgus monkeys. *J Reprod Dev*, Vol. 50, pp. 639-645

Tuohy, PG. (2003). Soy infant formula and phytoestrogens. *J Paediatr Child Health*, Vol. 39, pp. 401-405

Udagawa, N., Takahashi, N., Jimi, E., Matsuzaki, K., Tsurukai, T., Itoh, K., Nakagawa, N., Yasuda, H., Goto, M., Tsuda, E., Higashio, K., Gillespie, MT., Martin, TJ. & Suda, T. (1999). Osteoblasts/stromal cells stimulate osteoclast activation through expression of osteoclast differentiation factor/RANKL but not macrophage colony-stimulating factor. *Bone*, Vol. 25, pp. 517–523

Väänänen, HK., Zhao, H., Mulari, M. & Halleen JM. (2000). The cell biology of osteoclast function. *J Cell Sci*, Vol. 113, pp. 377-381

van der Deure, WM., Peeters, RP. & Visser, TJ. (2010). Molecular aspects of thyroid hormone transporters, including MCT8, MCT10, and OATPs, and the effects of genetic variation in these transporters. *J Mol Endocrinol*, Vol. 44, pp. 1-11

Van Wyk, JJ., Arnold, MB., Wynn, J. & Pepper, F. (1959). The effects of a soybean product on thyroid function in humans. *Pediatrics*, Vol. 24, pp. 752-760

Vandenput, L., Ederveen, AG., Erben, RG., Stahr, K., Swinnen, JV., Van Herck, E., Verstuyf, A., Boonen, S., Bouillon, R. & Vanderschueren, D. (2001). Testosterone prevents orchidectomy-induced bone loss in estrogen receptor-alpha knockout mice. *Biochem Biophys Res Commun*, Vol. 285, pp. 70-76

Vanderschueren, D., Van Herck, E., Suiker, AMH., Visser, WJ., Schot, LPC. & Bouillon, R. (1992). Bone and mineral metabolism in aged male rats: short- and long-term effects of androgen deficiency. *Endocrinology*, Vol. 130, pp. 2906–2916

Vanderschueren, D., Boonen, S. & Bouillon, R. (1998). Action of androgens versus estrogens in male skeletal homeostasis. *Bone*, Vol. 23, pp. 391-394

Vanvooren, V., Allgeier, A., Cosson, E., Van Sande, J., Defer, N., Pirlot, M., Hanoune, J. & Dumont, JE. (2000). Expression of multiple adenylyl cyclase isoforms in human and dog thyroid. *Mol Cell Endocrinol*, Vol. 170, pp. 185-196

Varga, F., Spitzer, S. & Klaushofer, K. (2004). Triiodothyronine (T3) and 1,25-dihydroxyvitamin D3 (1,25D3) inversely regulate OPG gene expression in dependence of the osteoblastic phenotype. *Calcif Tissue Int*, Vol. 74, pp. 382-387

Villa, I., Dal,Fiume, C., Maestroni, A., Rubinacci, A., Ravasi, F. & Guidobono, F. (2003). Human osteoblast-like cell proliferation induced by calcitonin-related peptides involves PKC activity. *Am J Physiol Endocrinol Metab*, Vol. 284, pp. E627–E633

Wangen, KE., Duncan, AM., Merz-Demlow, BE., Xu, X., Marcus, R., Phipps, WR. & Kurzer, MS. (2000). Effects of soy isoflavones on markers of bone turnover in premenopausal and postmenopausal women. *J Clin Endocr Metab*, Vol. 85, pp. 3043-3048

Watanabe, K., Takekoshi, S. & Kakudo, K. (1992). Effects of ipriflavone on calcitonin synthesis in C cells of the rat thyroid. *Calcif Tissue Int*, Vol. 51, pp. S27–S29

Weiner, KX. & Dias, JA. (1990). Protein synthesis is required for testosterone to decrease ornithine decarboxylase messenger RNA levels in rat Sertoli cells. *Mol Endocrinol*, Vol. 4, pp. 1791–1798

Williams, AJ., Robson, H., Kester, MH., van Leeuwen, JP., Shalet, SM., Visser, TJ. & Williams, GR. (2008). Iodothyronine deiodinase enzyme activities in bone. *Bone*, Vol. 43, pp. 126-134

Williams, JP., Jordan, SE., Barnes, S. & Blair, HC. (1998). Tyrosine kinase inhibitor effects on avian osteoclastic acid transport. *Am J Clin Nutr*, Vol. 68, pp. 1369S-1374S

Wong, C., Lai, T., Hilly, JM., Stewart, CE. & Farndon, JR. (2002). Selective estrogen receptor modulators inhibit the effects of insulin-like growth factors in hyperparathyroidism. *Surgery*, Vol. 132, pp. 998-1006

Wu, J., Wang, XX., Chiba, H., Higuchi, M., Takasaki, M., Ohta, A. & Ishimi, Y. (2003). Combined intervention of exercise and genistein preventedand rogen deficiency-induced bone loss in mice. *J Appl Physiol*, Vol. 94, pp. 335–342

Wu, J., Wang, X., Chiba, H., Higuchi, M., Nakatani, T., Ezaki, O., Cui, H., Yamada, K. & Ishimi, Y. (2004). Combined intervention of soy isoflavone and moderate exercise prevents body fat elevation and bone loss in ovariectomized mice. *Metabolism*, Vol. 53, pp. 942-948

Wu, J., Oka, J., Tabata, I., Higuchi, M., Toda, T., Fuku, N., Ezaki, J., Sugiyama, F., Uchiyama, S., Yamada, K. & Ishimi, Y. (2006). Effects of isoflavone and exercise on BMD and fat mass in postmenopausal Japanese women: a 1-year randomized placebo-controlled trial. *J Bone Miner Res*, Vol. 21, pp. 780–789

Yamagishi, T., Otsuka, E. & Hagiwara, H. (2001). Reciprocal control of expression of mRNAs for osteoclast differentiation factor and OPG in osteogenic stromal cells by genistein: evidence for the involvement of topoisomerase II in osteoclastogenesis. *Endocrinology*, Vol. 142, pp. 3632-3637

Yamaguchi, M. & Sugimoto, E. (2000). Stimulatory effect of genistein and daidzein on protein synthesis in osteoblastic MC3T3-E1 cells: activation of aminoacyl-tRNA synthetase. *Mol Cell Biochem*, Vol. 214, pp. 97-102

Yen, PM. (2001). Physiological and molecular basis of thyroid hormone action. *Physiol Rev*, Vol. 81, pp. 1097-1142

Zaidi, M., Datta, HK., Moonga, BS. & MacIntyre, I. (1990). Evidence that the action of calcitonin on rat osteoclasts is mediated by two G proteins acting via separate post-receptor pathways. *J Endocrinol*, Vol. 126, pp. 473–481

7

Studies of Osteoporosis in Cancer Patients in Slovakia – Experience from Single Institute

Beata Spanikova and Stanislav Spanik
St. Elisabeth Cancer Institute, Bratislava
Slovak Republic

1. Introduction

Osteoporosis is a metabolic skeletal disease characterized by low bone mineral density (BMD), damage of bone microstructure, bone fragility resulting in increase risk of bone fractures. Epidemiologic data are continuously showing rising number of newly diagnostic patients with osteoporosis. The expected number of bone fractures due to osteoporosis is to be 6. 26 million in 2050, growth from 1. 56 million in 1990 (Payer et al., 2007). The fractures are usually localized in lumbar spine (or other vertebra), hip and forearm (wrist), The most serious is the fracture of proximal femur (hip), beacuse approximately 20% of these pateints die within one year after the fracture and almost 80% become dependent on some kind of care (Cooper, 1997). The precise number of vertebral pathological fractures is difficult to assess, because many of these fractures are asymptomatic. Despite this they increase mortality by 23% (Cooper, 2007). The wrist fracture do not increase the mortality. The incidence is much more frequent in women than in men (4 : 1). The increased frequency of osteoporosis is partly due to increase in absolute number of new patients and partly due to continualy improving diagnostic procedures. The new generation of equipments and laboratory technics more precisely identify patients with bone loss. In the same time improvement in public information leads to increasing number of densitometric examinations.

Bone tissue is highly active metabolic organ. The bone tissue remodelation (formation of new bone tissue and its degradation) is active and continual process. Very important role in regulation of this process have hormones (estrogens and androgens). The mostly understood and resolved is postmenopausal osteoporosis and the most important risk groups and factors were identified (Rizzoli et al., 2005).

Cancer patients, especially those with „hormone dependent" disease (breast cancer, prostate cancer) or those with treatment interfering in hormonal metabolism (breast cancer, prostate cancer, thyroid cancer, ovarian cancer, germ cell tumor and others) are in inceased risk of disease or therapy induced osteoporosis. There are increased numbers of information and references on this topic.

The most advanced are data on patients with breast cancer, particularly those with early breast cancer (EBC) on adjuvant aromatase inhibitors (AI) therapy.

Women with breast cancer, especially those receiving aromatase inhibitors are at higher risk for bone loss and fracture. Postmenopausal women may already have multiple risk factors for fracture, and breast cancer therapies compound these risk (Hadji & Bundred, 2007). Fractures can have serious clinical consequences including need for major surgery, increased morbidity and mortality, increased cost of disease management, and reduced quality of the life for patients (Body, 2011).

Additional group of patients in risk are those with prostate cancer on hormonal therapy, thyroid cancer (TC) after total or nearly total thyroidectomy on whole-life substitution therapy by oral thyroxine (T_4) and patients with germ cell tumors (GCT) after surgery and radiotherapy and/or chemotherapy.

We have started to measure BMD in patients with breast cancer (BC), prostate cancer, thyroid cancer (TC) and germ cell tumors few years ago. Some of the results are nearly mature and ready to be publish (EBC, TC, GCT) others need more patients and time of follow-up (PC).

2. Breast cancer

2.1 Introduction

Postmenopausal breast cancer patients are in high risk of osteoporosis in many reasons – primary diagnosis of breast cancer, then side-effects of anticancer therapy, postmenopausal status. These factors mean not just elevated risk of bone loss, osteoporosis, but especially risk of patological fractures. Many of postmenopausal breast cancer patients, especially those with early stage, with aromatase inhibitors (AI) adjuvant therapy have very good prognosis. The elevated risk of osteoporosis can lead to patological fractures which may markedly worsen their quality of life (Coleman et al., 2008).

Antagonizing estrogen in hormone-dependent breast cancer is well-known method of reducing tumor growth. Five years of treatment with tamoxifen, an antiestrogen or selective estrogen-receptor modulator (SERM), has been shown to reduce the risk of recurrence and breast cancer mortality by 41% and 34% respectively and is still recommended as one of several options for early-stage hormone receptor-positive breast cancer.

New data from clinical trials comparing third-generation aromatase inhibitors (AI) with tamoxifen have confirmed that AI offer significant efficacy and tolerability advantage over tamoxifen. Aromatase inhibitors are recommended as adjuvant treatmen for postmenopausal women with hormone-receptor positive early breast cancer. The group of clinicaly used AI contains non-steroidal AI letrozole and anastrozole and steroidal-AI exemestane. The primary mechanism of action of AI is inhibition of aromatase activity. Aromatase is the most important enzyme responsible for conversion of androgens to estrogens, mainly in tissues outside endocrine system. This is the most important mechanism of estrogen production in postmenopausal women. Estrogen production blockade influences bone metabolism directly via osteoclastogenesis stimulation. Survival extension of osteoclasts is the main mechanism. Cytokines, interleukines 1 and 6, osteoprotegerin, bone resorption potentiation, osteocytes and osteoblasts apoptosis are other important mechanisms resulting in osteosynthesis inhibiton. AIs also play key role in calcium metabolism. Their action influence calcium absorption in small bowel and renal elimination. It is very similar to estrogens level decrease after menopause leading to postmenopausal osteoporosis (Rizzoli, 2005).

AIs in breast cancer treatment are used as adjuvant therapy – it means after radical surgery in early breast cancer, stages I - III or as palliative therapy of locally advanced or metastatic disease. Standard duration of adjuvant hormonal therapy is now 5 years. Recently published results of large international multicenter clinical studies (including more than 15 000 pacients) such as ATAC (Howell et al., 2005) and BIG (Coates et al., 2007) have shown that adjuvant hormonal therapy using AIs and lasting 5 years is more effective than adjuvant therapy using selective estrogen receptor modulators (SERMs), mainly tamoxifen. Substudies of these and many other similar studies dealing with bone mineral density (BMD) in early breast cancer patients on adjuvant hormonal therapy are consistently showing higher decrease of BMD during treatment with AIs than that with tamoxifen. This is the reason why regular BMD measurements at the beginning and during AIs adjuvant therapy were implemented into new recommendations for early breast cancer therapy published in July 2007 as results of consensus of panel of most important international leaders in the field during 10th St Gallen Conference (Goldhirsch et al., 2007).

2.2 Patients and methods

We started regular bone mineral density (BMD) measurement of postmenopausal early breast cancer patients treated either with aromatase inhibitors (AIs) or tamoxifen in St. Elisabeth Cancer Institute on September 2005. The most important goal of our study was to determine bone mineral density decrease in early breast cancer patients treated with (AIs). We measured BMD at the begining of treatment and during therapy (after one year or two depending on initial results) with AIs and a group of patients who have their hormonal therapy switched from tamoxifen do AIs for different reasons (intolerance or toxicity).

As an comparative groups we measured BMD in group of early breast cancer patients treated with tamoxifen and patients after finished hormonal therapy without any anticaner therapy, only on regular follow-up. The study is sitll active, in this preliminary evaluation we analysed group of 263 consecutive patients with early breast cancer, 42 on active AIs therapy - 22 on letrozole on oral daily dose 2,5 mg, 20 on anastrozole on oral daily dose 1 mg, 72 patients with „switched" therapy from tamoxifen to AIs, 69 on active tamoxife therapy on oral daily dose 20 mg and 80 patients just on follow-up after finishing active hormonal treatment.

In all our patients the BMD measurement was performed on total body densitometer Hologic Explorer. We measured and evaluated region of proximal femur and L spine. In cases of degenerative changes which overestimated results we measured and evaluated the region of forearm. For comparisons we evaluated T score. All patients included in our study have measured height, weight, assessed age, duration of menopause, hormonal replacement therapy and history of other risk factors and previous fractures. All patients have measured calcium blood level. We also measured markers of bone turnover, CTX (CrossLaps - C telopeptide of alfa chain 2(I) colagen) as marker of osteoporosis measured by ELISA method and isoensyme of ALP as marker of osteoproduction. In patients with BMD results on levels of osteoporosis we made differential diagnostic examinations to exclude secondary osteoporosis. This is important especially in patients with breast cancer to exclude bone marrow metastases, which are most frequent sites of generalised disease. We used cancer markers, RTG, CT, MRI or bone scan - sceletal gamagraphy

For the statistical analysis we used standard methods of descriptive statistics, test of data independence and multiple regression was used to verify influence of separate factors especially to exclude possible secondary influences in case of interactive correlation among parameters.

2.3 Results

From the whole study group of 263 postmenopausal early breast cancer patients, 114 patients in the group treated with AIs (72 of them switched from previous tamoxifen to AIs), 69 on tamoxifen therapy and 80 patients without hormonal therapy only on follow-up after finishing hormonal treatment (figure 1).

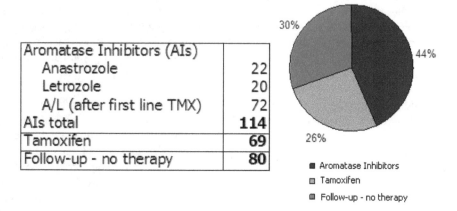

Aromatase Inhibitors (AIs)	
Anastrozole	22
Letrozole	20
A/L (after first line TMX)	72
AIs total	**114**
Tamoxifen	**69**
Follow-up - no therapy	**80**

Fig. 1. Patients Characteristics

We found normal BMD only in 13,31% among all evaluated patients, 43,35% of the whole analysed patients had BMD rate in levels of osteoporosis. Analysing the localisations of measured osteoporosis we found this in 5,25% in proximal femur, 63,1% in L spine and 31,58% in region of the forearm (figure 2) – those were patients with deformations or degenerative changes in region of spine, which overestimated the results.

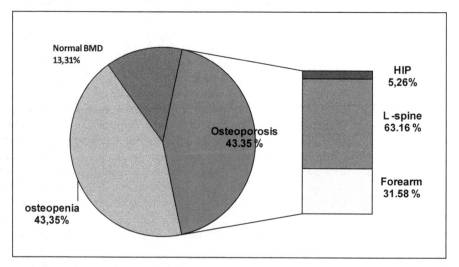

Fig. 2. BMD in Patients with Breast Cancer

Median of age of the whole group of patients was 61 years. The BMD loss to levels of osteoporosis was found in group of patients under 50 years of age in 26%, where 50% of them had osteoporosis in region of L spine, 38% in region of proximal femur and only 13% in region of forearm. The rate of osteoporosis was higher in the group of patients older than 70 years - 73% and most of them had osteoporosis in the region of forearm – 49%. The region of L spine was overestimated by degenerative and deformative changes in this age group of patients. Group of patients in age between 50 to 70 years had BMD levels of osteoporosis in 34%, most frequently in region of L spine – 80%. These findings are in correlation with many clinical studies confirming rising incidence of osteoporosis with rising age. We confirm influence of menopause duration on osteoporosis as well as negative correlation of weight and osteoporosis in our study. All this findings are in consensus with literature data.

We also analysed impact of therapy on BMD loss. In the group of patients with AI therapy BMD loss to level of osteoporosis was diagnosed in 43,86% and normal BMD had 13,16% of patients, in the group with tamoxifen therapy the rate of osteoporosis was 30,43% and normal BMD had 18,84% of patients, in the group on follow-up without hormonal therapy the rate of osteoporosis was 53,75% and normal BMD had 8,7% of patients. The correlation between BMD loss and hormonal therapy was not proven statistically significant despite trend of tamoxifen protective effect on BMD maintenance. This was not statistically significant - (p=0,0610). In subanalysis, where we correlate BMD loss only in subgroup of patients treated by AIs at least one year and patients treated less than 1 year or just on follow-up without hormonal therapy (figure 3), the difference was statistically significant. The rate of BMD loss to level of osteoporosis was 53,13% in the first group and only 40,2% in the letter and normal BMD rate was only 3,13% in the first group versus 16,58% in second one - (p=0,0150).

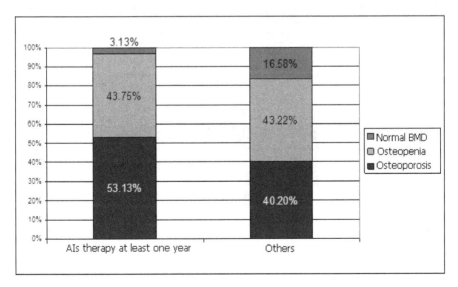

Fig. 3. BMD in Patients with Aromatase Inhibitors Therapy and Others

We analysed other risk factors and we found highest rate of patients with diabetes mellitus among those risk factors (33 patients) but we did not confirm statistical significant influence of diabetes mellitus on BMD loss - (p=0,816).

Correlation of BMD loss and increase levels of CTX as a marker of bone resorption was not confirmed in our study.

We tested all above mentioned risk factors statistically also (figure 4) using method of multiple linear regression to eliminate potential secondary influences in cross interactions among factors. Correlations BMD level to age (p<0,0001 and weight (p<0,0001) were confirmed by multiple linear regression. Borderline statistical significance was shown in correlation to AIs therapy (=0,0476). The influence of time from menopause (p=0,3410) seemed to be secondary regarding to high correlation to age of patients (r=0,89, p< 0,0001).

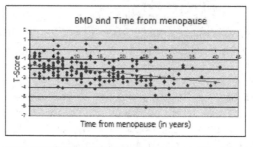

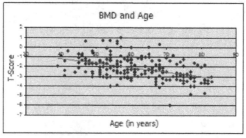

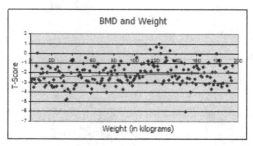

Correlation coefficients:

(BMD,Age) = -0.44 (p<0.001)
(BMD,Weight) = 0.43 (p<0.001)
(BMD,Time from menopause) = -0.39 (p<0.001)

Fig. 4. Correlation of BMD with Age, Weight and Time from Menopause

The rate of pathological fractures was analysed also (figure 5). The most frequent incidence was in group of patients with osteoporosis. Wrist fracture was found in 10 patients and 5 had fractures in region of L spine. In the group of patients with BMD on level of osteopenia, 5 patients had pathological fractures, 3 of them were wrist fractures and 2 in region of L spine. There were only 2 pathological fractures in patients with normal BMD levels, both were wrist fractures. The whole group of patients we considered to be too small to make statistical analysis of risk factors of pathological fractures.

The last was the analysis of influence of antiresorptive therapy on BMD changes (figure 6). The analysis seemed to be preliminary as in the control group (control BMD measurement after 1 year of duration of antiresorptive therapy) were only 53 patients. This did not allow us to make relevant statistical analysis, although we found trend toward protective effect of antiresorptive therapy in this group of patients.

Osteoporosis	
Wrist	10
Spine	5
Hip	0
Osteopenia	
Wrist	3
Spine	2
Hip	0
Normal BMD	
Wrist	2
Spine	0
Hip	0

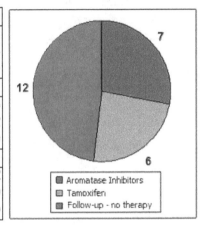

Fig. 5. Patological Fractures Rate

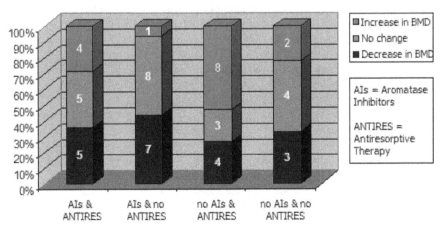

Fig. 6. Impact of Antiresorptive Therapy on BMD in patients with Breast Cancer

2.4 Discussion

The AIs are new standard in adjuvant hormonal therapy of early breast cancer postmenopausal patients. As the results of many large international multicentre clinical trials are more mature and results of substudies focused on BMD loss more and more consistant, new standards for BMD examination are evolving. The prognosis of early breast cancer patients is continually improving. BMD loss means increasing risk of osteoporosis and it means increasing risk of pathological fractures. There are many risks factors for this group of patients - age, postmenopausal status, breast cancer, AIs therapy. Adjuvant hormonal therapy is one of the most important factors leading to significant improvement in patient survival and the same important is quality of life which may be markedly decreased by pathological fractures from osteoporosis.

Identification of all risk factors of origin and progression of osteoporosis as well as exact examination procedures to find them is as important as prevention and therapy of BMD loss. Generally confirmed risk factors for pathological fractures of osteoporosis in breast cancer patients are:

AIs therapy
T-score < 1. 5
Age > 65 years
Low body mass index (BMI < 20 kg/m²)
Family history of hip fracture
Personal history of fracture from osteoporosis after age of 50
Oral corticosteroid therapy lasting > 6 months
Smoking (in present or in past)

Table 1. Risk factors for pathological fractures of osteoporosis in breast cancer patients

In multicenter international clinical trial „ATAC", where the postmenopausal early breast cancer patients were randomised (final design) to AI anastrozole (A) versus tamoxifen (T) showed that after 5 years of therapy (Howell et al., 2005) there were significantly more bone fractures on arm A (11% versus 7%; $p < 0.001$). In clinical trial „BIG 1-98" the same postmenopausal early breast cancer patients were randomised to AI letrozole (L) versus tamoxifen (T). With median of follow-up of 26 months (Thurliman et al., 2005) there were significantly more bone fractures on arm L (5.7% versus 4.0%; $p < 0.001$). Very similar results were reached in the clinical study „IES" where the postmenopausal early breast cancer patients were randomised to AI exemestane (E) versus tamoxifen (T) and with median of follow-up ~ 56 months (Coombes et al., 2007) there were significantly more bone fractures on arm E (7% versus 4. 9%; $p = 0.003$). In combined clinical study „ABCSG-8 and ARNO 95" the patients were „switched" after anastrozole (A) therapy to tamoxifen (T) vs continuing T therapy. With median of follow-up of 28 months (Jakesz et al., 2005) there was similar significant difference against arm A (2% versus 1%; $p = 0. 015$). In the clinical study „MA.17" were the patients after 5 years on tamoxifen (T) therapy randomised to „switch" to anastrozole (A) versus only follow-up without hormonal treatment. With median of follow-up of 30 months (Goss et al., 2005), there were more patients with newly diagnostic osteoporosis on arm A (8. 1% versus 6. 0%; p = 0. 003), and more bone fractures (5. 6% versus 4. 6%, this difference was however not statistically significant p = 0. 25).

In comparison of patients on AI anastrozole (A) therapy from the clinical study „ATAC" to their healthy counterparts matched in age, postmenopausal status, with osteopenia, the incidence of bone fractures were nearly doubled.

We confirmed the prognostic importance of age, duration of menopause, AIs treatment in comparison to tamoxifen treatment or no therapy in follow-up group in our clinical observation. All these results are in concordance with world scientific literature.

According to WHO and NOF (National Osteoporotic Foundation) guidelines is the value of T-score in BMD measurement critical in distribution to normal BMD (T-score ≥ - 1. 0), osteopenia (T-score between – 1. 0 and – 2. 5) and osteoporosis (T-score ≤ - 2.5) (Kanis et al., 2008). According to international general guidelines is this classification universally accepted and it is recognised that with decreasing BMD level the risk of pathological bone fractures is rising. That is why the results and observations of the clinical study NORA (National Osteoporosis Risk Assessment) are so interesting. They observed > 200 000 healthy postmenopausal women and found that 82% pathological bone fractures happened in women with T-score > - 2. 5, which means that they did no have osteoporosis and 52% fractures were in women with osteopenia (T-score – 1. 0 to – 2.5).

All these results and findings confirm the importance of BMD measurement before AIs therapy initiation and importance of preventive measurements as components of adjuvant AIs therapy as well. Calcium and vitamin D supplementation and appropriate physical activity are standard components of these recommendations (Goldhirsch et al., 2007). Preventive bisphosphonates application is being evaluated in many running clinical studies. Especially zoledronic acid is showing excellent results and it seems to be incorporated into standard combination with AIs in adjuvant therapy of postmenopausal early breast cancer patients very soon as osteoporosis and bone fracture prevention (Gnant et al., 2007).

There was observed protective effect against bone loss, longer period to bone metastases occurence and suspected direct anticancer effect as well. These results will probably lead very soon to change today ´s standards and bisphosphonates will be used together with AIs in adjuvant therapy of early breast cancer patients (Gnant et al., 2007).

The influence of antiresorptive therapy on BMD was part of our study as well. This analysis is difficult to interpret as our control group (control BMD measurement after 1 year of duration of antiresorptive therapy) was very small (only 53 patients) and median of follow-up very short. This did not allow us to make relevant statistical analysis but we found trend toward protective effect of antiresorptive therapy in this group of patients.

We did not confirm correlation of BMD decrease and CTX elevation. Probably the reason was small analysed group of patients and low specificity of CTX as osteoporosis marker (S.Špánik & B. Špániková, 2010).

2.5 Conclusions and future directions

The most important goal of our study was to confirm the importance of BMD measurement and evaluation in group of postmenopausal early breast cancer patients on AIs therapy. Even the study group is not very large, all the patients are from single institute and we have planned to follow-up them throughout the AIs therapy and thereafter. Preliminary analysis of our data confirmed significant BMD loss in this group of patients. The AIs therapy influence on BMD loss was statistically significant after one year of therapy. For more valid data we need more patients and longer time of follow-up. Our plan is to continue in evaluation of influence of antiresorptive therapy on BMD as we observed trend of protection of BMD. Evaluation of importance of BMD loss for increase risk of pathological bone fractures also needs more patients and longer time of follow-up (Hadji et al., 2011).

Our observational study confirmed importance of BMD measurement and evaluation in postmenopausal early breast cancer patients on AIs therapy. This is in concordance with new recommendations for early breast cancer therapy published in July 2007 as a result of consensus conference (10th St Gallen Conference) and other important international guidelines.

3. Testicular cancer

3.1 Introduction

Testicular cancer (TC) is still being serious disease although when the patients are correctly diagnosed and treated the cure rate is about 90%. Testicular cancer make about 1% of malignant tumors in men, the incidence in recent years is going up. The incidence in Slovak Republic in 2003 was 7,3/100000 men and during last 30 years has increased almost 5-times.TC appear mostly in men from 20 to 40 years of lilfe. (D. Ondruš & M. Ondrušová, 2008). According to international classification more than 95% of TC are germ cell tumors (GCT), which are classified into two major subgroups: seminoma and non-seminoma GCT. Nonseminomatous GCT comprises approximately 50% of all GCT. Most tumors are mixed, consisting of two or more cell types (embryonal carcinoma, choriocarcinoma, yolk sac tumor, teratoma or their mixtures). The rest of testicular tumors are rare - Leydig cell tumors, Sertoli cell tumors, granulosa cell tumors, gonadoblastoma, sarcomas, lymphomas and others).

The diagnosis of GCT is based on clinical picture – painless testicular mass, symptoms of epididymitis or orchitis, less frequently occurs testicular pain.

For pretreatment staging we use ultrasound, computed tomography (CT) of chest, abdomen and pelvis and serum tumor markers (alfa-fetoprotein, human chorionic gonadotropin, lactate dehydrogenase).

The standard therapeutic procedure is surgery, radical orchiectomy and retroperitoneal lymph node dissection (according to histological type and stage of the disease). Other therapeutic options are radiotherapy and chemotherapy (again according to histological type and stage of the disease).

During recent decades the survival rate of patients with testicular cancer or germ cell tumors (GCT) has substantially improved. Consequently the long-term side effects of treatment of GCT have gained attention, including accelerated bone loss leading to increased risk of osteoporosis. Treatment-related bone loss is well recognized in breast and prostate cancer, but there has been little information in long-term survivors from other tumors (Marcus et al., 2008).

We have a large group of GCT patients in our registry at the Department of Urology of St. Elisabeth Cancer Institute with a long duration follow-up. It is already known that androgens influence bone modelling and remodelling acting on osteoblasts, osteocytes and pluripotent stem cells through androgen receptors. They also act indirectly via estrogen receptors. The combined influence of androgens and estrogens is even stronger. We suppose that patients after unilateral orchiectomy (OE) or bilateral orchiectomy and consecutive radiotherapy and/or chemotherapy should have lower levels of testosterone. Literature sources on this issue are scarce and conflicting. There are numerous animal studies proving the effect of androgens on bone and also proving much stronger effect of androgen and estrogen combination (Ondruš et al., 2007).

3.2 Patients and methods
Our aim was to determine BMD and serum bone turnover markers in survivors from GCT. We included 719 patients with GCT into the study. We measured BMD in GCT patients from 2005.

BMD was measured by dual-energy X-ray absorptiometry using osteodenzitometer Holgic Discovery in the lumbar spine and hips. BMD was classified as osteopenia (T score ranging from –2, 5 to –1.0) and osteoporosis (T score less than –2. 5). Latter according to WHO recommendation for men under 50 years of age we use Z score (comparison of detected BMD to healthy bone of comparable age group).

C-terminal cross-linked telopeptides of type I collagen (CTX) were measured using Enzyme-Linked Immunoabsorbent Assay (ELISA). Additionally serum total testosterone was measured.

Comparison was made with matched healthy control group from Ministery of health registry. Relationships between baseline characteristics (age, treatment type and time from orchiectomy) and BMD were assessed using univariate and multivariate analysis tools.

The data was evaluated using Microsoft Excel 2003 software and its built-in statistical functions and data analysis tools. We used standard uni-, bi- and multivariate statistical methods as appropriate throughout data analysis. Association between two nominal variables was tested using the Chi-squared test of independence. Association between an interval variable and a nominal one was tested using ANOVA or Kruskal-Wallis test, depending on the distribution of the interval variable; in case of a dichotomous variable, t-test was applied instead of ANOVA and Mann-Whitney test instead of Kruskal-Wallis test. A multiple linear regression was performed to test for association between an dependent interval variable and several predicting interval variables (Mardiak et al., 2007)

3.3 Results
We included 719 patients into the study (21 – 76 yrs old, median: 39 yrs) who were treated for GCT since 1982. In this group, 663 pts (92%) were treated by unilateral orchiectomy (OE) and 56 pts (8%) by bilateral OE. The further treatment was radiotherapy of retroperitoneal lymph nodes (RPLND) in 124 pts (17%), chemotherapy in 405 pts (57%), radiotherapy and chemotherapy in in 16 pts (2%), the rest 174 pts (24%) did not receive any adjuvant therapy (fig. 7). Median time since OE was 6. 5 yrs, average time was 8. 1 yrs.

We have proved a significant difference between BMD patients with GCT compared to the healthy population ($p < 0.0001$) with more osteopenia and osteoporosis in GCT patients.

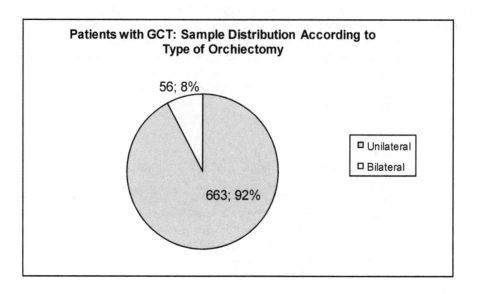

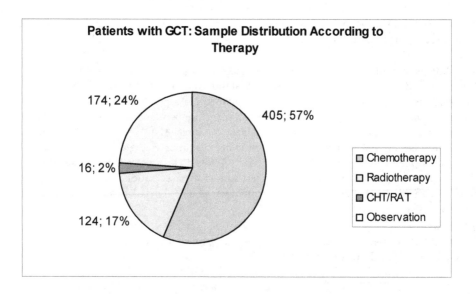

Fig. 7. Patients characteristics

We have made comparisons between the group of GCT patients and the healthy match control group according to type of surgery and subsequent therapy (fig. 8)

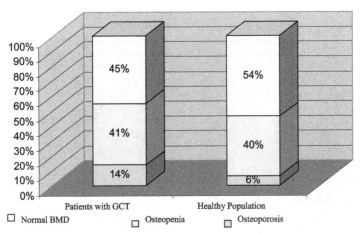

Fig. 8. Comparison of GCT group to healthy match control group

We made comparison of BMD and the type of orchiectomy (fg. 9)

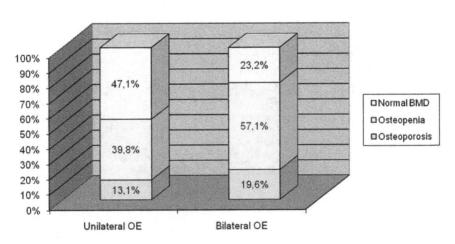

Fig. 9. Comparison of BMD and type of OE

Comparison was made between the subgroup of patients with unilateral orchiectomy and a the subgroup of those treated with bilateral orchiectomy. While the incidence of osteoporosis has not proved to be significantly different in the two subgroups (p=0.1725), patients treated with bilateral OE have significantly higher incidence of osteopenia (p=0.0116).

We also made comparisons of BMD of patients with GCT and different types of OE to healthy match control group (fig. 10)

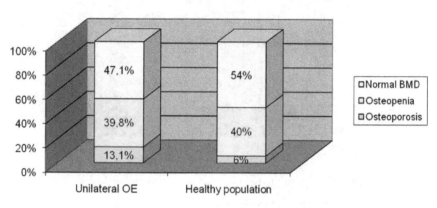

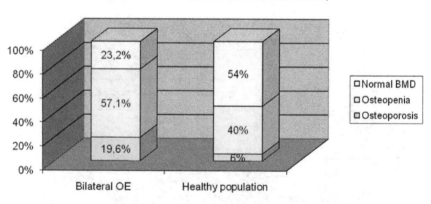

Fig. 10. Comparisons of BMD of patients with GCT and different types of OE to the healthy match control group

In a separate comparison of the subgroup of patients treated with bilateral orchiectomy to the healthy population we have concluded not only a significantly higher incidence of osteoporosis in the former (p<0.0001), but also a significantly higher incidence of osteopenia in those patients treated with bilateral OE (p=0.0114). Patients treated with unilateral OE compared to the healthy population have a significantly higher incidence of osteoporosis (p<0.0001) We also made comparisons of BMD according to time from primary therapy

BMD and Median Time since Orchiectomy in Patients with GCT

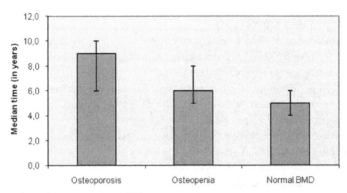

Fig. 11. BMD and median time since OE

All the most important results are summarized in table 2.

	Total	Osteoporosis		Osteopenia		Normal BMD		P value
Number of patients:	719	98 /	14%	296 /	41%	325 /	45%	
Treatment:								
Unilateral OE	663	87 /	13%	264 /	40%	312 /	47%	
Bilateral OE	56	11 /	20%	32 /	57%	13 /	23%	
Chemotherapy	405	48 /	12%	172 /	42%	185 /	46%	
Radiotherapy	124	19 /	15%	48 /	39%	57 /	46%	
Chemo- and Radiotherapy	16	3 /	19%	10 /	63%	3 /	19%	
Characteristics (Risk Factors):								
Fractures	98	10 /	10%	47 /	48%	41 /	42%	
Demographics:								
Median age		43,0		39,0		37,0		(<0.0001)
Average age		43,8		39,5		37,7		(<0.0001)
Baseline Characteristics (medians):								
Time since OE	702	9,0		6,0		5,0		(0.0049)
Testosterone (nmol/l)	478	16,8		16,6		16,3		(0.6887)
Free Testosterone (pg/ml)	132	7,0		8,3		8,3		(0.3526)
CTX (scale 1: ng/ml)	137	0,4		0,5		0,4		(0.5545)
CTX (scale 2: pM)	287	3341,0		4175,5		3941,5		(0.2101)
LH		4,6		4,6		4,6		(0.3602)

Table 2. Patients with GST – characteristics and results

3.4 Conclusions and future directions

- We have proved a significant difference between BMD patients with GCT and healthy population (p<0.0001).
- The incidence of osteoporosis is significantly higher in patients with GCT compared to the healthy population (p<0.0001).
- While the incidence of osteoporosis has not proved to be significantly different in the two subgroups (p=0.1725), patients treated with bilateral OE have significantly higher incidence of osteopenia (p=0.0116).
- Comparing the minimum T-score between the two subgroups, we have concluded significantly lower median T-score in patients with bilateral OE compared to those treated with unilateral OE (p=0.0148).
- We have come to the conclusion of no significant association between BMD and type of therapy in patients with GCT (p=0.287).
- There is no significant association between BMD and CTX level (p=0.1600).
- Correlation between T-score and testosterone also free testosterone level in patients with GCT, the correlation coefficient of 0.0881, did not prove as significant (p=0.3263).

We did not find any significant differences between GCT and matched control data regarding the incidence of osteopenia and bone turnover marker, but the incidence of osteoporosis was considerably higher in GCT patients. The incidence of osteopororsis appeared to increase with age and to slightly correlate with time since OE, particularly after 10 years following OE. Type of therapy did not prove to have significant impact on the appearance of osteoporosis. Serum testosterone level did not correlate with BMD. We recommend BMD measurement and evaluation in GCT patients after therapy (Ondrušová et al., 2009).

4. Bone mineral density in thyroid cancer (TC) patients on suppresive therapy after total thyroidectomy

4.1 Introduction

Thyroid cancer (TC) is another type of cancer which should be associated with decrease of BMD after total thyreoidectomy and subsequent suppressive therapy. Although TC comprises only 1. 1 – 1. 9% of all cancers it is the most frequent endocrine tumor making around 90% of them. It is 3-times more frequent in women than in men. The most frequent types are well-differentiated cancers – papillary (80 – 85%) and less frequent follicular (5 – 10%) thyroid carcinoma.

The standard therapy of thyroid carcinomas (TC) consists of total or nearly total thyroidectomy. Then the whole-life substitution therapy by oral thyroxine (T4) is given. Another goal of this therapy is to suppress serum thyroid stimulating hormone (TSH) to prevent the growth factor-like effect of TSH on well-differentiated TC cells. The recommendation is to administer supraphysiologic amounts of oral T4. This leads to hyperthyroidism, which is subclinical. The influence of thyroid hormones on bone tissue is well known (Altabas et al., 2007). In hyperthyreosis the acitivty of osteoblasts and osteoclasts is increased, but the influence of osteoclasts is dominating leading to bone resorption and osteoporosis. The longstanding subclinical hyperthyroidism may result in increased bone turnover and decreased bone mineral density (BMD). The aim of the study was to assign the damage of bone metabolism in TC patients.

4.2 Patients and methods

Bone mineral density (BMD) was measured by dual energy photon x-ray absorptiometry BMD using osteodenzitometer Holgic Discovery in the lumbar spine and hips. In cases with arteficialy increased bone density caused by degenerative bone changes we measured BMD also in forearm. BMD was classified using T score in postmenopausal women and more than 50 years old men . We classified Z score in premenopausal women and younger than 50 years men. C-terminal cross -linked telopeptides of type I collagen (CTX) were measured using ELISA. Additionally serum TSH and fT_4 (free T_4) were measured. Relationships between baseline characteristics (age, menopausal status in women, TSH levels and duration of substitutional therapy) and BMD were assessed using univariate and multivariate analysis tools.

Association between two nominal variables was tested using the Chi-squared test of independence. Association between an interval variable and a nominal one was tested using ANOVA or Kruskal-Wallis test, depending on the distribution of the interval variable; in case of a dichotomous variable, t-test was applied instead of ANOVA and Mann-Whitney test instead of Kruskal-Wallis test. A multiple linear regression was performed to test for association between an dependent interval variable and several predicting interval variables.

We analysed BMD data from 165 TC patients after total tyroidectomy on supportive therapy in our study. There were 13 men and 152 women, 94 were postmenpausal (postMP), 44 premenopausal (preMP), in 14 the menopausal sattus was unknown. The mean age was 51 years. Age characteristics are in table 3.

Age characteristics:				
	All	Men	PostMP women	PreMP women
Min	21	29	34	21
Max	78	77	78	55
Mean	53	49	59	39
Median	54	50	58	41
Standard deviation	12.65	14.21	8.25	8.45

Table 3. Age characteristics

4.3 Results

We included 165 TC patients in the study. There were 13 men a 152 women, the mean duration of thyroid suppressive therapy was 7. 2 years (0 – 24 years). The patients exhibit osteporosis in 31%, 39% had osteopenia, whereas 30% had normal BMD (fig. 12).

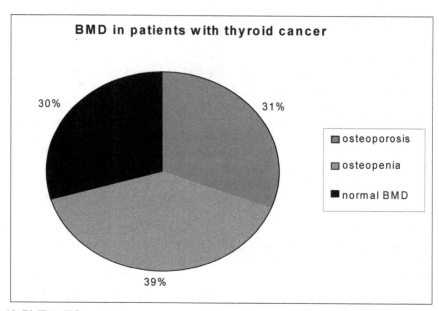

Fig. 12. BMD in TC patients

The BMD changes were localised in different sites (fig. 13)

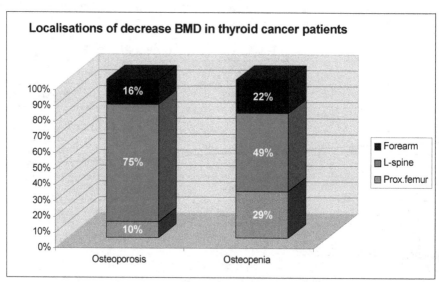

Fig. 13. Localisations of BMD decresae in TC paients

The incidence of osteoporosis appeared to increase with age but did not correlated with duration of thyroid suppressive therapy (fig. 14)

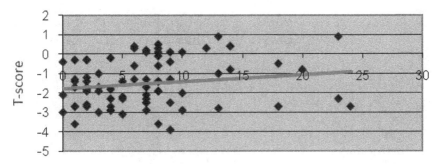

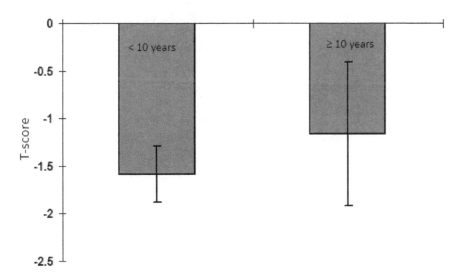

Fig. 14. Duration of suppressive therapy and BMD

We confiirmed higher incidence of osteoporosis in postMP women and in the small subgroup of postMP women on antiporotic therapy we confirmed efficacy of this therapy (fig.15). But the gorup was very small and we cannot make any conclusuions.

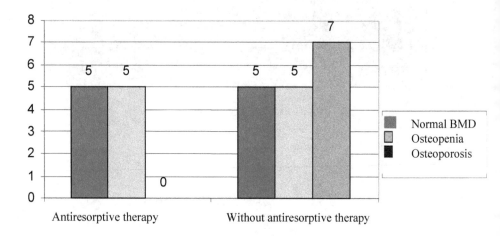

Fig. 15. Comparison of BMD changes in controlled group with/without antiresorpitve therapy

We confirmed 10 pathological fractures in our study (tab. 4)

Fractures

10 pathological fractures

Site
- wrist 3
- spine 3
- others 4

Table 4. Pathological fractures in TC patients

The pathological fractures were in correlation with decreased BMD to osteopenia or osteoporosis (fig. 16)

BMD (T-score) and compressive fractures CF) in TC pacients (p=0.048)

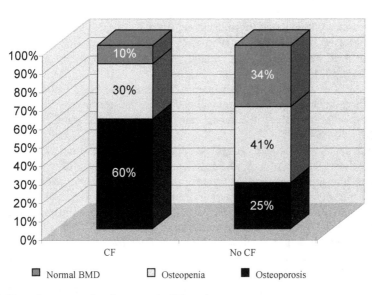

Fig. 16. BMD and compressive fractures in TC patients

4.4 Discussion

Published data on this topic are scarce and conflicting. Some of them did not prove correlation between subclinical hyperthyreosis and decrease in BMD (S. I. Greenspan & F. S. Greenspan, 2005). Others have found, that if suppressive therapy does not suppress the TSH below normal value it does not decrease BMD and does not worsen the prognosis of TC (Biondi & Cooper, 2010). Similar results were published also in the past (Shomon, 1995). Some on the other hand has confirmed that long term suppressive therapy affects bone turnover and bone mineral density in pre and postmenopausal women with TC (Heijekmann et al., 2005). Decrese in BMD as a result of suppressive therapy in TC was confirmed but this effect was ameliorated by preventive substitution of calcium and calcitonin (Mikosch et al., 2006). In this metaanalysis of 8 studies the influence of thyreoidal suppression on BMD in postmenopausal women was confirmed. It was not confirmed in men and premenopausal women. The limitation was a substantial inhomogeneity of patients groups and uneveness in calcium supplementation.

4.5 Conclusions and future directions

The long term survivors from TC after total thyroidectomy on thyroid suppressive therapy have higher risk of osteoporosis and therefore we recommend BMD testing and appropriate measures according to results. The BMD decrease may be a risk factor for pathological fractures and as the TC has very good prognosis, it does matter (B. Špániková.& S. Špánik, 2011)

5. References

Altabas, V., & Berkovič, M., & Bečejac, B., & Solter, M.: Bone Remodeling and Thyroid Function, Acta Clin Croat 2007; 46: 41-47

Biondi, B., & Cooper, D.S.: Benefits of thyreotropin suppresion versus the risk of adverse effects in differentiated thyroid cancer, Thyroid 2010; 20, 135-146.

Body, J. J. Increased Fracture Rate in Women With Breast Cancer: a Review of the Hidden Risk. BMC Cancer. 2011 Aug 29; 11 (1): 384. http://www.biomedcentral.com/1471-2407/11/384

Coates, A.S., & Keshaviah, A., & Thurlimann, B., et al.: Five years of letrozole compared with tamoxifen as initial adjuvant therapy for postmenopausal women with endocrine-responsive early breast cancer: update of study BIG 1-98, J Clin Oncol 2007; 25, 486-492

Coleman, R.E., & Banks, L.M,, & Girgis, S.I., & Kilburn, L.S., & Vrdoljak, E., & Fox, J., & Cawthorn, S.J., & Patel, A., & Snowdon, C.F., & Hall, E., & Bliss, J.M., & Coombes, R.C.: Intergroup Exemestane Study group.Skeletal effects of exemestane on bone-mineral density, bone biomarkers, and fracture incidence in postmenopausal women with early breast cancer participating in the Intergroup Exemestane Study (IES): a randomised controlled study, Lancet Oncol 2007 Feb:8(2),119-27

Coleman, R.E., & Body, J. J., & Gralow, Jr, Lipton A: Bone loss in patients with breast cancer receiving aromatase inhibitors and associated treatment strategies. Cancer Treat Rev 2008;34:S1–S18. July 2008

Coombes, R.C., & Kilburn, L.S., & Snowdon, C.F., et al. Survival and safety of exemestane versus tamoxifen after 2 – 3 years tamoxifen treatment (Inergroup Exmestane Study): a randomized controled trial. Lancet 2007; 369: 559 – 570.

Cooper, C. The crippling consequences of fractures and their impact on quality of life. Am J Med 1997 Aug 18;103(2A):12S-17S; discussion 17S-19S.

Gnant M, et al.: Adjuvant ovarian suppression combined with tamoxifen or anastrozole, alone or in combination with zoledronic acid, in premenopausal women with hormone-responsive, stage I and II breast cancer: First efficacy results from ABCSG-12. ASCO 2008. Abstract LBA4

Goldhirsch, A., & Wood, W.C., & Gelber, R.D., & Coates, A.S., & Thurlimann, B., & Senn, H.J, - Panel Members: Progress and promise: highlights of the internqational expert consensus on the primary therapy of early breast cancer 2007. Ann Oncol 2007; 18: 1133 – 1144

Goos, P.E., & Ingle, J.N., & Martino, S., et al: Random.trial of letrozol tamoxifen as extended adjuvant therapy in receptor-positive breast cancer. Update findings from MA 17. J.Nat.Cancer Inst 2005; 97:1262-1271

Greenspan, S.I., & Greenspan, F.S.: The effect of tyroid hormone on skeletal integrity. Horm Res 2005; 64(6), 293-8

Hadji, P., & Aapro, M.S., & Body, J.J.: Management of aromatase inhibitor-associated bone loss in postmenopausal women with breast cancer: practical guidance for prevention and treatement Annals of Oncol. Advance Access; 2011, doi:10.1093/annonc/mdr017

Hadji, P & Bundred, N.: Reducing the risk of cancer treatment-associated bone loss in patients with breast cancer. Semin Oncol 2007; Dec: 34 (6 Suppl 4): S4-10

Heijekmann, A.C., & Huijberts, M.P., & Geusens, P., & Vries, J., & Menheere, P., & Wolffenbuttel, B.: Hip bone mineral density, bone turnover and risk of fracture in patiens on long-term suúúressive L-thyroxine therapy for differentiared toroid carcinoma Eur J Endocrinol 2005; 153, 23-29

Howell, A., & Cuzick, J., & Baum, M., & Buzdar, A., & Dowsett, M., & Forbes, J.F., & Hoctin-Boes, G., & Houghton, J., & Locker, G.Y., & Tobias, J.: Results of the ATAC (Arimidex, Tamoxifen, Alone or in Combination) trial after completion of 5 years' adjuvant treatment for breast cancer. Lancet. 2005 Jan 1-7;365 (9453), 60-2.

Jakesz, R., et al: Switching of postmenopausal women with endocrine-responsive early beast cancer to anastrozole after two years adjuvant tamoxifen: Combine results of ABCSG trial 8 and ARNO 95 trial. Lancet 2005;366: 455 – 462

Kanis, J. A., & Johnell, O., & Oden,.A., & Johansson, H., & Closkey, E.Mc.: Frax™ and the assessment of fracture probability in men and women from the UK. Osteoporos Int. 2008; 19, s. 385–397

Marcus, R., & Feldman, D., & Nelson, D.A., & Rosen, C.J.: Osteoporosis, Elsevier AP, Burlington MA, 2008: 1939

Mardiak, J., & Ondrus, D., & Spanikova, B., & Ostatnikova, B.: Damage of bone metabolism and osteoporosis in testicular cancer patients. J Clin Oncol (Meeting Abstracts) June 2007 vol. 25 no. 18_suppl 5052

Mikosch, P., & Igerc, I., & Kudlacek, S., & Woloszczuk, W., & Kresnik, H., et al: Receptor activator of nuclear factor kappa B ligand and osteoprotegerin in men with thyroid cancer. Eur J Clin Invest 2006; 36, 8, 566-73

Ondruš, D., & Ondrušová, M.: Testicular cancer – diagnostic and therapy. Onkológia 2008; 3 (3): 170–174

Ondruš, D., & Špániková, B., & Ondrušová, M., & Mardiak, J.: Damage of hormonal function and bone metabolism in long term survivors of testicular cancer. European Andrology, 2007; 1,1, 36-37

Ondruš, D., & Špániková, B., & Ondrušová, M., & Mardiak, J.: Testosteron deficiency and bone metabolism damage in testicular cancer survivors. Urology 2007; 70, 3A, 166

Ondrušová, M., & Ondruš, D., & Dušek, L., & Špániková, B.: Damage of hormonal function and bone metabolism in long –terma survivors of testicular cancer. Neoplasma 2009; 56, 6 473-479

Payer, J., & Rovensky, J., & Killinger, Z. Lexikon of osteoporosis. Slovak Academic Press 2007; Bratislava, 75 pp., ISBN: 80809

Rizzoli, R, & el. Atlas of postmenopausal osteoporosis. 2nd ed. London: Current Medicine Group, 2005:25-46.

Shomon, M.: The tyroid treatement osteoporosis Controversy. Does the tyroid treatement contribute to los soft bone density? Thyroid 1995; 5(1):13-7

Špánik, S., & Špániková, B.: Bone mineral density in early brest cancer patients. Bratisl Lek Listy 2010; 111(1) 27-32

Špániková, B., & Špánik, S.: Changes in bone mineral density in breast cancer patients. Osteolog bulletin 2010; 15,3,127-8

Špániková, B., & Špánik, S.: Bone mineral density in patients with thyroid cancer on suppressive therapy after total thyroidectomy. J Clin Oncol 29:2011 (suppl; abstr e 19739)

Thürlimann, B., & Keshaviah, A., & Coates, A.S., & Mouridsen, H., & Mauriac, L., & Forbes, J.F., & Paridaens, R., & Castiglione-Gertsch, M., & Gelber, R.D., & Rabaglio, M., & Smith, I., & Wardley, A., & Price, K.N., & Goldhirsch, A.: Breast International Group (BIG) 1-98 Collaborative Group, A comparison of letrozole and tamoxifen in postmenopausal women with early breast cancer .N Engl J Med. 2005; Dec 29, 353(26), 2747-57

Part 2

Pediatric Issues in Osteoporosis

8

Physical Activity Interactions with Bone Accrual in Children and Adolescents

Izabella A. Ludwa and Panagiota Klentrou
Brock University,
Canada

1. Introduction

1.1 Osteoporosis and peak bone mass

Osteoporosis is a skeletal disease characterized by low bone mass and the deterioration of the micro architecture of bone tissue resulting in bone fragility and susceptibility to fractures (Gordon, 2003). According to the World Health Organization, osteoporosis is estimated to affect approximately 200 million women worldwide (Kanis, 2007) with the burden of osteoporosis being felt both personally and economically. Although the prevalence of fractures is higher is women, the mortality rate related to fragility fractures is higher in men (Center et al. 1999; Hasserius et al., 2003). Moreover, the annual cost of treating fractures in the United States is projected to increase to $25 billion in 2025 from $17 billion in 2005 (Burge et al., 2005).

Achieving peak bone mass (PBM) during adolescence and the subsequent rate of bone loss are major determinants of bone mass later in life (Hansen et al., 1991). The amount of bone mass achieved early in life has been shown to predict the level of bone mass and the incidence of fracture later in life suggesting that a primary risk factor for the development of osteoporosis is the inability to attain high PBM (Hansen et al., 1991; Heaney et al., 2000). PBM is generally defined as the highest level of bone mass achieved as a result of normal growth and seems to be established, for most sites of the skeleton, by late adolescence (Matkovic et al., 1994). Previous studies (Bonjour et al., 1991; Bailey et al., 1996) have demonstrated the period between 9-20 years of age to be critical in building peak bone mass as 90% of total body bone mineral content (BMC) is accrued by the age of 16 (Elgan et al., 2003; Stager et al., 2006), with the remaining 5-10% of total body bone mass achieved in the third decade (Cadogan et al, 1998). In fact, the most rapid bone mineral accumulation occurs approximately 1 year after the age of peak linear growth (Bailey et al., 1996); around the time of menarche for females (Cadogan et al., 1998). With considerable increases in bone mass occurring during puberty, maximizing PBM during this time is often advocated as the best way to delay age-related bone loss and prevent osteoporotic fractures (Fulkerson et al., 2004; Molgaard et al., 1999; Valimaki et al., 1994).

It appears, therefore, as though there is a critical period, a 'window of opportunity' (MacKelvie et al., 2002), in which we can influence the amount of bone mass we attain. However, bone development is the product of complex interactions between genetic and environmental factors including diet, hormonal influences, and mechanical stimuli (Gordon, 2003; Steelman & Zeitler, 2001). Permanent deficits in PBM are the result of any process that interferes with normal bone mineral accretion during adolescence, such as inadequate calcium intake, physical inactivity, and poor lifestyle choices (related to smoking, alcohol consumption, carbonated beverages) (Javaid & Cooper, 2002). As a result, research in bone growth and development in youth has endeavoured to ascertain the factors important to increasing bone mineral accretion.

1.2 Physical activity

The use of physical activity (PA) in maintaining bone health throughout the lifespan and ultimately preventing osteoporosis has been the focus of considerable research in improving PBM in order to minimize later bone loss (Beck & Snow, 2003). It is generally accepted that engaging in PA during growth enhances bone development (Boot et al., 1997; Janz et al., 2001; Janz et al., 2006). Habitual PA has been shown to enhance lean mass (Baxter-Jones et al., 2008) and bone accrual (Baxter-Jones et al., 2003) in youth, both of which are believed to promote bone health and muscle function in older age (Lefevre et al., 1990). Furthermore, 'when' activity occurs during the lifespan is important as PA at a young age can account up to 17% of the variance in bone mineral density (BMD) seen in individuals in their late 20s (Davies et al., 2005).

In addition to the timing of PA, the method by which PA imparts its benefits on bone is also important. Mechanical loading of sufficient intensity to promote increases in skeletal mass during growth require maximal strains to be greater than those of normal everyday living. If the bone is properly overloaded the load will elicit a modeling response making the bone susceptible to new levels of mechanical demand (Bailey et al., 1996). Some of the largest loads placed on the skeleton are physiological ones resulting from muscle contractions (Rauch et al., 2004; Scheonau & Frost, 2002). Furthermore, gravitational or ground reaction forces are also capable of generating the loads necessary to elicit a favourable response in bone. These two loading methods have lead to investigations of bone responses to different forms of PA with comparisons between athletes and non-athletes. Studies have demonstrated athletes involved in high-impact weight-bearing activities such as gymnastics and running have higher BMD (Lehtonen-Veromaa et al., 2000b, 2000c) than athletes participating in low-impact sports such as swimming; with such athletes exhibiting lower or normal bone densities than non-active youth (Bellew & Gehrig, 2006; Cassell et al., 1996; Courteix et al., 1998). Resistance training and simple jumping exercises have also been shown to have positive effects on femoral BMD in adolescent females and as such can be useful in promoting bone growth and maintaining acquired gains (Fuchs & Snow, 2002; Kato et al., 2006; Nichols et al., 2001). Therefore, different forms of PA, such as resistance training (Nichols et al., 2001) and weight-bearing exercise (Fuchs & Snow, 2002; Lehtonen-Veromaa et al., 2000c) have been shown to have positive effects on the developing skeleton through ground reaction forces and muscle contraction.

Various studies have examined the relationship between PA and markers of bone metabolism (Creighton et al., 2001; Lehtonen-Veromaa et al., 2000a), with little research conducted on markers of bone formation and resorption in relation to different types of sports, particularly in children and adolescents. In female athletes between the ages of 18-26, Creighton et al. (2001) found bone formation to be lower and resorption similar in swimmers compared to basketball, volleyball, and soccer players. In a younger population of boys and girls, ages 9-16 years, no differences were found in any markers of bone metabolism between gymnasts (Lehtonen-Veromaa et al., 2000a), swimmers (Derman et al.,

2008) and controls. Therefore, research investigating the relationship regarding bone markers and different PA types is limited and ambiguous, but even more so in children and adolescents, making it difficult to ascertain the effect of sport on bone. The examination of biochemical measurements of bone turnover, in addition to static measures of bone, is advantageous in the study of skeletal metabolism and growth as they provide an understanding of the dynamic course of bone remodelling. To date, the use of biochemical marks of bone turnover in PA interventions on bone in youth has been extremely limited.

Difficulties in comparing and assessing the benefits of PA on bone during growth reflect the varying methodologies used between studies. PA interventions aimed at improving bone health in youth have been subject to limited maturational comparisons as the majority of interventions have been conducted in one distinct pubertal group. Furthermore, the types of PA interventions that have been applied have varied greatly between studies. Discrepancies in results are due in part to the varying bone assessment techniques that are used across cross-sectional and intervention studies. Many of the aforementioned studies measured improvements in BMD using dual-energy x-ray absorptiometry (DXA). The use of DXA to interpret and evaluate BMD in the growing years can be difficult as there are considerable changes to the size and shape of bone (Bailey et al., 1996; Gordon, 2003; Schoenau et al., 2004), making comparisons between youth problematic. Furthermore, the measurements provided by DXA fail to account for the architecture, organization of tissues, mechanical properties and other factors known to impart bone strength. In addition, the bone assessment techniques used in majority of these studies have provided a static rather than dynamic picture of bone, which could in fact allow for more comparisons across studies.

Evidence supporting the role of PA on bone health has been accumulated from a wide range of studies investigating different activity methods using athletes, non-athletes and inactive individuals. Although these studies contribute to the literature they do not provide us with causality that PA does impart benefits to bone health. In response, there has been an increase in the number of intervention studies conducted, particularly in the school setting. PA interventions in schools are in many ways ideal places to intervene as they allow for a large population of children and adolescents to be targeted in a somewhat controlled environment, regardless of socioeconomic status, in a location where youth already spend a majority of their day during their most skeletally responsive years (Hughes et al. 2007).

2. Methods

Therefore, the primary objective of this chapter is to conduct a systematic review on the effectiveness of exercise and PA interventions to improve bone accrual in children and adolescents. Key finding from controlled intervention trials using various techniques to assess bone mineral density, content and strength changes will be discussed and be grouped according to maturity status. This will hopefully help to shed light on the best time during growth and development to influence bone health and to ascertain if there is indeed a window of opportunity for bone response.

We will also discuss and compare the different types of interventions used to affect changes in bone properties in youth, to determine if there is a modality that is best suited to improving bone development and to what degree these interventions influence changes in bone. Furthermore, we will address the characteristics of loading that have been shown to be best associated with particular structural improvements as interventions can be designed to impart mechanical loading on bone by jumping or by resistance training where the weight-bearing load on bone is applied through muscle. As majority of interventions measure only static properties of bone, this chapter will also be used to discuss bone remodelling parameters influenced by such exercise interventions. To our knowledge there has not been any studies examining the effects of PA interventions on bone remodelling.

2.1 Eligibility criteria and search strategy

The aim of the literature search was to find all available randomized control trials and controlled studies that examined the effects of any type of exercise or PA intervention trial on bone status in healthy (non-clinical, non-athletes) children and adolescents between 6 and 17 years of age. For this review we included all types of bone parameters from various bone assessment techniques (DXA, pQCT, QUS etc.) to be used as primary outcome measures as long as there were at least two measurement time points. Primary outcome measures included areal bone mineral density (aBMD), volumetric bone mineral density (vBMD), bone mineral content (BMC), bone area (BA), cortical thickness, bone strength index (BSI), stress-strain index (SSI), maximal moment of inertia (I^{mas}), section modulus (SM), speed of sound (SOS), broadband ultrasound attenuation (BUA), and markers of bone metabolism.

A computerised search of the MEDLINE and PubMed databases was performed on articles up till 2011 using a comprehensive combination of keywords to describe exercise, bone and participant parameters. The keywords used to describe exercise included: intervention and intervention studies, training, exercise, resistance training, physical education and physical education training, physical activity and motor activity. Bone parameter keywords included: bone mineral, bone density, bone and bones, bone strength, bone accrual and development, bone turnover, resorption, modelling and metabolism. For the participants, keywords such as children, adolescents, boys and girls were used. A total of 2728 were found, their titles and abstracts reviewed to determine if they met the inclusion criteria. Papers from all journals were considered and retrieved electronically or by interlibrary loan.

After screening the articles a total of 35 studies met the criteria and were used for the current review. Studies were grouped according to the maturity status of their participants based on Tanner Staging of development (Tanner, 1962). Participants were grouped as either prepubertal (Tanner 1), early pubertal (Tanner 2 and 3), and pubertal (Tanner 4 and 5) to maintain consistency with other literature review groupings. Studies in which authors provided results for more than one maturity group were divided into two parts (A and B).

3. Results

Table 1 represents the numerical breakdown of all the intervention studies reviewed into particular categories based on the type of intervention that was used, the method in which bone parameters were assessed, the maturity and sex of the population measured. Studies were included more than once if more than one measurement technique was used and if results were separated by sex or maturity group. Table 2 is a detailed summary of the design and outcomes of all the PA intervention studies reviewed, and are grouped according to the participants' maturity status. The results presented in Table 2 express the percentage difference in gain between the experimental groups participating in the intervention in comparison to controls. The results presented in the Table 2 are the final finding after any statistical adjustments have been made.

Type of Intervention		Measurement Technique		Maturational Status		Gender	
School Based		SXA	1	Prepubertal	16	Boys	12
Part of PE Class	23	DPA	1	Early Pubertal	16	Girls	24
At the School	5	DXA	33	Pubertal	7	Boys + Girls	7
Outside School	7	HSA	4	Multi Pubertal^{separate}	4		
Jumping	18	pQCT	5	Multi Pubertal^{together}	5		
General WBPA	14	QUS	3				
Resistance Training	3	Bone Markers	1				

Table 1. Numerical Breakdown by Category of Exercise Interventions for Bone in Youth

Prepubertal corresponds to Tanner Stage 1, early pubertal Tanner Stages 2-3, and pubertal Tanner Stages 4-5. Multi pubertal *separate* are studies with results separated by maturity, with *together* being studies that averaged data for more than one maturity group. Boys + girls reflect studies that did not separate results by sex. PE: physical education; WBPA: weight-bearing physical activity; SXA: single energy x-ray absorptiometry; DXA: dual energy x-ray absorptiometry; DPA: dual photon absorptiometry; pQCT; peripheral QCT; HSA: hip structural analysis; QUS: quantitative ultrasound.

Majority of the intervention studies were school based with 23 of the studies being conducted as part of a regular physical education class and 5 at some point within the school day. Approximately half (51%) of the studies utilized specific jumping interventions that relied on ground reaction forces in order to elicit a positive response on bone. Fourteen studies consisted of general weight bearing types of activities such as running, volleyball, aerobics etc., with only 3 studies specifically using resistance training with free or machine assisted weights. Significant increases in primary bone outcomes were found in 16 jumping interventions, 14 WBPA interventions, and 1 resistance training study. This translated into 79.5% of physical activity interventions positively influencing some form of bone strength parameter in children and adolescents. Furthermore, 5 studies also included calcium interventions which demonstrated benefits to bone in addition to physical activity.

Of the 35 studies reviewed 24 presented results separately for girls, 12 for boys, with 7 studies presenting data for boys and girls together. Moreover, 16 studies conducted interventions in prepubertal and early pubertal children. The smallest number of studies was performed in pubertal youth with a total of 7. All the pubertal interventions were completed on a population of girls, with 1 study (Weeks et al., 2008) including boys in their sample. Based on pubertal groups, an even number of boys and girls were represented in the results of prepubertal youth with 8 studies separately reporting results for boy and girls and 2 grouping results together. In early pubertal children, a larger number of studies were conducted on and included girls. Ten studies reported results separately for girls, 3 for boys and 5 did not distinguish results between genders.

DXA was the measurement technique predominantly used (94%) to assess bone, followed by pQCT (14%) and then QUS (8.5%). In total, 5 studies used more than one technique to determine changes in bone and these were all done in conjunction with DXA measurements. Four studies using DXA also performed hip structural analysis (HSA), which is a new application for DXA allowing for the estimation of geometric contributions to bone strength in the proximal femur and may potentially provide a better representation of bone strength (Bonnick, 2007). It is surprising that such a large percentage of studies utilized DXA given the known methodological issues with assessing changes in bone during growth. Until recently, we had thought no intervention studies had used biochemical markers of bone metabolism. Our extensive literature search found 1 study (Schneider et al., 2007) that measured serum markers of bone formation and resorption in adolescents. As static measures require longer durations for differences to be found, measuring biochemical markers of bone turnover to assess dynamic properties of bone could be advantageous in detecting changes sooner and allow for better comparisons of results between studies.

3.1 Prepubertal interventions

Positive effects of exercise on bone indices were found in 13 of 16 studies (81%), with overall effects ranging from 0.6% to 9.5% depending on the skeletal location and the type of measure (BMC, BMD, etc) taken for studies 7-36 months in duration. The average percent improvements for BMC included 4.5%, 4%, 2%and 1.5% at the lumbar spine (LS), femoral neck (FN), femur and total body (TB) respectively. BMD gains across studies were between 0.6-3% for the LS, FN and TB. The largest gains in girls was in BMC and area of the forearm (12.5% and 13.2% respectively) using peripheral DXA after 36 months of increased physical education class time (Hasselstrom et al., 2008). The one study that used pQCT in this group (Macdonald et al., 2007) was also the study that exhibited the largest bone gains in boys after 16 months of jump training, finding an increase of approximately 25% in BSI (an index of bone structural strength) of the distal tibia. MacKelvie et al. (2004) also presented large gains using HSA, with boys seeing a 12% increase in FN cross-sectional moment of inertia.

Despite the bone gains being similar between boys and girls, the number of studies that reported significant findings differed (4 vs. 7 out of 8 for girls vs. boys respectively). These discrepancies can largely be explained by the differences in the length and type PA intervention employed. MacKelvie et al. (2001) and (2002) were studies that utilized 7 months of school based physical education classes to employ a jump circuit intervention eliciting ground reaction forces 3-5 times one's body weight and demonstrated favourable gains in bone in boys but not girls. Fuchs et al. (2001) also found 7 months of jump training to be favourable to improvements in LS and FN BMC and BMD in prepubertal boys and girls. In fact the gains demonstrated in Fuchs et al. (2001) were greater than those in the MacKelvie et al. (2001, 2001) studies, most likely due to the larger ground reaction forces generated (8.8 vs. 3.5-5 x body weight). Studies at 12 months (Alwis et al., 2008b; Linden et al., 2007) utilizing a weight bearing physical education intervention follow a similar trend with improvements being seen in boys but not girls. The extra intervention time has not helped to elicit a significant positive bone response in the young girls. It is not till 24 months of the same type of weight bearing PA intervention that positive gains are found in girls (Linden et al., 2006). It would therefore appear that improvements in bone as a result of a PA intervention would more likely occur in prepubertal boys than girls. This is particularly true after 7 months of jumping training (MacKelvie et al., 2001, 2002) and 12 months of weight bearing PA (Alwis et al., 2008b; Linden et al., 2007). Improvements in prepubertal girls were seen in studies lasting 24 months in duration (Linden et al. 2006) and any studies demonstrating bone gains in a mixed gendered population (Fuchs et al., 2001; McKay et al., 2000) could be due to greater changes in the boys than the girls.

Reference	Population	Intervention	Measures	Results	Limitations
Pre Pubertal (Tanner Stage 1)					
Alwis et al. (2008a)	Boys, White Ex: n=80, Con: n=57 Age range: 6.7-9 yrs All remained TS 1 Randomized by school: 1 Ex + 3 Con.	24 Months Typical PE class: ball games, running jumping, climbing Ex: 40min/day (200min/wk) Con: 60min/wk Compliance: Con 84%, Ex 95%	DXA BMC: total body and L3 vertebra L3 vertebral width HSA of femoral neck	BMC L3: +3% L3 width: +1.3%	Uneven sample size between Ex and Con. Accelerometers captured only 4 days of 2-yr intervention Compliance not reported
Alwis et al. (2008b)	Girls, White Ex: n=53, Con: n=50 Age range: 6.7-9 yrs All remained TS 1 Randomized by school: 1Ex + 3 Con.	12 Months Typical PE class: ball games, running jumping, climbing Ex: 40min/day (200min/wk) Con: 60min/wk Compliance: Con 76%, Ex 95%	DXA and HSA BMC, aBMD, periosteal and endosteal diameter, cortical thickness, CSMI section modulus, and CSA of FN	No significant between group differences were found	Follow up periods varied Higher spare time activities in control group.
Bass et al. (2007)	Boys, White + Asian Total n=88, 7-11 yrs Ex Placebo: n=21 Ex Ca: n=20 No Ex Ca: n=21 No Ex Placebo: n=26 Randomized groups Ca: double blind	8.5 Months Part of PE class: 20min 3x week Hopping jumping, skipping moderate or low impact Ex: Ground rx forces 2-8 x BW No Ex: Ground rx forces 1 x BW Ca: 800mg Ca/day Compliance 86%	DXA BMC: total body, lumbar spine, femur, tibia-fibula, humerus, radius-ulna	Femur BMC: +2% Ex+Ca > all other grps Tibia-fibula BMC: +2% ExCa>Ex Placebo +3% Ex Ca> No ExCa and No Ex Pl NS for BMC in arms	Low sample sizes in each of the groups Control grp participated in low impact exercise making possible differences between groups smaller Population not all TS1 61% TS 1, 39% TS 2
Bradney et al. (1998)	Boys, White N=20 Ex, m=20 Con Age range: 8.4-11.8 All remained TS 1 Randomized by school: 1 Ex + 1 Con	8 Months Program outside of school: aerobics, soccer, volleyball, dance, gymnastics, basketball, weight training 30 minutes, 3 x week	DXA aBMD: total body and lumbar spine, femur, Femoral Midshaft BMC, aBMD and vBMD, and cortical thickness	aBMD TB: +1.2% aBMD LS: +2.8% BMC and aBMD femoral midshaft: +5.6% cortical thickness: +6.4%	Low sample sizes in each of the groups volumetric bone densities were derived/estimated
Fuchs et al. (2001)	Boys and Girls, Asian and White Age range: 5.9-9.8 yrs n=45 Ex, n=41 Con Randomized 1 school All remained TS 1	7 Months Activities added to PE classes: 10 min 3x week jumping 50-100 high box jumps, 2 footed Ground rx forces = 8.8 x BW 90% Compliance	DXA BMC and aBMD: lumbar spine and femoral neck BA: femoral neck	BMC LS: +3% BMC FN: +4.5% aBMD LS: +2% aBMD FN: NS BA FN: +2.9%	cannot distinguish results between boys and girls

Table 2. Randomized and Non-Randomized Controlled Studies on the Effects of Exercise on Bone Indices in Youth

Pre Pubertal (Tanner Stage 1)

Reference	Population	Intervention	Measures	Results	Limitations
Hasselstrom et al. (2008)	Boys and Girls, White (Ex: n= 135 and 108) (Con: n= 62 and 76) Age Range: 6-8 No Randomization TS 1 and 2	36 Months School based curriculum, time increased: 4 classes 180 min/wk Con: regular school curriculum 90min/wk Activities conducted in classes not mentioned	Peripheral DXA BMC and BMD: Calcaneus and distal forearm	Girls: NS changes in calcaneal and distal forearm BMD BMC forearm: +12.5% forearm area: +13.2% Boys: NS changes in all measures	Non-randomized study design allowing for selection bias DXA locations measured less studied Possible differences in standard anatomical region measured due to growth
Linden et al. (2006)	Girls, White Ex: n=49, Con: n=50 Age range: 7-9 All remained TS 1 Randomized by school: 1 Ex + 3 Con.	24 Months Typical PE class: ball games, running jumping, climbing Ex: 40min/day (200min/wk) Con: 60min/wk Ex. Attendance: 90%	DXA BMC and aBMD: TB, LS L2-L4 and L3, FN, and Leg vBMD, bone size: L3 and FN	BMC: L2-L4 +3.8%, L3 +7.2%, Leg +3.0% aBMD: TB +0.6%, L2-L4 +1.2%, L3 +1.6%, Leg +1.2% Bone Size: L3 +1.8%, and FN +0.3%	Differences in leisure time PA Compliance not reported
Linden et al. (2007)	Boys, White Ex: n=81, Con: n=57 Age range: 7-9 All remained TS 1 Randomized by school: 1 Ex + 3 Con.	12 Months Typical PE class: ball games, running jumping, climbing Ex: 40min/day (200min/wk) Con: 60min/wk Ex. Attendance: 90%	DXA BMC and aBMD: TB, L3 vertebra, FN Bone Width: L3 and FN	BMC, aBMD, bone width L3: +5.9%, +2.1% and +2.3%	Uneven sample size between Ex and Con. Compliance in Con Low Only assessed duration of PA, not intensity or effort
Macdonald et al. (2007) (Part A)	Boys and Girls Asian and White Ex: n=140, Con: n=72 Age range: 9.6-10.8 Randomized by school: 7 Ex. + 3 Con.	16 Months Ex: 15 min/day PA 5 x week, 5-36 jumps/day 4 x week Con: regular school curriculum Compliance 74%	pQCT BSI distal tibia SSI tibial midshaft	Boys: BSI distal tibia increased ~+25% Girls: NS changes in all measures	Low Compliance Potential bias for school selection
MacKelvie et al. (2001) (Part A)	Girls, White + Asian Ex: n=44, Con: n=26 Age range: 9.4-10.6 Randomized by schools: 7 Ex + 7 Con	7 Months Activity added to regular PE class: 10min, 3 x week 50-100 jumps and circuit training, progressing w/jumps Jumping = 3.5-5 x BW Compliance 80% across schools	DXA BMC and aBMD: TB, LS, PF, FN vBMD: FN	NS differences in any of the bone variables measured	Low Compliance Uneven sample sizes and distribution of sexes vBMD measurements were derived/estimated Uneven sample size between Ex and Con. More Ex's advances from TS 1 to TS2

Table 2. Continued – Studies on the Effects of Exercise on Bone in Youth

Pre Pubertal (Tanner Stage 1)

Reference	Population	Intervention	Measures	Results	Limitations
MacKelvie et al. (2002)	Boys White + Asian; Ex: n=61, Con: n=60; Age range: 9.7-10.9; Randomized by schools: 7 Ex + 7 Con	7 Months; Activity added to regular PE class: 10min, 3 x week; 50-100 jumps and circuit training, progressing w/jumps; Jumping = 3.5-5 x BW; Compliance 80% across schools	DXA; BMC and aBMD: TB, LS, PF, FN; vBMD: FN	BMC TB: +1.6%; aBMD PF: +1%	vBMD measurements were derived/estimated
MacKelvie et al. (2004)	Boys, White + Asian; Ex: n=31, Con: n= 33; Age range: 9.6-10.7; Randomized by schools: 7 Ex + 7 Con	20 Months; Activity added to regular PE class: 10min, 3 x week; 50-100 jumps and circuit training, progressing w/jumps; Jumping = 3.5-5 x BW	DXA and HSA; BMC and BA: TB, LB, PF, FN, and TR; HAS: PF, NN, TR, FN; SM: FN	BMC FN: +4.3%; Cross-sectional moment of inertia: +12.35%; SM: +7.4%	Study compliance: Ex 39% and Con 42%; More Con remained TS 1 and more Ex's advanced to TS 3
McKay et al. (2000)	Boys and Girls; White and Asian; Ex: n=63, C: n=81; Age range: 6.9-10.2; School randomized	8 Months; Part of PE classes: jumping, hopping, skipping 2 x week; 3 x week 10 tuck jumps; Con: regular PE classes	DXA; aBMD: TB, LS, PF, FN, and trochanter (TR)	aBMD TR: +1.2%	All boys remained TS 1, with some girls maturing to TS 2; Compliance not reported
Petit et al. (2002) (Part a)	Girls, Asian + White; Age range: 9.4-10.6; Ex: n=43, Con: n=25; Randomized by schools: 14 schools ethnic stratification	7 Months; Part of PE classes: 10-12 min; 3x week: 5 x diverse jumping exercise stations; Con: regular PE classes; Ground rx forces=3.5-5 x BW	DXA and HSA; aBed: TB, LS, TR, PF; cortical thickness, area; and SM: PF	NS differences in any of the bone variables measured	Compliance not reported; Errors related to method of measurement
Valdimarsson et al. (2006)	Girls, White; Ex: n=53, Con: n=50; Age range: 7-9 yrs; Ex group come from one school	12 Months; Typical PE class: ball games, running jumping, climbing; Ex: 40min/day (200min/wk); Con: 60min/wk. 90% Attendance	DXA; BMC and aBMD: TB, LS (L2-L4), L3, FN, leg; vBMD: L3 and FN	BMC LS: +4.7%; BMC L3: +9.5%; aBMD LS: 2.8%; aBMD L3: 3.1%; Bone width L3: +2.9%	No randomization; Compliance low in controls; volumetric bone densities were derived/estimated

Table 2. Continued – Studies on the Effects of Exercise on Bone in Youth

Reference	Population	Intervention	Measures	Results	Limitations
Pre Pubertal (Tanner Stage 1)					
Van Langendonck et al. (2003)	Girls, Ethnicity not reported, Ex: n=21, Con: n=21, 21 pairs of monozygotic twins, Age range: 8-9yrs	9 Months, Ex: 3x week: hopping/jumping, Progression: removal of shoes different stimulus, Ground rx forces not measured, Compliance: Ex 91%	DXA, BMC, aBMD, BA: FN and PF	BMC PF: +2.5%, aBMD PF: +1.3%, BMC FN: +2.0%, aBMD FN: +2.4%	Some of the girls participated in high impact sports during their leisure time - separate analysis conducted
Early Pubertal (Tanner Stage 2-3)					
Barbeau et al. (2007)	Girls, Black, n=77 Ex., n=83 Con. Age range: 8-12 yrs, Recruited from 8 elementary schools	10 Months, After school intervention, 5 days/week, 80 min PA: 25min skills, 35min MVPA, 20min toning + stretching	DXA, Total body BMD, BMC	BMC TB: +4.0%, BMD TB: +2%	Examined girls who attended 40% of classes 2d/wk, Main focus was to improve cardiovascular fitness, Low compliance
Courteix et al. (2005)	Girls, White (n=85), Age range: 8-13 yrs, Ex Ca: n=12, Ex Placebo: n=42, No Ex Ca: n=10, No Ex Placebo: n=21, Randomized, Blinded	12 Months, Ex: 7.2h/week, No Ex: 1.2h/week, Ca: 800 mg/day, Compliance 75%, Ex: Participated in weight bearing physical activity	DXA, aBMD: TB, LS, FN, WT	aBMD TB: +6.3%, aBMD LS: +11%, aBMD FN: +8.2%, aBMD WT: 9.3% (all Ex Ca > No Ex Pl) NS differences between other groups	Uneven sample size distribution between groups, Type of exercise not controlled, Exercise based on habitual activity
Heinonen et al. (2000) (Part A)	Girls, White, Ex: n=25, Con: n=33, Age range: 10-12yrs, Selection to groups decided by teachers	9 Months, Step aerobic program: 50 min 2 x week: 20 min of jumping exercises: 100-200 jumps from box (two and one footed), Ground rx forces not measured, Compliance: Ex 73%, Study 92%	DXA and pQCT, BMC: LS, FN, and TR, Cortical area: tibial midshaft	BMC LS: +3.3%, BMC FN: +4.0%	Compliance low, Potential selection bias due to teachers selecting groups
Iuliano-Burns et al. (2003)	Girls, White + Asian, Total n=64, Age range: 8-9 yrs, Mod Ex. Ca: n=16, Mod Ex. Pl: n=16, Low Ex. Ca: n=16, Low Ex. Pl: n=16, Randomized groups	8.5 Months, Ex: 20 min 3 x week, Mod Ex. Impact: skipping, hopping, jumping. Used hand weights in final 8 weeks, Low Ex. Impact: stretching, Ca: average of 434 mg/day, Compliance: Ex 93%, Study 88%	DXA, BMC: LS, Femur, Tibia-Fibula	BMC tibia-fibula: +3% Mod ex>Low Ex. +7.1% Mod Ex Ca > Low Ex. No Pl.	Low sample sizes

Table 2. Continued – Studies on the Effects of Exercise on Bone in Youth

Reference	Population	Intervention	Measures	Results	Limitations
Early Pubertal (Tanner Stage 2-3)					
MacKelvie et al. (2001) (Part B)	Girls, White + Asian Ex: n=43, Con: n=64 Age range: 9.9-11.1 yr Randomized by schools: 7 Ex + 7 Con	7 Months Part of PE class: 10min 3x week 50-100 jumps and circuit training, progressing w/jumps Jumping = 3.5-5 x BW Compliance 80% across schools	DXA BMC and aBMD: TB, LS, PF, FN Volumetric BMD: FN	BMC LS +1.8% aBMD LS +1.7% BMC FN: NS aBMD FN: +1.6% vBMD FN: +3.1%	Volumetric bone densities were derived/estimated Uneven sample size between Ex and Con.
MacKelvie et al. (2003)	Girls, Asian + White Ex: n=33, C: n=43 Age range: 9.3-10.7 Randomized by schools: 7 Ex + 7 Con	20 Months Part of PE class: 10min 3x week 50-100 jumps and circuit training, progressing w/jumps Jumping = 3.5-5 x BW Compliance 42% over 20 Mos.	DX BMC: LS and FN	BMC LS: +3.7% BMC FN: +4.6%	Con group older and more mature Compliance not reported for Ex. Group
Macdonald et al. (2007) (Part B)	Boys and Girls Asian and White Ex: n=135, Con: n=57 Age range: 9.6-10.8 yrs Randomized by school: 7 Ex. + 3 Con.	16 Months Ex: 15 min/day PA 5 x week, 5-36 jumps/day 4 x week Con: regular school curriculum Compliance 74%	pQCT BSI distal tibia SSI tibial midshaft	NS changes in any of the measures	Low Compliance Potential bias for school selection Uneven sample sizes and distribution of sexes between groups
Macdonald et al. (2008)	Boys and Girls Asian and White Ex: n=140, Con: n=72 Age range: 9-11 yrs Randomized by school: 7 Ex. + 3 Con. TS 1-3	16 Months Ex: 15 min/day PA 5 x week, 5-36 jumps/day 4 x week Con: regular school curriculum Compliance 74%	DXA and HSA FN bone strength, geometry, and BMC BMC: TB, PF, LS	Boys: BMC LS: +2.7% BMC TB: +1.7% Girls: section modulus of FN: +5.4% (only in girls with 80% compliance)	Low teacher compliance Uneven sample sizes and distribution of sexes btw grps More boys prepubertal and girls early pubertal Results not separated by maturity status
Macdonald et al. (2009)	Boys, Asian + White Ex: m=139, Con: n=63 Age range: 9-11 yrs Randomized by school: 7 Ex. + 3 Con.	16 Months Ex: 15 min/day PA 5 x week, 5-36 jumps/day 4 x week Con: regular school curriculum Compliance 74%	pQCT Second moments of area, cortical area, cortical thickness of tibia	Max second moment of area: +3% Trends for increase in cortical area and thickness, but NS	Uneven sample sizes Higher percentage of TS2 in Ex Group compared to Con at baseline, with Con having more TS1

Table 2. Continued - Studies on the Effects of Exercise on Bone in Youth

Early Pubertal (Tanner Stage 2-3)

Reference	Population	Intervention	Measures	Results	Limitations
McKay et al. (2005)	Girls and Boys Asian and White Ex: n=51, Con: n=73 Age Range: 9.5-10.5 No Randomization	8 Months Program: Bounce at the Bell 10 counter movement jumps 3 min 3 x day each school day Ground Rx forces: 5 × BW Compliance: Ex 60%, study 100%	DXA and HSA BMC: PF and TR BA: PF and TR Cortical thickness and area: PF	BMC PF: +2.0% BMC TR: +2.7% BA PF: +1.3% BA TR: +2.0% Con > Ex: BMC and BA TB	Compliance Low Ex group participated in greater PA at baseline Con greater increase in TB BMC and BA
Meyer et al. (2011)	Boys and Girls, White Ex: n=297, Con: n=205 Age range: 6.6-11.7 yrs Randomized by classes: Ex: 16 classes/ 9 schools, Con: 12 classes/6 schools TS 1-3	12 Mos School based program Ex: regular PE class + 2 extra PE classes that include 10 min jumping activities. 2-5min jumping/balancing tasks through out day Con: regular PE classes	DXA BMC and aBMD: TB, FN, L2-L4	BMC TB: +5.5% BMC FN: +5.4% BMC LS: +4.7% aBMD TB: +8.4% aBMD LS:+7.3% Pubertal stage*group interaction favored prepubertal children	Has distinct pubertal groups but results not separated by maturity. Maturity used to adjust for variables Small sample size of pre pubertal Con grp (loss of data) Compliance not reported
Morris et al. (1997)	Girls, Ethnicity not given, but schools stratified according to ethnicity Ex: n=38, Con: n=33 Age range: 8.6-10.4 yrs No randomization Grouped by teachers	10 Months Activity added to regular PE class: 30 min 3 x week Aerobics, skipping, dance, ball games, progressing to weight training Ground rx forces not measured Compliance: Ex 92%, Study 97%	DXA and BMAD BMC: TB, LS, FN, PF aBMD: TB, LS, PF BMAD: LS, FN	BMC TB and LS: +5.5% BMC FN: +4.5% BMC PF: +8.3% aBMD TB: +2.3% aBMD LS: +3.6% aBMD FN: +10.3% aBMD pF: +3.2% BMAD LS: +2.9%	Potential selection bias as teachers selected groups Maturity greater in Ex than control (due to drop outs) and could contribute to the greater gains seen
Nemet et al. (2006)	Boys and Girls, Ethnicity not given Ex: n=12, Con: n=12 Age range: 6-16 yrs Obese participants Randomized groups	3 Months Structured activities to mimic PE classes. Mainly endurance: 50% sports, 50% running and games: 1 hour 2 x week Received nutrition counseling	QUS SOS of left tibia	SOS: +2.9% Difference due to significant SOS decrease (-2.6%) in Con, and NS increase in Ex. (+0.6%)	Small sample size Population spans a large age range Compliance not reported

Table 2. Continued - Studies on the Effects of Exercise on Bone in Youth

Reference	Population	Intervention	Measures	Results	Limitations
Early Pubertal (Tanner Stage 2-3)					
Nichols et al. (2008)	Boys and Girls, White Total n=112 Age range: 9-10yrs Ex only: n=61 Nutrition only: n=9 Ex + nutrition: n=14 Con: n=28 4 schools randomized 85% TS1 at baseline	20 Months Activity added to PE classes: 8-12min 2 x week: of jumping and skipping Ground Rx forces 2-3 x BW Nutrition: 45min biweely clases to improve Ca intake Compliance: 80% at 8 months, 73% at 20 months	DXA BMD: TB, LS (L2-L4), PF, and FN BMC: TB, LS, FN, PF Measures taken twice: 8 and 20 months	NS differences between groups for any of the bone measurements taken at 8 and 20 months	Uneven sample size distribution between groups TS estimated based on height velocity Leisure PA not controlled: 59% reported participating in organized sports/activities Ground rx forces estimated
Petit et al. (2002) (Part B)	Girls, Asian + White Age range: 9.9-11.1yrs Ex: n=43, Con: n=63 Randomized by schools: 14 schools stratified by ethnic composition	7 Months 10-12 min 3x week 5 x diverse jumping exercise stations Activities done in addition to regular PE classes Con: regular PE classes Ground rx forces=3.5-5 x BW	DXA and HSA aBMD: TR and FN SM: FN cortical thickness: FN	aBMD TR: +1.7% aBMD FN: +2.6% SM FN: +4.0% cortical thickness FN: : +3.2%	Compliance not reported Errors related to method of measurement
Sundberg et al. (2001)	Boys and Girls, White Ex Boys: n=40 Ex Girls: n=40 Con Boys: n=82 Con Girls: n=66 Age range: 12-16 yrs 2 Schools (1 Ex, 1 Con) Recruited grade 6,7 (12-13yrs), follow up grade 9 (15-16yrs) TS 2,3 start TS 4,5 end	3-4 Years Additional time in PE classes Ex: 40min 4 x week 3 of 4 classes: weight bearing activities, jumping, running, gymnastics, ball games 1 of 4 classes: swimming Con: regular PE classes of 60 min 2 x week Compliance: Ex 93%, Con 91%	DXA: BMC, aBMD, vBMD, and bone size: TB, LS, FN SXA: BMC and aBMD: distal radius and ulna ultradistal radius QUS: BUA, SOS, and SI: calcaneus (heel)	3/4 Years Boys: BMC FN: +8% / 0% aBMD FN: +9% / +14% vBMD FN: 9% / +15% BMC LS: +9% / 0% aBMD LS: 0% / +10% SOS Heel: +1% / +11% SI Heel: +7% / +2% 3-4 Years Girls: aBMD distal/ultra-distal radius: -6-7%	vBMD and BA was derived Con girls had high levels of leisure PA, bone mass, Ca intake and earlier menarche than Ex girls, which may have masked effects of intervention Ex program not specific to building bone Control group not from the same school
Pubertal (Tanner Stage 4-5)					
Blimkie et al. (1996)	Girls Ethnicity not reported Ex: n=16, Con: n=16 Age range: 15.9-16.3 All postmenarcheal	6.5 Months Machine assisted weight training 3 x week 4 sets of 12 reps each, with progression every 6 weeks	DPA BMC: TB and LS aBMD: TB and LS	NS differences in any of the bone variables measured	Compliance was no clear The duration/length of each session was not clear

Table 2. Continued - Studies on the Effects of Exercise on Bone in Youth

Pubertal (Tanner Stage 4-5)

Reference	Population	Intervention	Measures	Results	Limitations
Heinonen et al. (2000) (Part B)	Girls, White Ex: n=39, Con: n=29 Age range: 12.8-15yrs Selection to groups decided by teachers	9 Months Step aerobic program: 50 min 2 x week with 20 min of jump exercises: 100-200 jumps from box (two and one footed) Ground rx forces not measured Compliance: Ex 65%, Study 92%	DXA and pQCT BMC: LS and FN Cortical area: tibial midshaft	NS differences in any of the bone variables measured	Compliance low Potential selection bias due to teachers selecting groups
Nichols et al. (2001)	Girls Ethnicity not reported Ex: n=5, Con: 11 Age range: 14-17 yrs All postmenarcheal Randomized groups	15 Months Resistance training program weights and machines: 30-45 min, 3 x week of 15 Progression: weight increase Compliance: Ex. 73%, Study 15%	DXA BMC and aBMD: TB, LS, FN, WT, and TR BMAD: LS and FN	aBMD WT: +3.2% aBMD FN: +2.3%	Large dropout rate resulting in small sample size (originally Ex=46, Con=21)
Schneider et al. (2007)	Girls, White, Hispanic, Asian Ex: n=63, Con: n=59 Age range: Randomized two schools: 1 Ex + 1 Con All given 500mg Ca/d	10 Months, 2 school semesters School based program: 60 min 5 x week (~40min activity time) Variety of aerobic (3 x week), strength building (1 x week), educational (1 x week) activities	DXA + bone turnover BMC and BMD: TB, LS, Hip, thoracic spine, FN and TR Bone formation: OC, BSAP, and CICP Bone resorption: PYD	Thoracic BMC: +4.9% NS differences in BMD measurements or markers of bone turnover	Compliance not reported Population may not be generalizable as proactive approach to attrition taken and terminated participation Duration of study time points is unclear
Stear et al. (2003)	Girls, White Total n=144 Age range: 16-18 yrs Ca Ex: n=37 Ca No Ex: n=28 Placebo Ex: n=38 Placebo No Ex: n=28 All postmenarcheal Randomized, double blinded 2 schools	15.5 Months Lunch + after school program 45min 3 x week of aerobic to music: moderate to vigorous high impact movements Ground rx forces not measured Ca: 1000mg/day Ex attendance: 36% Ca compliance: 70%	DXA BMC and BA: TB, LS, FN TR, hip, nondominant total, ultradistal and distal third radius	Ca Ex > Placebo No Ex BMC TB: +0.8% BMC LS: +1.9% BMC FN: +2.2% BMC Hip: +2.7% BMC TR: +4.8% Ex > No Ex BA LS: +0.7% BMC Hip: +1.4% BMC TR: +2.6%	Poor Ex attendance Decreased BA in the hip which may suggest reorientation of the hip with increasing age, redistribution of mineral, or alternation in bone-edge detection of DXA Results based on good compliance (smaller sample)

Table 2. Continued - Studies on the Effects of Exercise on Bone in Youth

Table 2. Randomized and Non-Randomized Controlled Studies on the Effects of Exercise on Bone Indices in Youth

Reference	Population	Intervention	Measures	Results	Limitations
Pubertal (Tanner Stage 4-5)					
Weeks et al. (2008)	Boys and Girls Total n=81 Ex Boys: n=22 Con Boys: n=15 Ex Girls: n=21 Ex Girls: n=23 Age range: 13.5-14.5 Randomized 1 school	8 Months Ex: 10 min 2x week jumping activities as warmup in PE class worked up to ~300 jumps at 1-3 Hz, height 0.2-0.4m Con: 10min 2x week of regular PE class warmup Compliance Ex 80% Study dropout rate 18%	DXA and QUS BMC, BMD, and BA: TB, FN, LS, TR BMAD, CSMI, IBS, and cortical wall thickness BUA: nondominant calcaneus	Boys: BMC TB: +4.3% NS increases Ex boys: BUA calcaneus: +3.6% FN area: +1.1% Girls: NS differences NS increases Ex girls: BMC FN: +9% BMAD LS: +3.7% LS area: +2.9%	Volumetric bone densities were derived/estimated Small sample size for between group sex differences
Witzke & Snow. (2002)	Girls, White Ex: n=25, Con: n=28 Age range: 14-15 yrs All postmenarcheal No randomization	9 Months Ex: 30-45 min 3 x week of resistance and plyometrics training with increasing intensity over 9 months Ground rx forces not measured	DXA BMC: TB, LS, FN, TR	NS differences in BMC between groups However, increases in BMC for TB, LS, FN, TR ranged +0.1-2.1% in Ex group	Compliance not reported Potential selection bias

Ex: exercise group; Con: control group; BMC: bone mineral content; aBMD: areal bone mineral density; vBMD: volumetric BMD; BA: bone area; BMAD: bone mineral apparent density (BMD adjusted for BA); TB: total body; LS: lumbar spine; FN: femoral neck; NN: narrow neck; PF: proximal femur; WT: wards triangle; TR: trochanter; SXA: single energy x-ray absorptiometry; DXA: dual energy x-ray absorptiometry; DPA: dual photon absorptiometry; QCT: qualitative computed tomography, pQCT; peripheral QCT; HSA: hip structural analysis; QUS: quantitative ultrasound; SOS: speed of sound; SM: section modulus; CSMI: cross-sectional moment of inertia; IBS/BSI: index of bone structural strength; SSI: strength strain index; BUA: broadband ultrasound attenuations; OC: osteocalcin; BSAP: bone-specific alkaline phosphatise; CICP: c-terminal procollagen peptide; PYD: deoxypyridinoline; Ca: calcium; Rx: reaction; BW: body weight; PE: physical education; TS: Tanner stage; Pl: Placebo; Grps: Groups; NS: no significant.

3.2 Early pubertal interventions

Eighty-three percent of the PA interventions were capable of creating a positive effect on bone strength parameters in pubertal boys and girls. Study durations ranged from 3 months to 4 years, with both the average and median duration being 12 months. The percent gains in bone ranged anywhere between 1.3-15%; again depending on the measurement location and the technique employed. Of the 16 studies conducted in this group 12 utilized DXA, 3 pQCT, 2 QUS, and 1 SXA. Three of the DXA studies also conducted HSA with 2 of the overall studies employing more than one technique to assess experimental effects on bone. The largest improvements in bone for girls was a 10.3% change in aBMD at the FN following 10 months of a mixed program using jumping, weight bearing exercise and weight training (Morris et al, 1997). This large improvement, however, could be the result of a potential selection bias. In boys, the greatest improvements were in the double digits at 10%, 11%, 14% and 15% for LS aBMD, calcaneal SOS, FN aBMD and vBMD, respectively (Sundberg et al., 2001). These finding in boys were demonstrated after 4 years of increased physical education classes that involved a mixed program of weight bearing and jumping activities. In addition to a PA intervention, 2 of the studies also employed a calcium intervention (Courteix et al., 2005; Iuliano-Burns et al., 2003). These studies (Courteix et al., 2005; Iuliano-Burns et al., 2003) demonstrated calcium supplementation in addition to PA can elicit greater responses in bone than with exercise alone, highlighting the importance of monitoring calcium intake during intervention studies particularly during puberty.

The number of interventions conducted in boys and girls was not equal as it was in the prepubertal group making the discussion on gender differences and effects of PA on bone in this group problematic. Three studies in early pubertal children by the same author (Macdonald et al., 2007, 2008, 2009) incorporated 16 months of 60 minute weekly classroom PA including a bone building program of 5-36 jumps per day 4 times a week. Using pQCT, DXA and HSA these studies demonstrated no significant changes in bone strength in the tibia, but improvements in tibial geometry and bending resistance in boys (Macdonald et al., 2007, 2009). Boys also experienced improvements in lumbar spine BMC and whole body BMC, with girls seeing increases in section modulus (a measure of bending resistance) of the femoral neck (Macdonald et al., 2008). These results imply there may be gender differences in the properties of bone that improve following an exercise intervention. There are 3 reasons why the trends shown by Macdonald et al. (2007, 2009) failed to reach significance. Firstly, there was an uneven distribution of sample size, maturity status and gender between groups making some of the groups underpowered. Secondly, as ground reaction forces were not reported it is possible that external loads applied during the intervention was not high enough to instigate a loading response in bone. Third and most likely, the benefits of the jumping intervention could have been attenuated due to the low compliance to the program. In fact, Macdonald et al. (2008) reported significant findings for individuals with 80% compliance. This notion is supported by 3 studies that (MacKelvie et al., 2001, 2003; Petit et al., 2002) demonstrated improvements in BMC, aBMD and vBMD in girls following a shorter jumping program (7 months) eliciting larger ground reaction forces (3.5-5 x body weight) and for whom study compliance was 80% (MacKelvie et al., 2001).

Not only does it appear that larger loading responses are needed to elicit positive changes in bone, but also the way in which that load is applied to bone matters. A large number of studies (69%) employed specific jumping exercises as part of their intervention demonstrating that short, irregular, diverse large loads at varying times of the day are sufficient to instigate bone responses (Heinonen et al., 2000; MacKelvie et al., 2001; McKay et al. 2005, Meyer et al., 2011; Petit et al., 2002). Unlike the studies conducted in prepubertal youth, interventions prescribing weight bearing activities do not need to be conducted over long periods of time to see similar responses in bone. Barbeau et al. (2007), Courteix et al. (2005), and Morris et al. (1997) demonstrated such improvements in 7-12 months time. Interventions in which there were no improvements in bone parameters attributed this to higher levels of leisure PA in the non-experimental groups, increased bone mass at baseline, and earlier menarcheal status (Petit et al., 2002; Sundberg et al., 2001). All of these factors would contribute to bone indices being elevated prior to the intervention allowing for only small changes to occur and in turn masking any effects of the intervention program.

3.3 Pubertal interventions

The fewest PA interventions were conducted in pubertal youth, with all 7 involving girls and 1 including boys. The types of interventions included resistance training (Blimkie et al., 1996; Nichols et al., 2001; Witzke & Snow, 2002), jumping trials (Weeks et al., 2008), and those with a variety of different weight-bearing activities (Heinonen et al., 2000, Schneider et al., 2007, Stear et al., 2003). DXA was the predominant method used to asses bone in this population, with one study using DPA (Blimkie et al., 1996). Three of the studies that used DXA also used an alternate method such as pQCT (Heinonen et al. 2000), QUS (Weeks et al., 2008) and serum biochemical markers of bone turnover (Schneider et al., 2007). Half of the trials demonstrated significant changes (0.7-4.9%) in bone following their interventions, with 3 of the studies demonstrating non-significant trends (Schneider et al., 2007; Weeks et al., 2008, Witzke & Snow, 2002). Of those studies that reported significant trends, one included both an exercise and calcium intervention and observed bone mineral advantages at the femoral neck, lumbar spine and total body in adolescent girls receiving both interventions (Stear et al., 2003). Albeit the combination of calcium and exercise generated greater improvements, those girls receiving just the exercise also demonstrated significant changes at the hip. Schneider et al. (2007) provided all pubertal girls with 500mg of calcium per day and unlike Stear et al. (2003) only observed significant changes in thoracic BMC despite improved trends in BMD and markers of bone turnover. It is possible that these results failed to reach significance as the intervention by Schneider et al. (2007) was shorter in duration than Stear et al. (2003), 10 vs. 15.5 months respectively. Moreover, as everyone in Schneider et al.'s (2007) study was taking calcium the room for improvements may have been smaller than Stear et al.'s (2003) who observed the greatest differences between exercising calcium takers and non- exercising non-calcium consuming controls. Regardless of these discrepancies, the one thing that is clear from these two studies and those described in the early pubertal section (Courteix et al., 2005; Iuliano-Burns et al., 2003), is that calcium is important to bone health and its use during PA interventions will greatly affect results.

Three investigations of the effects of resistance training on bone mineral accrual in pubertal girls were completed, with only 1 reporting significant changes in bone indices (Nichols et al., 2001). A major difference between the studies that did not find significant changes (Blimkie et al., 1996; Witzke & Snow, 2002) and the one that did (Nichols et al., 2001) was the duration of the intervention trial. It appears that with resistance training a longer trial of approximately 15 months is necessary to demonstrate significant improvements in bone, similarly to the 15.5 months of WBPA in Stear et al. (2003). In addition to resistance training Witzke & Snow (2002) used plyometric training and the utilization of this may have resulted in the strong non-significant trends, demonstrating that perhaps shorter trials that include ground reaction forces can be efficacious at improving bone. Results from studies examining jumping trials (Heinonen et al., 2000; Weeks et al., 2008) 8-9 months in duration have been ambiguous. Heinonen et al. (2000) failed to measure significant changes in bone; however, Weeks et al. (2008) did observe improved total body BMC in pubertal boys but not girls. Interestingly, Weeks et al. (2008) did measure large percent changes, albeit non-significant trends, in many different parameters of bone strength in both boys and girls. These trends could be the result of the greater ground reaction forces used in this study compared to that of Heinonen et al. (2000) and could possibly have reached significant if the length of the trial were longer. A common theme in all of these studies not having significant findings or 'almost' measuring differences is poor compliance. If it were not for the issues with compliance, there is a large probability these studies would have found significant results.

Another important factor as to why very few studies reported changes in pubertal youth is due to how bone is accrued in this maturity group. According to Bailey et al. (1996, 1999) peak velocity of BMC accrual for the whole body occurs approximately 0.7-1 year after peak linear growth around the time of menarche, which corresponds to approximately 12-13 years of age in girls. The pubertal girls in the 7 studies reviewed were between the ages of 13 and 18, putting them after the point of peak BMC velocity accrual where the velocity at which they are accruing bone is actually decreasing. The schematic representation of PBM and the rate at which bone mass is accrued over time resembles a dose response curve. It would appear that the pubertal girls in these studies are nearing their PBM, putting them near the plateau of the accrual process, and therefore both the rate and amount of BMC that can be accrued during this time is less. As a result, detecting significant changes will be difficult. Just because these percent gains are small and non-significant statistically does not mean that they are not meaningful. Turner and Robling (2003) demonstrated that a 5.4% and 6.9% gain in aBMD and BMC respectively, translated into a 64% and 94% increase in the amount of force and energy a bone could absorb before failure. This suggests that even small changes in bone mass, which are marginally detectable by DXA can significantly improve bone strength. Therefore a little bone goes a long way.

4. Discussion

4.1 The window of opportunity for bone adaptations

The early pubertal period may be the best time to generate skeletal adaptations to PA. Studies conducted in more than one maturity group demonstrated positive bone gains in early pubertal girls with no significant increases in prepubertal (MacKelvie et al., 2001; MacKelvie et al., 2003; Petite et al., 2002) or pubertal (Heinonen et al., 2000) girls. When reviewing all of the intervention studies the greatest gains in bone on average, regardless of sex, skeletal location and type of activity used, was during the early pubertal years. These results are more definitive in girls as a larger proportion of intervention studies have been conducted on females across puberty, with the sample of boys decreasing with maturity. Despite this trend, longer duration intervention studies where boys most likely transitioned from pre- to early puberty also demonstrate larger gains in bone than in just prepubertal boys (MacKelvie et al., 2004). Larger skeletal gains were also observed in interventions trials that supplemented with calcium during early puberty (Courteix et al., 2005; Iuliano-Burns et al., 2003) compared to those supplementing in prepubertal (Bass et al., 2007) and pubertal

(Schneider et al., 2007; Stear et al., 2003) stages. Moreover, the velocity for BMC accrual is highest in early puberty prior to menarche (in girls) (Bailey et al., 1996, 1997; Cadogan et al., 1998, after which accrual rates decrease with age plateauing in late adolescence upon achieving PBM (Davies et al., 2005). Therefore, the 'window of opportunity' to impart the largest influences on bone development may be during early puberty.

4.2 Optimal physical activity interventions for bone adaptations
Based on our systematic review of the literature we can deduce that regular exercise can be an effective way to improve bone density, size, and shape; in turn improving the mechanical strength of bone. With the variability in the types of interventions used and how they were employed there is no clear consensus on exactly how we should prescribe exercise in order to see the greatest returns in terms of bone health. However, in reviewing the literature, regardless of pubertal stage, the duration of the trial and the intensity in which it was employed appeared to matter. If interventions were short in duration (8-10 months) those that utilized jumping activities with high ground reaction forces received the most positive results (Bass et al. 2007; Fuchs et al., 2001; MacKelvie et al., 2001, 2002; McKay et al., 2005; Petit et al., 2002; Weeks et al., 2008). If weight bearing PA or resistance training was utilized the length of the intervention needed to be longer (10-24 months depending on maturity), in order to see significant gains in bone (Alwis et al., 2008a; Courteix et al., 2005; Linden et al., 2006, 2007; Morris et al., 1997; Nichols et al., 2001; Stear et al., 2003; Valdimarsson et al., 2006). In terms of frequency of exercise, Turner & Robling (2003) suggest it is better to shorten each individual exercise session than to reduce the number of sessions, as jump training has been shown to improve BMC when performed at least 3 time per week but not when reduced to 2 time per week, with gains increasing up to 5 days a week with 2 shorter session in one day. This is reflected in the interventions reviewed with significant gains in bone indices being observed in trials occurring 3-5 times per week. The most recent intervention study reviewed (Meyer et al., 2011) is a good example of these last two concepts by demonstrating that a variety of different activities in one intervention at random times of the day can be effective in eliciting bone gains. Therefore, PA is beneficial for bone health and irregular activities utilizing jump and resisting training to weight bearing activities are some of the best ways to elicit an adaptive response in bone. Not only is the variety beneficial for bone but it can also help to alleviate the boredom that accompanies exercise regimens. Remember that in terms of bone change really is good!

4.3 Methodological issues
DXA was the technique most often used in the PA intervention trials reviewed, and was used to measure BMC and BMD in various skeletal regions of the body. However, BMD assessed using DXA is an estimation of 'true' bone density and the areal density that is expressed is affected by bone size making it difficult to interpret, evaluate and compare BMD in the growing years when there are considerable changes to the size and shape of bone in children (Bailey et al., 1996; Fulkerson et al., 2004; Gordon, 2003; Schoenau et al., 2004). Moreover aBMD is a surrogate measure for bone strength and even though BMC and BMD are related to bone strength inferring information regarding strength from studies using these measures can be misleading. This fact is represented in the many studies citing increases in BMD and BMC that were not always significant. It is possible that DXA may not be sensitive enough to detect small changes in bone particularly at a time in development

when small changes are difficult to come by, like later in puberty when the rate of BMC accrual is decreasing. However, even these small detectable changes in bone mass using DXA can signify improvements in bone strength most likely by favourably altering bone geometry (Turner & Robling, 2003). Therefore the best parameter for assessing the effectiveness of PA interventions on bone would be to use a technique that includes measures of bone strength but also bone shape and size.

pQCT is a method that can be used to detect true vBMD, bone strength, shape and size. Unfortunately, only 5 of the studies that we reviewed utilized this method. An advantage of using pQCT to compare bone structural differences is that it has the capability to demonstrate bone strength adaptations in bone size via changes in cortical thickness or area through investigation of periosteal or endocortical expansion (Haapasalo et al., 2000; Kontulainen et al., 2002; Nikander et al., 2009). Moreover, these measurements indirectly provide an idea of the dynamic course of bone and how bone is metabolized to infer strength. However, to date only 1 study has directly measured biochemical markers of bone turnover in response to a PA intervention (Schneider et al., 2007). Measuring bone turnover would allow for detection of potential exercise effects sooner, as gains in bone markers have been demonstrated after 8 weeks of resistance training in women 20 years of age (Lester et al., 2009). Moreover, reference values for many of the markers have been set within the literature allowing for comparison across studies; something that is difficult to do for static measures of bone as the standards and definitions defining low bone mass are available only for postmenopausal women and not youth.

One way of avoiding this issue is to cease relating bone mass and strength to age, and relate it instead to muscle function (Schoenau & Fricke, 2008). This new methodological concept is based on the thought that the critical property of bone is strength rather than weight and that what influences bone strength are the mechanical loads it must endure either through PA or muscle contraction. Regardless of the mode of mechanical load the stability of the bone must be adapted to muscle strength, in a sense creating a functional muscle-bone unit (Schoenau & Fricke, 2008). Such an analysis removes the concept of a 'peak bone mass', which in fact is something we are not capable of measuring for an individual. Instead this approach allows for determination and comparison of bone deficits irrespective of age as bone strength is related to the strength and function of muscle (Schoenau & Fricke, 2008). Moreover, this approach moves away from looking at bone as a separate entity but as functionally linked system.

4.4 Psycho-social factors

It is also important to consider the psycho-social factors that are believed to affect bone health; these include osteoporosis beliefs, knowledge and practises. Women's willingness to adopt healthy behaviors depends on their level of knowledge of osteoporosis (Cook et al., 1991; Jamal et al., 1999). Majority of research examining calcium intake and PA with respect to osteoporosis knowledge and beliefs, and as preventative behaviours have been investigated in post menopausal women (Tudor-Locke & McColl, 2000). A few researchers have examined these criteria in younger women (Kasper et al., 1994, 2001; Wallace, 2002), let alone in adolescents (Anderson et al., 2005; Schrader et al., 2005). A lack of knowledge about osteoporosis risk factors (insufficient calcium intake and daily PA), as well as perceptions of low risk for developing osteoporosis, has been reported among college women (Kasper et al., 2001) and adolescent females (Anderson et al., 2005). Moreover, studies have suggested exercise self-efficacy and barriers to exercise are the best predictors of weight bearing exercise and dietary intake (Wallace, 2002), with educational interventions targeting youth demonstrating improvements in bone health knowledge, increases in intake of calcium rich foods and calcium self-efficacy (Schrader et al., 2005; Sharma et al., 2010). Therefore, knowing which factors will help children and adolescents adopt healthy 'bone' behaviors is important to making the exercise interventions we reviewed a reality.

Based on our literature review we know that structured and controlled PA interventions are effective in eliciting bone gains in youth. In order for youth to get involved in osteoporosis preventative behaviors such as PA they need to be able intervene in their daily lives on their own. McWannell et al. (2008) conducted a study to determine whether a structured high impact exercise program would be more effective in improving BMC and BMD than a lifestyle intervention program promoting PA in middle school children 10-11 years of age. This study demonstrated that the structured high impact PA program significantly improved total body BMC and BMD compared to controls after 9 weeks, with the lifestyle intervention seeing insignificant trends for bone gains. Moreover, a health plan-based lifestyle intervention designed at improving both diet and PA in adolescent girls outside of school demonstrated significant improvements in BMD and bone metabolism due to greater consumption of calcium and vitamin D (DeBar et al., 2006). However, when a larger focus was placed on PA and the adolescent girls taught how to properly conduct exercises a self-led PA program proved to be just as significant in improving bone strength parameters as a structured teacher-led PA program (Murphy et al., 2006). More importantly, those girls involved in the self-led PA program continued to exercise after the intervention had ceased, whereas the teach-led group did not. Therefore, it is not only important to get youth physically active in order to improve bone health, it is just as important to develop the personal skills necessary to direct their own activity.

5. Conclusions

With the current growing inactivity and unhealthy dietary habits, the body composition of youth is changing making this systemic review regarding the different types of exercise interventions, those utilizing resistance training vs. ground reaction forces, relevant. For long-term gains, it appears that short-term high-impact exercises undertaken early in childhood (pre and early puberty) if sustained into adulthood has a persistent effect over and beyond that of normal growth and development. Benefits in total body, lumbar spine, thoracic and femoral neck BMC (2.3-4.4%) as well as BMC at the hip (1.4%) have respectively been observed 3 (Gunter et al., 2008b) and 5 years (Gunter et al., 2008) following the jumping intervention by Fuchs et al. (2001). It is therefore redundant in some respect to conduct more PA interventions, unless more advanced techniques of measuring bone are used, as it is apparent from this review that PA in a structured controlled environment is effective in creating positive gains in bone. The next step is to influence change by schools either adopting these activities into their physical education curriculums or providing youth with the tools to administer this change on their own. Therefore, the examination of behavioral, social-psychological variables in addition to physical determinants of skeletal development provides a holistic multi-faceted conceptual framework of bone health that will provide the tools to better disseminate knowledge on positive bone building activities in hopes of creating life-long PA practices.

6. References

Alwis, G.; Linden, C.; Ahlborg, H.G.; Dencker, M.; Gardsell, P. & Karlsson, M.K. (2008a). A 2-year school-based execise programme in pre-pubertal boys induces skeletal benefits I lumbar spine. *Acta Pediatrica*, Vol. 97, (July 2008), pp. 1564-1561

Alwis, G.; Linden, C.; Stenevi-Lundgren, S.; Ahlborg, H.G.; Besjakov, J.; Gardsell, P. Karlsson, M.K. (2008b). A one-year exercise intervention program in pre-pubertal girls does not influence hip structure. *BMC Musculoskeletal Disorders*, Vol. 9, No. 9,

Anderson, K.D., Chad, K.E. & Spink, K.S. (2005). Osteoporosis knowledge, beliefs, and practices among adolescent females. *Journal of Adolescent Health*, Vol. 36, No. 4, (April 2005), pp. 305-312

Bailey, D.A. (1997). The Saskatchewan Pediatric Bone Mineral Accrual Study: Bone mineral acquisition during the growing years. *Journal of Sports Medicine*, Vol. 18, Suppl. 3, pp. S191-S194

Bailey, D.A.; Faulkner, R.A. & McKay, H.A. (1996). Growth, physical activity, and bone mineral acquisition. *Exercise & Sport Sciences Review*, Vol. 24, No. 1, (January 1996), pp. 233-266

Barbeau, P.; Johnson, M.; Howe, C.; Allison, J.; Davis, C.L.; Gutin, B. & Lemon, C.R. (2007). Ten months of exercise improves general and visceral adiposity, bone, and fitness in black girls. *Obesity*, Vol. 15, No. 8, (August 2007), pp. 2077-2085

Bass, S.L.; Naughton, G.; Saxon, L.; Iuliano-Burns, S.; Daly, R.; Briganti, E.M.; Hume, C. & Nowson, C. (2007). Exercise and calcium combined results in a greater osteogenic effect than either factor alone: a blinded randomized placebo-controlled trial in boys. *Journal of bone and Mineral Research*, Vol. 22, No. 3, (Dec 2006), pp. 458-465

Baxter-Jones, A.D.; Eisenmann, J.C.; Mirwald, R.L.; Faulkner, R.A. & Bailey, D.A. (2008). The influence of physical activity on lean mass accrual during adolescence: a longitudinal analysis. *Journal of Applied Physiology*, Vol. 105, No. 2, (August 2008), pp. 734-741

Baxter-Jones, A.D.; Mirwald, R.L.; McKay, H.A. & Bailey, D.A. (2003). A longitudinal analysis of sex differences in bone mineral accrual in healthy 8-19-year-old boys and girls. *Annals of Human Biology*, Vol. 30, No. 2, (March 2003), pp. 160-175

Beck, B.R. & Snow, C.M. (2003). Bone health across the lifespan – exercising our options. *Exercise and Sport Sciences Reviews*, Vol. 31, No. 3, (July 2003), pp. 117-122

Bellew, J.W. & Gehrig, L. (2006). A comparison of bone mineral density in adolescent female swimmers, soccer players, and weight lifters. *Paediatric Physical Therapy*, Vol. 18, No. 1, (Spring 2006), pp. 19-22

Blimkie, C.J.; Rice, S.; Webber, C.E.; Martin, J.; Levy, D. & Gordon, C.L. (1996). Effects of resistance training on bone mineral content and density in adolescent females. *Canadian Journal of Physiology and Pharmacology*, Vol. 74, No. 9, (April 1996), pp. 1025-1033.

Bonjour, J.P.; Theintz, G.; Buchs, B.; Slosman, D. & Rizzoli, R. (1991). Critical years and stages of puberty for spinal and femoral bone mass accumulation during adolescence. *Journal of Clinical Endocrinology and Metabolism*, Vol. 73, No. 3, (September 1991), pp. 555-563

Bonnick, S.L. (2007). Beyond BMD with DXA. *Bone*, Vol. 41, No. 1, (July 2007), pp. S9-S12

Boot, A.M.; De Ridder, M.A.J.; Pols, H.A.P.; Krenning, E.P. & de Muink Keizer-Schrama, S.M.P.F. (1997). Bone mineral density in children and adolescents: relation to puberty, calcium intake, and physical activity. *Journal of Clinical Endocrinology and Metabolism,* Vol. 82, No. 1, (January 1997), pp. 57-62

Bradney, M.; Pearce, G.; Naughton, G.; Sullivan, C.; Bass, S.; Beck, T.; Carlson, J. & Seeman, E. (1998). Moderate exercise during growth inprepubertal boys: changes in bone mass, volumetric density and bone strength: a controlled prospective study. *Journal of Bone and Mineral Research,* Vol. 13, No. 12, (December 1998), pp. 1814-1821

Burge, R.; Dawson-Hughes, B.; Solomon, D.H.; Wong, J.B.; Kind, A. & Tosteson, A. (2007) Incidence and economic burden of osteoporosis-related fractures in the United States, 2005-2025. *Journal of Bone and Mineral Research,* Vol. 22, No. 3, (March 2007), pp. 465-475

Cadogan, J.; Eastell, R.; Jones, N. & Barker, M. (1997). Milk intake and bone mineral acquisition in adolescent girls: randomized, controlled intervention trial. *British Medical Journal,* Vol. 315, No. 7118, (November 1997), pp. 1255-1260

Cadogan, J.; Blumsohn, A.; Barker, M.E. & Easterll, R. (1998). A longitudinal study of bone gain in pubertal girls: anthropometric and biochemical correlates. *Journal of Bone and Mineral Research,* Vol. 13, No. 10, (October 1998), pp. 1602-1612

Cassell, C.; Benedict, M. & Specker, B. (1996). Bone mineral density in elite 7- to 9-yr-old female gymnasts and swimmers. *Medicine and Science in Sports and Exercise,* Vol. 28, No. 10, (October 1996), pp. 1243-1246

Center, J.R.; Nguyen, T.V.; Schneider, D.; Sanbrook, P.M. & Eisman, J.A. (1999) Mortality after all major types of osteoporotic fracture in men and women: an observational study. *Lancet,* Vol. 353, No. 9156, (March 1999), pp. 878-882

Cook, B.; Noteloviz, M.; Rector, C. & Krischer, J.P. (1991). An osteoporosis patient education and screening program: Results and implications. *Patient Education and Counselling,* Vol. 17, Vol. 2, (April 1001), pp. 135-145

Courteix, D. ; Jaffre, C. ; Lespessaille, E. & Benhamou, L. (2005). Cumulative effects of calcium supplementation and physical activity on bone accretion in premenarchal children: a double-blind randomised placebo-controlled trial. *International Journal of Sports Medicine,* Vol. 26, No. 5, (September 2004), pp. 332-338

Courtiex, D.; Lespesailles, E.; Loiseau-Peres, S.; Obert, P.; Germain, P. & Benhamou, C.L. (1998). Effect of physical training on bone mineral density in prepubertal girls: a comparative study between impact-loading and non-impact loading sports. *Osteoporosis International,* Vol. 8, No. 2, (March 1998), pp. 152-158

Creighton, D.L.; Morgan, A.L.; Boardley, D. & Brolinson, G. (2001). Weight-bearing exercise and markers of bone turnover in females and athletes. *Journal of Applied Physiology,* Vol. 90, No. 2, (February 2001), pp. 565-570

Davies, J.H.; Evans, B.S. & Gregory, J.W. (2005). Bone mass acquisition in healthy children. *Archives of Disease in Childhood,* Vol. 90, No. 4, (April 2005), pp. 373-378

DeBar, L.L.; Ritenaugh, C.; Aickin, M.; Orwoll, E.; Elliot, D.; Dickerson, J.; Vuckovic, N.; Stevens, V.J.; Moe Esther, and Irving, L.M. (2006). A health plan-based lifestyle intervention increases bone mineral density in adolescent girls. *Archives of Pediatric and Adolescent Medicine,* Vol. 160, Vol. 12, (December 2006), pp. 1269-1276

Derman, O.; Cinemre, A.; Kanbur, N.; Dogan, M.; Kilic, M. & Karaduman, E. (2008). Effect of swimming on bone metabolism in adolescents. *Turkish Journal of Pediatrics*, Vol. 50, No. 2, (March 2008), pp. 149-154

Elgan, C.; Samsioeb, G. & Dykesa, A. (2003). Influence of smoking and oral contraceptives on bone mineral density and bone remodeling in young women: a 2-year study. *Contraception*, Vol. 67, No. 6, (June 2003), pp. 439-447

Fuchs, R.K.; Bauer, J.J. & Snow, C. (2001). Jumping improves hip and lumbar spine bone mass in prepubescent children: a randomized controlled trial. *Journal of Bone and Mineral Research*, Vol. 16, No. 1, (January 2001), pp. 148-156

Fuchs, R.K. & Snow, C.M. (2002). Gains in hip bone mass from high-impact training are maintained: A randomized controlled trial in children. *Journal of Pediatrics*, Vol. 141, No. 3, (September 2002), pp. 357-362

Fulkerson, J.A.; Himes, J.H.; French, S.A.; Jensen, S.; Petit, M.A.; Stewart, C.; Story, M.; Ensrud, K.; Fillhouer, S. & Jacobson, K. (2004). Bone outcomes and technical measurement issues of bone health among children and adolescents: considerations for nutrition and physical activity intervention trials. *Osteoporosis International*, Vol. 15, No. 12, (December 2004), pp. 929-941

Gordon, C.M. (2003). Normal bone accretion and effects of nutritional disorders in childhood. *Journal of Women's Health*, Vol. 12, No. 2, (February 2003), pp. 137-142

Gunter, K.; Baxter-Jones, A.D.G.; Mirwald, R.; Amstedt, H.; Fuches, R.K.; Durski, S. & Snow, C. (2008). Impact exercise increases BMC during growth: an 8-year longitudinal study. *Journal of Bone and Mineral Research*, Vol. 23, No. 7, (Dec 2007), pp. 986-993

Gunter, K.; Baxter-Jones, A.D.G.; Mirwald, R.; Amstedt, H.; Fuller, A.; Durski, S. & Snow, C. (2008b). Jumping skeletal health: a 4-year longitudinal study assessing the effects of jumping on skeletal development in pre and circum pubertal children. *Bone*, Vol. 42, No. 4, (April 2008), pp. 710-718

Haapasalo, H.; Kontulainen, S.; Sievan, H.; Kannus, P.; Jarvinen, M. & Vuori, I. (2000). Exercise-induced bone gain is due to enlargement in bone size without a change in volumetric bone density: a peripheral quantitative computed tomography study of the upper arms of male tennis players. *Bone*, Vol. 27, Vol. 3 (Sept 2000), pp. 351-357

Hansen, M. A.; Overgaard, K.; Riis, B.J. & Christiansen, C. (1991). Role of peak bone mass and bone loss in postmenopausal osteoporosis: 12 year study. *British Medical Journal*, Vol. 303, No. 6808, (October 1991), pp. 961-964

Hasselstrom, H.A.; Karlsson, M.K.; Hansen, S.E.; Gronfeldt, V.; Froberg, K. & Anderson, L.B. (2008). A 3-year physical activity intervention program increases the gain in bone mineral and bone width in prepubertal girls but not boys: the prospective Copenhagen School Child Interventions Study (CoSCIS). *Calcified Tissue International*, Vol. 83, No. 4, (October 2008), pp. 243-250

Hasserius, R.; Karlsson, M.K.; Nilsson, B.E.; Redlund-Johnell, I. & Johnell, O. (2003) Prevalent vertebral deformities predict increased mortality and increased fracture rate in both men and women: a 10-year population-based study of 598 individuals from the Swedish cohort in the European Vertebral Osteoporosis Study. *Osteoporosis International*, Vol. 14, No. 1, (January 2003), pp. 61-68

Heaney, R.; Abrams, S.; Dawson-Hughes, B.; Looker, A.; Marcus, R. Matkovic, V. & Weaver, C. (2000). Peak bone mass. *Osteoporosis International* , Vol. 11, No. 12, pp. 985-1009

Heinonen, A.; Sievanen, H.; Kannus, P.; Oja, P.; Pasanen, M. & Vuori, I. (2000). High-impact exercise and bone of growing girls: a 9-month controlled trial. *Osteoporosis International*, Vol. 11, No. 12, (June 2000), pp. 1010-1017

Hughes, J.M.; Novotny, S.A.; Wetzsteon, R.J. & Petit, M.A. (2007). Lessons learned from school-based skeletal loading intervention trials: putting research into practice. *Medicine and Sport Science*, Vol. 51, pp. 137-158

Iuliano-Burns, S.; Saxon, L.; Naughton, G.; Gibbons, K. & Bass, S.L. (2003). Regional specificity of exercise and calcium during skeletal growth in girls: a randomized controlled trial. *Journal of Bone and Mineral Research*, Vol. 18, No. 1, (January 2003), pp. 156-162

Jamal, S.A., Ridout, R.; Chase, C.; , Fielding, L.; Rubin, L.A. & Hawker, G.A. (1999). Bone mineral density testing and osteoporosis education improve lifestyle behaviors in premenopausal women: a prospective study. *Journal of Bone Mineral Research*, Vol. 14, No. 12, (December 1999), pp. 2143-2149,

Janz, K.F.; Burns, T.L.; Torner, J.C.; Levy, S.M.; Paulos, R.; Willing, M.C. & Warren, J.J. (2001). Physical activity and bone measures in young children: the Iowa bone development study. *Pediatrics*, Vol. 107, No. 6, (June 2001), pp. 1387-1393

Janz, K.F.; Gilmore, J.; Burns, T.; Levy, S.; Torner, J.; Willing, M. & Marshall, T. (2006). Physical activity augments bone mineral accrual in young children: the Iowa bone development study. *Journal of Pediatrics*, Vol. 148, No. 6, (June 2006), pp. 793-799

Janz, N.K.; Champion, V.L. & Stretcher, V.J. (2002). The health belief model. In: *Health Behaviour and Health Education: Theory, Research and Practice*, Glanz, K., Rimer, B. K., & Lewis, F. M. (Eds), pp. 45-63, John Wiley and Sons Inc., San Francisco, Ca.

Javiad, M.K. & Cooper, C. (2002). Prenatal and childhood influences on osteoporosis. *Best Practice & Research Clinical Endocrinology & Metabolism*, Vol. 16, No. 2, (June 2002), pp. 349-367

Kanis, J.A.; on behalf of the World Health Organization Scientific Groups. (2007). Assessment of osteoporosis at the primary health-care level. Technical Report. World Health Organization Collaborating Centre for Metabolic Bone Diseases, University of Sheffield, UK

Kasper, M.; Peterson, M. & Allegrante, J. (2001). The need for comprehensive educational osteoporosis prevention programs for young women: results from a second osteoporosis prevention survey. *Arthritis and Rheumatism*, Vol. 45, No. 1, pp. 28-34

Kasper, M.; Peterson, M.; Allegrante, J.; Galsworthy, T. & Gutin, B. (1994). Knowledge, beliefs, and behaviors among college women concerning the prevention of osteoporosis. *Archives of Family Medicine*, Vol. 3, No. 8, (August 1994), pp. 696-702

Kato, T.; Terashima, T.; Yamashita, T.T.; Hatanaka, Y.; Honda, A. & Umemura, Y. (2006). Effect of low-repetition jump training on bone mineral density in young women. *Journal of Applied Physiology*, Vol. 100, No. 3, (March 2006), pp. 839-843

Kontulainen, S.; Sievanen, H.; Kannus, P.; Pasanen, M. & Vuori, I. (2002). Effect of long-term impact-loading on mass, size and estimated strength of humerus and radius of female racquet-sports players: a peripheral quantitative tomography study between young and old starters and controls. *Journal of Bone and Mineral Research,* Vol. 17, No. 12, (December 2002), pp. 2281-2289

Lefevre, J.; Beunen, G.; Steens, G.; Claessens, A. & Renson, R. (1990). Motor performance during adolescence and age thirty as related to age at peak height velocity. *Annals of Human Biology,* Vol. 17, No. 5, (September 1990), pp. 423-435

Lehtonen-Veromaa, M.; Mottonen, T.; Irjala, K.; Nuotio, I.; Leino, A. & Viikari, J. (2000a). A 1-Year prospective study on the relationship between physical activity, markers of bone metabolism, and bone acquisition in peripubertal girls. *The Journal of Clinical Endocrinology and Metabolism,* Vol. 85, No. 10, (Oct 2000), pp. 3736-3732

Lehtonen-Veromaa, M.; Mottonen, T.; Nuotio, I.; Heinonen, O.J. & Viikari, J. (2000b). Influence of physical activity on ultrasound and dual-energy x-ray absorptiometry bone measurements in peripubertal Girls: A Cross-Sectional Study. *Calcified Tissue International,* Vol. 66, No. 4, (April 2000), pp. 248–254

Lehtonen-Veromaa, M.; Mottonen,T.; Svedstrom, E.; Hakola, P.; Heinonen, O.J. & Viikari, J. (2000c). Physical activity and bone mineral acquisition in peripubertal girls. *Scandinavian Journal of Medical Science and Sports,* Vol. 10, No. 4, (August 2000), pp. 236–243

Lester, M.E.; Uros, M.L.; Evans, R.K.; Pierce, J.R.; Spiering, B.A.; Maresh, C.M.; Hatfield, D.S.; Kraemer, W.J. & Nindl, B.C. (2009). Influence of exercise mode and osteogenic index on bone biomarker responses during short-term physical training. *Bone,* Vol. 45, No. 4, (June 2009), pp. 768-776

Linden, C.; Alwis, G.; Ahlborg, G.; Gardsell, P.; Valdimarsson, O.; Stenevi-Lundgren, S.; Besjakov, J. & Karlsson, M.K. (2007). Exercise, bone mass and bone size in prepubertal boys: one-year data from pediatric osteoporosis prevention study. *Scandinavian Journal of Medicine in Science and Sports,* Vol. 17, No. 4, (August 2006), pp. 340-347

Linden, C.; Ahlborg, G.; Besjakov, J.; Gardsell, P. & Karlsson M.K. (2006). A school-curriculum-based exercise program increases bone mineral accrual and bone size in prepubertal girls: two-year data from the pediatric osteoporosis prevention (POP) study, *Journal of bone and Mineral Research,* Vol. 21, No. 6, (May 2006), pp. 829-835

Macdonald, H.M.; Cooper, D.M. & McKay, H.A. (2009). Anterior-posterior bending strength at the tibial shaft increase with physical activity in boys: evidence for non-uniform geometric adaptation. *Osteoporosis International,* Vol. 20, No. 1, (Jan 2009), pp. 61-70

Macdonald, H.M.; Kontulainen, S.A.; Khan, K.M.; Khan, H.M. & McKay, H.A. (2007). Is a school-based physical activity intervention effective for increasing tibial bone strength in boys and girls? *Journal of Bone and Mineral Research,* Vol. 22, No. 3, (March, 2007), pp. 434-446

Macdonald, H.M.; Kontulainen, S.A.; Petit, M.A.; Beck, T.J.; Khan, K.M. & McKay, H.A. (2008). Does a novel school-based physical activity model benefit femoral neck bone strength in pre- and early pubertal children? *Osteoporosis international,* Vol. 19, No. 10, (October 2008), pp. 1445-1456

MacKelvie, K.J.; Khan, K.M. & McKay, H.A. (2002). Is there a critical period for bone response to weight-bearing exercise in children and adolescents? A systematic review. *British Journal of Sports Medicine*, Vol. 36, No. 4, (August 2002), pp. 250-257

MacKelvie, K.J.; Khan, K.M.; Petit, M.A.; Janssen, P.A. & McKay, H.A. (2003). A school-based exercise intervention elicits substantial bone health benefits: a 2-year randomised controlled trial in girls. *Pediatrics*, Vol. 112, No. 6, (December 2003), pp. e447-e452,

MacKelvie, K.J.; McKay, H.A.; Khan, K.M. & Crocker, P.R.E. (2001). A school-based exercise intervention augments bone mineral accrual in early pubertal girls. *Journal of Pediatrics*, Vol. 139, No. 4, (October 2001), pp. 501-508

MacKelvie, K.J.; MckKay, H.A.; Petit, M.A.; Moran, O. & Khan, K.M. (2002). Bone mineral response to a 7-month randomised controlled school-based jumping intervention in 126 prepubertal boys: associations with ethnicity and body mass index. *Journal of Bone and Mineral Research*, Vol. 17, No. 5, (May 2002), pp. 834-844

MacKelvie, K.J.; Petit, M.A.; Khan, K.M.; Beck, T.J. & McKay, H.A. Bone mass and structure are enhanced following a 2-uyear randomised controlled trial of exercise in prepubertal boys. *Bone*, Vol. 34, No. 4, (December 2003), pp. 755-764

Matkovic, V.; Jelic, T.; Wardlaw, G.; Ilich, J.; Goel, P.; Wright, J.; Andon, M.B.; Smith, K.T. & Heaney, R.P. (1994). Timing of peak bone mass in Caucasian females and its implication for the prevention of osteoporosis. Inference from a cross-sectional model. *Journal of Clinical Investigation*, Vol. 93, No. 2, (February 1994), pp. 799-808

McKay, H.A.; MacLean, L.; Petit, M.; MacKelvie O'Brien, K.; Janssen, P.; Beck, T. & Khan, K.M. (2005). 'Bounce the bell': a novel program of short bouts of exercise improves proximal femur bone mass in early pubertal children. *British Journal of Sports Medicine*, Vo. 39, No. 8, (August 2005), pp. 521-526

McKay, H.A.; Petit, M.A.; Schutz, R.W.; Rior, J.C.; Barr, S.I. & Khan, K.M. (2000). Augmented trochanteric bone mineral density after modified physical education classes: a randomised school-based exercise intervention study in prepubescent and early pubescent children. *Journal of Pediatrics*, Vol. 136, No. 2, (February 2000), pp. 156-162

McWhannell, N.; Henaghan, J.L.; Foweather, L.; Doran, D.A.; Batterham, A.M..; Reilly, T. & Stratton, G. (2008). The effect of a 9-week physical activity programme on bone and body composition of children aged 10-11 years: an exploratory trial. *International Journal of Sports Medicine*, Vol. 29, No. 12, (December 2008), pp. 941-947

Meyer, U.; Romann, M.; Zahner, L.; Schindler, C.; Puder , J.J.; Kraenzlin, M.; Rizzoli, R. & Kriemler, S. (2011). Effect of a general school-based physical activity intervention on bone mineral content and density: a cluster-randomized controlled trial. *Bone*, Vol. 48, No. 4, (April 2011), pp. 792-797

Molgaard, C.; Thomsen, B.L. & Michaelsen, K.M. (1999). Whole body bone mineral accretion in healthy children and adolescents. *Archives of Disease in Childhood*, Vol. 81, No. 1, (July 1999), pp. 10-15

Morris, F.L.; Naughton, G.; Gibbs, J.L.; Carlson, J.S. & Wark , J.D. (1997). Prospective ten-month exercise intervention in premenarchal girls: positive effects on bone and lean mass. *Journal of Bone and Mineral Research*, Vol. 12, No. 9, (September 1997), pp. 1453-1462

Murphy, N.M.; Dhuinn, M.N.; Brown, P.A. & ORathaille, M.M. (2006). Physical activity for bone health in inactive teenage girls: is a supervised ,teacher-led program or self- led program best? *Journal of Adolescent Health*, Vol. 39, No. 4, (Oct 2006), pp. 508-514

Nemet, D.; Berger-Shermech, E.; Wolach, B. & Eliakim, A. (2006). A combined dietary-physical activity intervention affects bone strength in obese children. *International Journal of Sports Medicine*, Vol. 27, No. 8, (August 2005), pp. 666-671

Nichols, D.L.; Snaborn, C.F.; Essery E.V.; Clark R.Al & Letendre, J. (2008). Impact of curriculu-based bone loading and nutrition education program on bone accrual in children. *Pediatric Exercise Science*, Vol. 20, No. 4 (November 2008), pp. 411-425

Nichols, D.L.; Sanborn, C.F. & Love, A. (2001). Resistance training and bone mineral density in adolescent females. *Journal of Pediatrics*, Vol. 139, No. 4, (Oct 2001), pp. 494-500

Nikander, R.; Kannus, P.; Rantalainen, T.; Uusi-Rasi, K.; Heinonen, A. & Sievanen, H. (2009). Cross-sectional geometry of weight-bearing tibia in female athletes subjected to different exercise loadings. *Osteoporosis International*, Vol. 21, No. 10

Nikander, R.; Sievanen, H.; Heinonen, A.; Daly, R.M.; Uusi-Rasi, K. & Kannus, P. (2010). Targeted exercise against osteoporosis: a systematic review and meta-analysis for optimising bone strength throughout life. *BMC Medicine*, Vol. 8, No. 1, pp. 47

Petit, M.A.; McKay, H.A.; MacKelvie, K.J.; Heinonen, A.; Khan, K.M. & Beck, T.J. (2002). A randomised school-based jumping intervention confers site and maturity-specific benefits on one structural properties in girls: a hip structural analysis study. *Journal of Bone and Mineral Research*, Vol. 17, No. 3, (March 2002), pp. 363-372

Rauch, F.; Bailey, D.A.; Baxter-Jones, A.; Mirwald, R. & Faulkner R. (2004). The 'muscle-bone unit during' the pubertal growth spurt. *Bone*, Vol. 34, No. 5, (May 2004), pp. 771-75

Schoenaue, E. & Fricke, O. (2008). Mechanical influences on bone development in children. *European Journal of Endocrinology*, Vol. 159, pp. S27-S31

Scheonau, E. & Frost, H.M. (2002). The "muscle-bone unit" in children and adolescents. *Calcified Tissue International*, Vol. 70, No. 5, (April 2002), pp. 405-407

Schoenau, E.; Saggese, G.; Peter, F.; Baroncelli, B.I.; Shaw, N.J.; Crabtree, N.J.; Zadik, Z.; Neu, C.M.; Noordam, C. & Radetti, G. (2004). From bone biology to bone analysis. *Hormone Research*, Vol. 61, No. 6, (February 2004), pp. 257-269

Schneider, M.; Dunton, G.F.; Bassin, S.; Graha, D.J.; Eliakim, A.F. & Cooper, D.M. (2007). Impact of a school-based physical activity intervention on fitness and bone in adolescent females. *Journal of Physical Activity & Health*, Vol. 4, No. 1, (January 2007), pp. 17-29

Schrader, S. L.; Blue, R. & Horner, A. (2005). Better bones buddies: an osteoporosis prevention program. *The Journal of School Nursing*, Vol. 21, No. 2, (April 2005), pp. 106-114

Sharma, S.V.; Hoelscher, D.M.; Kelder, S.H.; Diamon, P.; Day, R.S. & Hergenroeder, A. (2010). Psychosocial factors influencing calcium intake and bone quality in middle school girls. *Journal of the American Dietetic Association,* Vol. 110, No. 6, (June 2010), pp. 932-936

Stager, M.; Harvey, R.; Secic, M.; Camlin-Shingler, K. & Cromer, B. (2006). Self-reported physical activity and bone mineral density in urban adolescent girls. *Journal of Pediatric and Adolescent Gynecology,* Vol. 19, No. 1, (February 2006), pp. 17-22

Stear, S.J.; Prentic, A.; Jones, S.C. & Cole, T.J. (2003). Effect of a calcium and exercise intervention on the bone mineral status of 16-18-y-old adolescent girls. *American Journal of Clinical Nutrition,* Vol. 77, No. 4, (April 2003), pp. 985-992

Stager, M.; Harvey, R.; Secic, M.; Camlin-Shingler, K. & Cromer, B. (2006). Self-reported physical activity and bone mineral density in urban adolescent girls. *Journal of Pediatric and Adolescent Gynecology,* Vol. 19, No. 1, (February 2006), pp. 17-22

Steelman, J. & Zeitler, P. (2001). Osteoporosis in pediatrics. *Pediatrics in Review,* Vol. 22, No. 2, (February 2001), pp. 56-65

Stillman, R.J.; Lohman, T.G.; Slaughter, M.H. & Massey, B.H. (1986). Physical activity and bone mineral content in women aged 30 to 85 years. *Medicine and Science in Sports and Exercise,* Vol. 18, No. 5, (October, 1986), pp. 576-580

Tanner J.M. (1962). *Growth at Adolescence.* (2nd ed). Blackwell Scientific Publications, Oxford.

Tudor-Locke, C. & R. S. McColl. (2000). Factors related to variation in premenopausal bone mineral status: a health promotion approach. *Osteoporosis International,* Vol. 11, No. 1, pp. 1-24

Turner, C.H. & Robling, A.G. (2003). Designing exercise regimens to increase bone strength. *Exercise Sport Science Review,* Vol. 31, No. 1, (September 2002), pp. 45-50

Valdimarsson, O.; Linden, C.; Johnell, O.; Gardsell, P. & Karlosson, M.K. (2006). Daily Physical Education in the school curriculum in prepubertal girls during 1 year is followed by increases in bone mineral accrual and bone width – data from the prospective controlled Malmo Pediatric Osteoporosis Prevention Study. *Calcified Tissue International,* Vol. 78, No. 2, (February 2006), pp. 65-71

Valimaki, M. J.; Karkkainen, M.; Lamberg-Allardt, C.; Laitinen, K.; Alhava, E.; Heikkinen, J.; Impivaara, O.; Makela, P.; Palmgren, J.; Seppanen, R.; Vuori, I. & the Cardiovascular Risk in Young Finns Study Group. (1994). Exercise, smoking, and calcium intake during adolescence and early adulthood as determinants of peak bone mass. *British Medical Journal,* Vol. 309, (July 1994), pp. 230-235

Van Langendonck, L.; Classens, A.L.; Vleintinck, R.; Derom, C. & Beunen, G. (2003). Influence of weight-bear exercises on bone acquisition in prepubertal monozygotic female twins: a randomised controlled prospective study. *Calcified Tissue International,* Vol. 72, No. 6, (June 2003), pp. 666-674

Wallace, L.S. (2002). Osteoporosis prevention in college women: application of the expanded health belief model. *American Journal of Health Behavior,* Vol. 26, No. 3, (May 2002), pp. 163-172

Weeks, B.K.; Young, C.M. & Beck, B.R. (2008). Eight months of regular in-school jumping improves indices of bone strength in adolescent boys and girls: the POWER PE study. *Journal of Bone and Mineral Research,* Vol. 13, No. 7, (Feb 2008), pp. 1002-1011

Witzke, K.A. & Snow, C.M. (2000). Effects of plyometric jump training on bone mass in adolescent girls. *Medicine and Science in Sports and Exercise*, Vol. 32, No. 6, (June 2000), pp. 1051-1057

Wyshak, G. & Frisch, R.E. (1994). Carbonated beverages, dietary calcium, the dietary calcium/phosphorus ratio, and bone fractures in boys and girls. *Journal of Adolescent Health*, Vol. 15, No. 3, (May 1994), pp. 210-215

9

Osteoporosis in Pediatric Patients and Its Clinical Management

Emilio González Jiménez
Departamento de Enfermería,
Facultad de Ciencias de la Salud, Universidad de Granada,
España

1. Introduction

The increase in longevity achieved at present, the population has determined a striking increase in the prevalence of certain diseases and in other cases, the emergence of new forms of illness and during different life stages (1).

Osteoporosis is defined as a decrease in bone mass associated with the deterioration of bone tissue architecture and increased fracture risk, has become a serious public health problem in our society that affects a wide strata of the population age variable, though increasingly common among younger (2). There are two types of osteoporosis, primary and secondary. Primary osteoporosis is rare affecting one case per 100,000 subjects. For high school, its frequency is higher, being secondary to diseases or drug therapies. Table 1 shows the main causes that can lead to a primary or secondary osteoporosis.

The bone will undergo changes during growth reaching its peak during the second decade. After the fourth decade, there is progressive increase in bone loss that mainly affects trabecular tissue at both the peripheral and axial. Accordingly, it is during childhood when determining events occur in the development of adequate bone mineralization and bone mass final (3).

It is now accepted that osteoporosis in the adult subject has its origins in childhood. Accordingly, the prevention of it would begin with the empowerment of those factors that promote the acquisition of optimal bone mass development. Now if we take into account the dietary habits and sedentary marking between the current youth population, we can glimpse the high risk of developing the disorder to an increasingly early age (3).

During the first decade of life, the appendicular skeleton is growing faster than the axial. Also, the bone mineralization process starts in utero found strongly influenced by calcium intake during growth. However, calcium requirements vary throughout life, being greatest during the first years of life and in times such as puberty, pregnancy and lactation. Moreover, the loss of bone mass increases with age and accelerates with menopause. In this sense, it is advisable to increase the intake of calcium from the perimenopause.

For pediatric patients, there is a relationship between bone mass and size. However, in periods like puberty and after the pubertal growth spurt can be established called an imbalance between the rate of bone growth rate and increased bone mass resulting from this transient increase in bone fragility (4).

Primary Osteoporosis	
Idiopathic juvenile osteoporosis	Marfan syndrome
Osteogenesis imperfecta	Homocystinuria
Ehler Danlos syndrome	
Bruck syndrome	
Secundary Osteoporosis	
Neuromuscular Disease	**Procesos Crónicos**
Cerebral Palsy	Leucemia
Duchenne Muscular Dystrophy	Fibrosis Quística
Prolonged Immobilization	Malabsorción intestinal
Endocrine Diseases	Talasemia
Hypogonadism	Cirrosis Biliar Primaria
Turner Syndrome	Nefropatías
Growth hormone deficiency	Anorexia Nerviosa
Hyperthyroidism	Trasplantes
hyperprolactinemia	Infección por VIH
Cushing Syndrome	**Yatrogenia**
Congenital Metabolic Disorders	**Corticosteroids**
Gaucher Disease	Metotrexate
	Cyclosporine
	Heparin
	Anticonvulsivants
	Radiotherapy

Table 1. Causes of primary and secondary osteoporosis in children

On the other hand, it is normal that there is a correlation between the stage of pubertal development and BMD at both the peripheral and axial. Among girls after menarche has been a significant increase in BMD. BMD in boys increases after puberty, with a more extended in time because their pubertal development is slower (5).

Genetic factors in turn, are equally important in the development of an adequate peak bone mass. Thus, a correlation in BMD between twins. For their part, black women have greater BMD and thus a lower incidence of osteoporosis when compared to white women. Also found lower BMD among women whose mothers had a post-menopausal status with osteoporosis compared to those other women the same age but without such a history. Accordingly, it should raise the transmission of genetic information is carried out mainly through the mother (6).

Analyzing the etiology of osteoporosis in children are significantly different from those in adulthood. Accordingly, the diagnostic approach would be completely different in children compared to adults. Among the risk factors associated with the occurrence of bone metabolism during childhood are processes that interfere with proper bone mineralization, the absence of positive stimulus of calcium and vitamin D from diet or exercise to obtain adequate bone mass. Other causes are disorders that cause interference in pubertal development as well as any conditions that cause increased bone loss. Finally, prolonged exposure to certain drugs that induce the development of osteoporosis.

Given the above should be considered the early diagnosis of osteoporosis in pediatric patients who have had one or more fractures are not preceded by trauma or as a result of minor trauma. Moreover, the development of significant angular deformities in the extremities and the presence of a marked kyphosis should guide the clinician to the presence of impaired bone quality.

This review aims to provide guidance on the characteristics of the process of normal and abnormal bone mineralization in the pediatric patient, the main factors involved and the existing prevention strategies.

2. Bone mass concept and assessment of their status

Bone mass is defined as the total amount of bone tissue in the organism including the extracellular matrix ossified. At present, it is accepted that the acquisition of appropriate peak bone mass is essential to prevent osteoporosis later in life. Since this formation and accumulation of bone mass occurs during the first decades of life, control of bone mineralization during childhood is a significant aspect to assess interest. This monitoring should aim to identify children at risk of developing osteopenia. Also, in the general population should implement measures to prevent the onset of the disease promoting lifestyles and measures to increase bone mass (7).

The development of an adequate level of bone mass is partly dependent on nutritional factors, so it is necessary to maintain an adequate nutrient supply during the growing season. Another aspect to consider genetic factors, accounting for 60% of total factors. In adulthood decreases the neo-bone formation after a period in which bone mass remains stable (8).

Puberty brings the largest increase in bone mineral density in both sexes, however, as in any period may generate changes to diet and exercise as much as 20% (9). Bone mass is increased from birth to be reduced by calcium deposition significantly as we approach the third decade or so. To three years increases to 30% after 20% and reach puberty about 40%. From the end of growth and to reach adulthood is increasing by 15%. Even 10 years ago mineralization at the same rate in both sexes. From this age is accelerated significantly in the girls (10).

The diagnosis and even prevention evaluation and therapy of osteoporosis may be jeopardized in a special way in the child all because of the need to use techniques which, although sensitive, reproducible and precise, resulting quick, painless, safe and non invasive.

Of all the methods proposed by the National Osteoporosis Foundation to assess the quality of bone, the most used technique is dual x-ray absorptiometry (DEXA). The basis of this technique in the study of attenuation is subjected to a dual X-ray beam through bone tissue (11). Although it can be done at different levels, the benchmarks for determining the criteria of normality, osteopenia or osteoporosis referred to data obtained at the height of the femoral neck or lumbar vertebrae (L2-L4) of the reference population. The interpretation of this technique has some difficulties in the child (12). There are already benchmarks (13-15), although obtained in cross-sectional studies.

The measures are available in axial regions (hip, spine) or peripheral (calcaneus, tibia, knee, radio and phalanges), but it has shown that measurements in predicting spinal fracture risk at that level, but not others, and so does the rest of the locations where BMD is measured.

In children, the area selection is further complicated because the timing and rate of mineralization depends on the biological age (13). Should be selected sufficiently vascularized bone, with good motility and under some pressure. In this regard, the determination in the calcaneus could induce excessive bias to withstand pressure, although some authors is the preferred (14).

Other recent application techniques are ultrasound imaging and computed tomography. It is noninvasive, excellent acceptance of any age which have been effective as bone assessment procedures in both the adult and the child (15). However, in the case of computed tomography to excessive cost limits their use as a technique for the prevention of osteoporosis.

3. Bone mineralization process

Bone mineralization is a complex process regulated by both genetic and hormonal factors, environmental and nutritional (16). From a genetic standpoint, the mineralization is controlled by a large group of genes. Among the most studied is the gene that controls vitamin D receptor, which depends on calcium absorption in the intestine. Hormonal level, there are several hormones involved in bone mineralization. These include parathyroid hormone which balances the mechanisms of formation and resorption of bone at the same time enhances the action of vitamin D. Calcitonin, which inhibits the action of osteoclasts, and growth hormone, HGH and IGF-1 that acts in the formation of cartilage and promotes the synthesis of the active metabolite of vitamin D (17).

Other molecules with activity on bone mass are the corticosteroids. They only act on bone mineralization when increased above normal levels, decreasing bone mass and bone growth. This is an important consideration in those children treated with corticosteroids. Thyroid hormones, in turn, are also involved in mineralization diminishing with increasing concentration. But all of these factors may also act on the environmental factors that can intervene by modifying diet and lifestyle (18).

4. Concept of osteopenia and osteoporosis

Osteopenia is defined by decreased bone mineral density between -1 and -2.5 SD for age, sex, height and pubertal stage. In cases where the decrease in bone mineral density is below 2 SD is considered osteoporosis (19).

Osteoporosis was defined in 1991 as a systemic skeletal disease characterized by low bone mass and microarchitectural deterioration of bone tissue, which leads to increased bone fragility with a consequent increase in fracture risk. This definition implies a qualitative concept of altered bone architecture and a quantity related to bone density (20). Both osteoporosis and osteopenia may be primary as in aging or menopause but may also result from inadequate nutrition, and hormonal disorders or diseases of the bone.

However, there are childhood diseases that may present with osteopenia thereby increasing the risk of osteoporosis in adulthood. Among the mechanisms of production of osteopenia could cite many, though, could be divided into three main groups. Those processes that occur with an inadequate intake of nutrients such as anorexia nervosa, bulimia, protein-calorie malnutrition or poorly controlled diets (21). A second group would be composed of those disorders with intestinal malabsorption boxes. Within this section as possible symptoms of osteopenia generators could include celiac disease, cystic fibrosis, intolerance to cow's milk proteins and inflammatory bowel disease. Other processes potentially involved in the development of osteopenia will neuropathy and liver disease that present with an impairment of the synthesis of active metabolites of vitamin D. Other processes involved will be the states of metabolic acidosis, prolonged administration of certain drugs such as anticonvulsants or corticosteroids and pictures of hypogonadism (22).

5. Nutritional factors

Proper nutrition is a key factor in maintaining adequate skeletal mineralization. In this process of bone mineralization energy and nutrients intervene in various ways, either by encouraging the development of cell mitosis, participating as visual elements, to be a source of vitamins which will involve regulating the synthesis of bone matrix and promoting the absorption level intestinal calcium or contributing to the synthesis of various hormones and factors crecimiento (23).

By feeding the body receives visual elements, vitamins intervene by regulating the synthesis of bone matrix and intestinal absorption of calcium and other minerals whose primary function is to act in the formation and consolidation of mineralized bone. Another essential aspect of bone remodeling in the child will be energy intake. This is an essential as the volume decreases in energy intake induce delays in growth, maturation and hence bone mineralization (24). Then in children with malnutrition by default is necessary to control the state of bone mineralization.

The bone mineralization process will necessarily regulated by protein intake through the diet. Its role essentially plastic makes these elements are essential for the synthesis of bone matrix. In this sense, the child, situations of inadequate intake may induce default to the emergence of problems of mineralization. On the contrary, when its contribution in the diet is excessive can cause hypercalciuria boxes, this is due to increased excretion of acid produced during protein catabolism. At present it is possible that the protein diet consumed in most developed countries it is closely linked with the increase in osteoporosis in the population (25).

Another aspect to consider is the ratio of sodium ingested with the level of calcium excretion by the kidney. Sodium and calcium share the same carrier at the proximal renal tubule. Although and yet there is no need to adjust the contribution of calcium to sodium intake through the diet in children (26). Calcium is an essential pillar in the prevention of osteoporosis. In our body and especially in the bones is deposited as hydroxyapatite crystals. Your deposit varies throughout life from 30 grams at birth to about 1.300 grams in adulthood (27).

Given the above will be necessary to modulate calcium intake during periods of increased growth and, especially during adolescence. During adolescence tends to accumulate 40% of total bone mass produced throughout life. Several studies have shown that calcium supplementation during adolescence increases bone mineral density (28). After administering 500 ml of milk per day during childhood will ensure intake of about 400mg of calcium, equivalent to 60% of the recommended daily amount.

Moreover, we have to take into account the bioavailability of calcium in food. The presence of phytates inhibit absorption and therefore vegetables, legumes and cereals despite containing high levels of calcium, it is not as comparable as that of milk. Similarly oxalates, alcohol, caffeine and phosphates hinder calcium absorption even when present in the diet (29, 30). Finally, pictures of obesity and overweight in children have been associated with increased bone density. However there is evidence linking these situations with a higher incidence of fractures (31).

Vitamin D is another factor regulating the homeostasis calcium / phosphorus. Its main sources are dairy products. Exposure to sunlight or UV light promotes the metabolism of it. However, alterations in intestinal absorption mechanism and factors affecting their metabolism at the level of the skin should be considered as processes that alter bone formation and thus risk factors for developing osteoporosis (32).

6. Idiopathic juvenile osteoporosis

In some pediatric patients (usually young) are not able to establish any risk factors for osteoporosis. In these cases must be considered the possibility of presenting idiopathic juvenile osteoporosis. Its etiology is unknown, manifesting itself in some cases for an accidental radiological finding which may also require a significant osteopenia, short stature and kyphosis (secondary to vertebral crush fractures) (32). Generally do not exhibit any endocrine abnormality nor metabolism of calcium/ phosphorus. The levels of vitamin D and calcitonin are variable in these patients. For bone biopsy, this is not conclusive proof but often shows an increase of osteocytes in trabecular bone as well as signs of increased bone resorption. In general, treatment consists of substitution of calcium and calcitriol, tending to improve spontaneously in the post pubertal period by several authors due to the effect of gonadal hormones (33).

7. Osteogenesis imperfecta

Osteogenesis imperfecta is a genetic disease, autosomal dominant, in which there is an abnormality in the formation of collagen type 1 (34). This disorder causes weakness and bone fragility of varying degrees of severity and subsequent pathological fractures, as well as affecting other tissues. The etiology of this disease lies in the mutation of genes that encode both qualitative and quantitative production of collagen fibers. In terms of prevalence in the world, this ranges from about 1 case per 30,000 live births (34). The continuous advances in diagnosis have created new expectations for subjects with the disease, greatly improving their quality of life. At present there is no effective treatment, healing, since it can not act directly on the formation of collagen type I (34). Throughout history have used various medical treatments (calcitonin, anabolic steroids, etc.) to try to increase bone mass, to no avail. Currently, treatment is symptomatic and should be approached in a multidisciplinary manner. The best results were achieved with growth hormone (GH) and bisphosphonates (34).

8. Osteopathy associated with use of drugs

Another group of pediatric patients at high risk for osteoporosis are those subjects taking medications which interfere with the normal process of bone mineralization. The drugs most commonly associated with the development of bone disease or iatrogenic demineralizantes include steroids, anticonvulsants, cyclosporine, anthracyclines, methotrexate, warfarin and agonists of gonadotropin-releasing hormone (35).

In the case of steroids, these lead to the development of osteoporosis secondary to increased bone resorption. In addition, they inhibit intestinal absorption of calcium, decreased tubular reabsorption of calcium and induce a secondary hyperparathyroidism. They also inhibit pituitary gonadotropin secretion and decrease the response of estrogen/testosterone to the follicle stimulating hormone (FSH). A level of osteoblasts caused a decrease in their ability to replicate, in turn stimulating the expression of collagenase by the osteoblast and thereby inducing the increase in bone matrix degradation with a decrease in the synthesis of growth factors (IGF1, IGF-2) (36).

Appropriate strategies to prevent osteoporosis from childhood: The prevention of osteoporosis to necessarily an assessment of bone mineralization status since early infancy, particularly in subjects at risk. In this sense, preterm infants, patients with malabsorption syndromes and corticosteroid therapy patients constitute the population most at risk of poor bone mineralization (37, 38).

The bioavailability of calcium in milk is far superior to commercial formulas, making it the leading source for calcium during breastfeeding. Only in the case of infants it should increase their calcium intake to the recommended supplementary with commercial formulas that have a higher calcium content (39).

In children aged 1 to 8 years there is no explicit consensus on the specific requirements of calcium. In any case, we recommend an intake of 500 mg per day for ages 1 and 3 years (40). This figure should be increased as they age and approach puberty. Thus, for ages 4 to 8 years the requirements will amount up to 800mg calcium per day. But have found no overt health benefits by increasing the daily amount (41). And at puberty, it is estimated that for every inch of growth are required calcio 20g (41).

Given the above, eating disorders, inflammatory bowel disease or the use of corticosteroids and prolonged rest in the minors are situations that require an attitude of monitoring and supervision by health staff (41).

It is estimated that the highest positive balance is achieved with an average daily intake of 1300mg. By contrast, those exposed to lower levels will have a negative impact on bone mineralization process (42). This corresponds to measurements made on white teens. In the case of blacks and adolescents have shown a better efficiency for the absorption of dietary calcium, can reach the same peak bone mass even with lower contributions of calcium (43).

Excess calcium in the diet, in turn, can cause a deficiency of iron and zinc, while favoring the formation of kidney stones (44). Similarly as phosphates present in carbonated drinks can also act by inhibiting the absorption of calcium in the intestine (45).

In cases of subjects with lactose intolerance, the simple addition of commercial lactase or ingestion of fermented dairy products like yogurt can remedy this situation (46).

The existence of toxic habits such as snuff or alcohol consumption can also interfere with the process of bone mineralization (47). But if there is a successful strategy to prevent osteoporosis from childhood this is the regular practice of exercise (48). The physical exercise from an early age not only ensure optimal weight status but also a formidable mineralization of our skeleton, reason is of great importance when the subject population are children and adolescents (49, 50). The continued practice of physical activity helps to acquire peak bone mass genetically determined (51). Although, to achieve these benefits, the current recommendations set out the need to practice a minimum of three days a week (52). Moreover, at present it is unknown whether calcium intake through diet may or may not alter the beneficial effect of exercise (52).

With regard to drug-induced osteoporosis, the most important preventive factor is the wise use and dosage of the same (53).

In summary, we conclude that the onset osteoporosis in children differs in its clinical management of osteoporosis in adults. In this sense, the early identification of risk grpos be a priority. Therefore it should be emphasized that during the first and second decade of life, events occur which are essential for the proper development of bone metabolism. On this basis, the prevention of osteoporosis in adults should begin as early as the early childhood.

9. References

[1] Nacional Institute of Health. Osteoporosis and related bone diseases-National Resources Center. www.osteo.org

[2] González Jiménez E, Álvarez Ferre J, Pozo Cano MD, Navarro Jiménez MC, Aguilar Cordero MJ, Tristán Fernández JM. Osteoporosis involutiva tipo I en la mujer posmenopáusica: diagnóstico y manejo clínico. Revista Española de Enfermedades Metabólicas Óseas 2009; 18 (4): 77 – 84

[3] Cooper C, Fall C, Eggerp, Hobbs R, Eastell R, Barker D. Growth in infancy and bone mass in later life. Ann Rheum Dis 1997; 56: 17-21.

[4] Frank GR. The role of estrogens in puberal skeletal physiology: ephyseal maturation and mineralization of the skeleton. Acta Pediatr 1995; 84: 627-630.

[5] Matovic V. Osteoporosis, as a pediatric disease: role of calcium and heredity. J Rheumatology 1992; 19 Suppl: 54-59.

[6] Riggs BL, Walhner HW, Dunn WL, Mazess RB, Offord KP, Melton LJ. differential changes of bone mineral density of the appendicular and axial skeleton. with aging. J Clin Invest 1981; 67: 328-335.

[7] Sluis IM, Muinck K. Osteoporosis in childhood: bone density of children in health and disease. J Pediatr Endocrinol Meta 2001; 14(7): 817

[8] Lonzer MD, Imrie R, Rogers D, Worley D, Licata A, Secie M. Effects of heredity,age, weight, puberty and calcium intake on bone mineral density in children. Clin Pediatr (Phila) 1996; 35 (4): 185

[9] Ballabriga A, Carrascosa A. (eds) Masa ósea y nutrición En Nutrición en la infancia y adolescencia. 3ª edición. Ergon. Madrid 2006

[10] Gil Campos M. Nuytrición y salud ósea en la infancia y la adolescencia En:Díaz Curiel M, Gil Hernández A, Mataix Verdú J (editores). Nutrición y Salud Osea. Puleva Granada 2004

[11] National Osteoporosis Foundation. Review of the evidence for prevention, diagnosis and treatment, and cost-effectiveness analysis. Osteoporosis Int 1998; 8: 1 – 88

[12] Gilsanz V. Bone density in children: A review of the available techniques and indications. Eur J Radiol 1998; 26: 177 – 82

[13] Yeste D, Del Rio L, Carrascosa A. Valores de contenido mineral óseo, densidad mineral ósea y densidad mineral ósea volumétrica en niños y adolescentes. En: Argente J, Carrascosa A, Gracia R, Rodríguez F, editores. Tratado de Endocrinología de la infancia y adolescencia. Barcelona: Doyma; 2000.p. 1501 – 12

[14] Carrascosa A, Ballabriga A. Patrones de crecimiento y composición corporal. En: Ballabriga A, Carrascosa A, editores. Nutrición en la infancia y adolescencia. 3ed. Madrid: Ergon; 2006 .p. 1289 – 1319

[15] Carrascosa A. Masa ósea y nutrición. En: Ballabriga A, Carrascosa A, editores. Nutrición en la infancia y adolescencia. 3 ed. Madrid: Ergon; 2006 .p. 919 – 49

[16] Bos S, Delmas PD, Pearce D. The differing tempo of grow thin bone size, mass and density in girls is region specific. J Clin Invest 1999; 104: 795 – 804

[17] Gregg EW, Kriska AM, Salamone LM. The epidemiology of quantitative ultrasound: Are view of the relations hip with bone mass, osteoporosis and fracture risk. Osteoporos Int 1977; 7: 89 – 99

[18] Polanco I, Hernández J, Scherer JI, Prieto G, Molina M, Sarria J. Curva de normalidad en población española de 4 a 22 años para un densitómetro óseo por ultrasonidos DBM Sonic 1200. Pediatrika 2000; 20 (2): 55 – 64

[19] Alonso Franch M, Redondo del Río MP. Nutrición y patología ósea en la infancia. En Ángel Gil Hernández (editor) Tratado de Nutrición. Acción Médica. Madrid 2005

[20] Creer FR, Krebs NF, Comité on Nutrition, Optimizing bone health and calcium intakes of infants, children and adolescents. Pediatrics 2006; 117: 578

[21] Morris RC, Frassetto LA, SchmidlinO, Forman A, Sebastián A. Expression of osteoporosis as determined by diet-disordered electrolyte and acid-base metabolism. En: Burckhardt P, Dawson-Hugues B, Heaney RP (eds). Nutrtional Aspects of Osteoporosis. CA Academic Press. San Diego 2001

[22] Winzenberg TM, Oldenburg B, Frendin S, De Wit L, Jones G. A mother-based intervention trial for osteoporosis prevention in children. Prev Med 2006; 42: 21

[23] Welten DC, Kemper HC, Post GB, et al. Weight-bearing activity during youth is a more important factor for peak bone mass than calcium intake. J Bone Miner Res 1994; 9: 1089

[24] Weaver CM, Hauney RP, Prouly WR, Choices for achieving adequate dietary calcium with a vegetarian diet. Am J Clin Nutr. 1999; 70: 534 - 38

[25] Stalling VA. Calcium and bone health in children: a review. Am J Ther. 1997; 4: 259

[26] Bishop NJ, King FJ, Lucas A. Increased bone mineral content of preterm infants fed with a nutrient enriched formula after discharge from hospital. Arch Dis Child. 1993; 68: 573.

[27] Hernández Rodriguez M. Alimentación y problemas nutricionales en la adolescencia. En: M Hernández Rodríguez Alimentación Infantil 2ª ed. Díaz de Santos. Madrid 1993

[28] Bryant RJ, Wastney ME, Martin BR, Wood O, McCabe GP, Morshidi M, Smith DL, Peacock M, Weaver CM. Racial differences in bone turnover and calcium metabolism in adolescent females. J Clini Endocrinol Metab 2003; 88: 1043 - 47

[29] Loud KJ, Gordon CM. Adolescence:bone disease. En: Walker, Watkins, Duggan (edditors) Nutrition in Pediatrics. Basic Science and Clinical Applications. 3th ed. Decker Inc Ontario 2003

[30] Díaz M, Riobo P, Esteban J, Rodríguez G. Nutrición en las enfermedades del tejido conectivo y del sistema óseo en el adulto. En: Gil A, editor. Tratado de Nutrición, T III. Madrid: Acción Médica; 2005 .p.1019 – 036

[31] Fernández I, Alobera MA, Del Canto M, Blanco L. Physiological bases of bone regeneration II. The remodeling process. Med Oral Patol Oral Cir Bucal. 11: E151 – E157

[32] Krall EA, Dawson-Hughes B. Osteoporosis. En: Shils ME, Olson JA, Ross AC (editores). Nutricion en Salud y Enfermedad. México: Interamericana. Pp: 1563 – 576

[33] Saggese G, Bertelloni S, Baroncelli GI, Perri G , Calderazzi A. Mineral metabolism and calcitriol therapy in idiopathic juvenile osteoporosis. Am J Diseases of Children 1991; 145: 457-462.

[34] Espallargues M, Sampietro-Colom L, Estrada MD. Osteoporosis: factores de riesgo y densitometría. Med Clin (Barc) 2002; 118: 319.

[35] Huth PJ, Dirienzo DB, Miller GD. Major scientific advances with dairy foods in nutrition and health. J Dairy Sci 2006; 89: 1207 - 221

[36] Hathcock JN, Shao A, Vieth R, Heaney R. Risk assessment for vitamin D. Am J Clin Nutr 2007; 85: 6 - 18

[37] Papierska L, Rabijewski M. Glucocorticoid induced osteoporosis. Pol Arch Med Wewn 2007; 117: 363 - 69

[38] Guéguen L, Pointillart A. The bioavailability of dietary calcium. J Am Coll Nutr 2000; 19: 119 - 136

[39] Food and Nutrition Board, Institute of Medicine. Dietary reference intakes for Arsenic, Boron, Calcium, Chromium, Copper, Fluoride , Ioride, Iron, Magnesium, Manganese, Molybdenum, Nickel, phosphorus, selenium, silicon, vanadium and zinc. Washington D.C.: National Academy Press: 2004 .p. 290 - 393

[40] Stevenson JC. Pathogenesis, prevention, and treatment of osteoporosis. Obstet Gynecol 1990; 75 (Suppl): 36 - 41

[41] Krassas GE. Idiopathic juvenile osteoporosis. Ann N Y Acad Sci 2000; 900: 409 - 12.

[42] Smith R. Idiopathic juvenile osteoporosis: Experience of twenty-one patients. Br J Rheumatol 1995; 34: 68 - 77

[43] Bacciottini L, Brandi ML. Foods and new foods: the role of nutrition in skeletal health. J Clin Gastroenterol. 38 (6): 115 - 17

[44] Ahmed SF, Elmantaser M. Secondary osteoporosis. Endocr Dev 2009; 16: 170 - 90

[45] Nikander R, Sievänen H, Heinonen A, Daly RM, Uusi-Rasi K, Kannus P. Targeted exercise against osteoporosis: A systematic review and meta-analysis for optimising bone strength throughout life. BMC Med 21 (8): 1 - 16

[46] Macdonald HM, Cooper DM, McKay HA: Anterior-posterior bending strength at the tibial shaft increases with physical activity in boys: evidence for non-uniform geometric adaptation. Osteoporos Int 2009; 20: 61 - 70

[47] Valimaki M, Karkkainen M, Lamberg-Allert C. Exercise, smoking and calcium intake during adolescence and early adulhood as determinants of peak bone mass. British Med J 1994; 309: 230-234.

[48] Macdonald HM, Kontulainen SA, Khan KM, McKay HA: Is a school-based physical activity intervention effective for increasing tibial bone strength in boys and girls?. J Bone Miner Res 2007; 22: 434 - 46

[49] Weeks BK, Young CM, Beck BR: Eight months of regular in-school dumping improves indices of bone strength in adolescent boys and Girls: the POWER PE study. J Bone Miner Res 2008; 23: 1002 - 11

[50] González I, Gracia R. Osteoporosis en la edad pediátrica. An Pediatr 2006; 64 (2): 85-91

[51] Bianchi ML. Osteoporosis in children and adolescents. Bone 2007; 41: 486-495

[52] Vainionpaa A, Korpelainen R, Sievanen H, Vihriala E, Leppaluoto J, Jamsa T: Effect of impact exercise and its intensity on bone geometry at weightbearing tibia and femur. Bone 2007; 40: 604 - 11

[53] Alonso Franch M, Redondo Del río MP, Suárez Cortina L. Nutrición infantil y salud ósea. Anales de Pediatría (Barc) 2010; 72 (1): 1 - 11

Permissions

The contributors of this book come from diverse backgrounds, making this book a truly international effort. This book will bring forth new frontiers with its revolutionizing research information and detailed analysis of the nascent developments around the world.

We would like to thank Yannis Dionyssiotis, MD, PhD, for lending his expertise to make the book truly unique. He has played a crucial role in the development of this book. Without his invaluable contribution this book wouldn't have been possible. He has made vital efforts to compile up to date information on the varied aspects of this subject to make this book a valuable addition to the collection of many professionals and students.

This book was conceptualized with the vision of imparting up-to-date information and advanced data in this field. To ensure the same, a matchless editorial board was set up. Every individual on the board went through rigorous rounds of assessment to prove their worth. After which they invested a large part of their time researching and compiling the most relevant data for our readers. Conferences and sessions were held from time to time between the editorial board and the contributing authors to present the data in the most comprehensible form. The editorial team has worked tirelessly to provide valuable and valid information to help people across the globe.

Every chapter published in this book has been scrutinized by our experts. Their significance has been extensively debated. The topics covered herein carry significant findings which will fuel the growth of the discipline. They may even be implemented as practical applications or may be referred to as a beginning point for another development. Chapters in this book were first published by InTech; hereby published with permission under the Creative Commons Attribution License or equivalent.

The editorial board has been involved in producing this book since its inception. They have spent rigorous hours researching and exploring the diverse topics which have resulted in the successful publishing of this book. They have passed on their knowledge of decades through this book. To expedite this challenging task, the publisher supported the team at every step. A small team of assistant editors was also appointed to further simplify the editing procedure and attain best results for the readers.

Our editorial team has been hand-picked from every corner of the world. Their multi-ethnicity adds dynamic inputs to the discussions which result in innovative outcomes. These outcomes are then further discussed with the researchers and contributors who give their valuable feedback and opinion regarding the same. The feedback is then collaborated with the researches and they are edited in a comprehensive manner to aid the understanding of the subject.

Apart from the editorial board, the designing team has also invested a significant amount of their time in understanding the subject and creating the most relevant covers. They scrutinized every image to scout for the most suitable representation of the subject and create an appropriate cover for the book.

The publishing team has been involved in this book since its early stages. They were actively engaged in every process, be it collecting the data, connecting with the contributors or procuring relevant information. The team has been an ardent support to the editorial, designing and production team. Their endless efforts to recruit the best for this project, has resulted in the accomplishment of this book. They are a veteran in the field of academics and their pool of knowledge is as vast as their experience in printing. Their expertise and guidance has proved useful at every step. Their uncompromising quality standards have made this book an exceptional effort. Their encouragement from time to time has been an inspiration for everyone.

The publisher and the editorial board hope that this book will prove to be a valuable piece of knowledge for researchers, students, practitioners and scholars across the globe.

List of Contributors

Bradley K. Weiner, Scott E. Parazynski and Ennio Tasciotti
Weill Cornell Medical College, Orthopaedic Surgery, Spinal Surgery, The Methodist Hospital, Orthopaedic Spine Advanced Technology Laboratory, The Methodist Hospital Research Institute, Houston, Texas, USA

Yannis Dionyssiotis
Physical and Social Rehabilitation Center Amyntæo, University of Athens, Laboratory for Research of the Musculoskeletal System, Greece

Geun-Young Park, Sun Im and Seong Hoon Lim
College of Medicine, The Catholic University of Korea, Republic of Korea

Marek W. Karwacki and Wojciech Wozniak
Nf-1 Outpatients Clinic & Department of Oncological Surgery for Children and Youth, Institute of Mother and Child, Poland

Federico G. Hawkins, Sonsoles Guadalix, Raquel Sanchez and Guillermo Martínez
Metabolic Unit, Endocrine Service, University Hospital 12 de Octubre, Faculty of Medicine University Complutense, Madrid, Spain

Branko Filipović and Branka Šošić-Jurjević
University of Belgrade, Institute for Biological Research"Siniša Stanković", Serbia

Beata Spanikova and Stanislav Spanik
St. Elisabeth Cancer Institute, Bratislava, Slovak Republic

Izabella A. Ludwa and Panagiota Klentrou
Brock University, Canada

Emilio González Jiménez
Departamento de Enfermería, Facultad de Ciencias de la Salud, Universidad de Granada, España

Printed in the USA
CPSIA information can be obtained
at www.ICGtesting.com
JSHW011401221024
72173JS00003B/373